The Christian Childbirth Handbook

The Christian Childbirth Handbook

By Jennifer Vanderlaan
foreword by Jan Tritten

Birthing Naturally ✦ 2008

The Christian Childbirth Handbook
© 2008 Jennifer Vanderlaan
www.birthingnaturally.net
All Rights Reserved

Published 2008 by Birthing Naturally, Colonie NY 12205
ISBN 10 0-9765541-2-7
ISBN 13 978-0-9765541-2-7

Scripture taken from the HOLY BIBLE, NEW INTERNATIONAL VERSION ®
Copyright © 1973, 1978, 1984 by International Bible Society
Used by permission of Zondervan Publishing House, All Rights Reserved.

The "NIV" and "New International Version" trademarks are registered in the United States Patent and Trademark Office by the International Bible Society. Use of either trademark requires the permission of International Bible Society.

Cover Photo Copyright ©2007 Christina Anne Pereira

DISCLAIMER: By reading this book, you agree to educate yourself about your options and be responsible for the choices you make. The author of this book is neither a physician nor a midwife. This book has been written to help you become educated and is intended to be used in consultation with your chosen health care provider. The publisher and author accept no responsibly for any loss, damage or injury alleged to be caused by the information contained in this book. This book is not a substitute for professional prenatal care or counseling.

For the mothers who have blazed a trail before me,
and for those who will travel the road after.
May God allow us to continue as a source of
wisdom, support and encouragement to each other.

*I myself am convinced, my brothers, that you yourselves
are full of goodness, complete in knowledge and
competent to instruct one another.
Romans 15:14*

Acknowledgments

Included in this volume are a number of articles, photographs and quotes from Christian families and childbirth professionals around the globe. The views expressed in those sections are the views of the individual authors and represent the wide variety of Christian beliefs about birth. For their assistance in this project, I am eternally grateful. You will find contact information for their ministries in the Appendix.

Pronoun Usage

The use of pronouns to refer to a baby is difficult. Newborns come in two varieties, he and she. But to use both pronouns is cumbersome to read, while the gender neutral pronoun "it" is too impersonal to refer to a human.

In the interest of ease in reading, your newborn baby will be referred to by male pronouns. To prevent confusion and be fair to the other half of newborns, older siblings will be referred to by female pronouns. Thank you for your understanding, and congratulations to your family whether you are expecting a "him" or "her."

Table of Contents

Foreword: Putting God into Your Birth	i
Christian Childbirth	**1**
What is Christian Childbirth?	3
How Faith Affects Labor	7
Biblical Principles for Pregnancy and Childbirth	12
Forming Opinions	15
Article: The Curse	20
Healthy Pregnancy	**23**
God's Design and Control	25
Stewardship of Good Nutrition	30
Stewardship of Adequate Exercise	36
Spiritually Healthy Pregnancy	42
Article: Making Positive Lifestyle Changes	50
Christian Childbirth	**53**
Overview of Pregnancy and Childbirth	55
Measuring Progress in Labor	58
Before Labor Begins	66
Early Labor	69
Active Labor	73
Transition	76
Second Stage	79
Third Stage	83
Article: Why We Labor	88

Birth Planning — 91

Birth Planning	93
Should I Write a Birth Plan?	95
Writing a Birth Plan	98
Using Your Birth Plan	102
Birth Planning and Guilt	105
Styles of Care	107
Article: Supportive Community	114

Childbirth Pain — 117

Why Pain in Labor	119
Factors That Affect Pain	126
Fear and Pain	130
Coping With Pain	134
Personal Pain Coping Strategies	139
Abnormal Pain in Childbirth	142
How Painful is Labor?	146
Article: More Than Conquerors!	152

Staying Comfortable — 155

Providing Comfort	157
Using Touch During Labor	160
Positions for Labor	167
Movement in Labor	174
Using Water in Labor	177
Relaxation for Labor	183
Comforting Environment	187
Article: Herbs for Labor	196

Options for Labor — 199

How and Why	201
Birth Place and Attendant	211
Routine Hospital Procedures	221
Induction Options	227
Pain Management Options	236
Newborn Care	248
From Decision to Reality	258
Making Decisions in Labor	263
Article: Home Birth	274

Labor Challenges — 277

Labor Challenges	279
Normal Variation or Emergency?	283
Before Labor Begins	285
During Labor	299
Cesarean Surgery	316
Article: The Miracle of Waterbirth	328

Getting to Know Your Newborn — 331

Your Newborn Baby	333
Your Baby as a Person	338
Feeding Your Baby	342
Parenting a Newborn	351
Article: The Baby God Gave You–Perfect?	358

Your New Family — 361

God's Design for Family	363
Mom's Needs Postpartum	366
Dad's Needs Postpartum	374
Sibling Adjustments	377
Article: Adjusting to Life with a New Baby	384

Appendices — 387

A1:	Sample Menus	389
A2:	Overcoming Fears	392
A3:	Birth Planning Checklist	393
A4:	Comfort Measures Checklist	394
A5:	Midwife Interview Questions	395
A6:	Birthplace Checklist	396
A7:	Breastfeeding Questions	397
A8:	Childbirth Verses	398
A9:	Global Birth Issues	399
A10:	Resources	400

References	405
Index	408

Foreword

Putting God into Your Birth

Jan Tritten
Founder, Editor-mother
Midwifery Today
www.MidwiferyToday.com

One of the most spiritual experiences in all of life is carrying and giving birth to a baby. A new person is formed and nurtured within your body. This is a stunning vantage point to see the face of God. How close you are to the Lord's presence and his ability to create. He is sharing that ability with you. The presence of God's new life within you for nine months then working his or her way onto this earth is truly Sacred Ground. You must be first born of flesh before you can be born again.

Joshua 5:15
Exodus 3:5

God is the perfect author of childbirth. He made a perfect God-breathed process of carrying, birthing and feeding his new children. It is my deepest desire that you experience the miracle of your labor and birth. Bringing forth your baby from inside you body is God created power and joy. This amazing process is one that will be the foundation of your entire life with your baby, with your new child of God. Birth is the foundation God created to launch you into motherhood. Jennifer does a magnificent job of explaining this to you in this incredibly sensitive book. I am so pleased you found it.

In Psalm 139:13-14 he says; "For you created my innermost being; you knit me together in my mother's womb. I praise you because I am fearfully and wonderfully made." Only God creates, but he has chosen you to co-create another human being with him. In essence for nine months you and your baby are one body. Wow, what a miracle you are chosen by God for, sharing this miracle of creation with him. God's design for childbirth is to bring babies on the earth in their first

Psalm 139:13-14

birth so they can also "be born again." It is a beautiful, miraculous design and you might even enjoy your pregnancy and birth process especially if you see and feel it as the spiritual experience it is meant to be. I certainly did. Indeed it was the highlight of my life—a joy beyond what words can express.

Romans 12: 1-2

As Romans 12: 1-2 says, "...offer your bodies as living sacrifices, holy and pleasing to God—this is your spiritual act of worship. Do not conform any longer to the pattern of this world, but be transformed by the renewing of your mind. Then you will be able to test and approve what God's will is—his good, pleasing and perfect will." Remember your baby is attached fully to you. He is probably feeling what you are feeling. This gives you responsibility to stay relaxed, calm, loving. "Fight fear" the Bible tells us this over and over. It is a command to fear not. Trust God not men, not medicine.

Please do not relinquish God's miracle to a fear-based, frantic medical culture. You know that when you are standing on Holy Ground, God has sent angels all around. You need to have faith. The spiritual voice is a quiet voice; easily drowned out by a large, noisy and fearful culture. Satan is waiting to rob you of your miracle. He has done this to nearly every family throughout the world today. It is time to reclaim the miracle and beat down evil and fear with faith and prayer. The Bible commands over and over "fear not."

You are at a most vulnerable time for spoiling your mind, heart and soul, which are all directly connected to your baby. Most often a woman has succumbed to one of Satan's lies transmitted by the culture or the doctor. This is a little like Eve eating the forbidden fruit. It starts with just one intervention like going into the hospital for an induction, that is not God's timing. You have already taken your birth out of God's hands and design and put it into man's and Satan's. You are given a possible array of dangerous drugs or procedures, usually both. At this point, actually with that first step into the hospital, the cascade of interventions has begun. It often leads to a cesarean which has many pitfalls and dangers. You and your baby are robbed of your miracle. Satan destroys women, babies and society in this way using the childbearing year of pregnancy, birth and breastfeeding. It is time to put God in the center of our childbearing.

Do you trust God with your baby? Placing this trust in doctors and medicine is like worshipping false gods. We are not to trust man and man made tests or ways. They interfere with God's plan and are very much designed to make money. Jennifer teaches you how to discern what is medically needed in this book. Remember, no procedure done to you or your baby is without risk including using a Doppler which is ultrasound. What is God's will for you and your baby is the question to discern.

We need to come out of medical bondage. We are women held in bondage, robbed of the miracle of birth. Birth is the most memorable life event along with being born again and finding our spouse. We are being robbed; held in fear, toil, pain and bondage that which God designed to be our greatest life experience our most beautiful miracle. Many suffer their entire lives with the pain incurred, foisted on them in the birth process. "Let my people go." — Exodus 5:1

Remember the battle is in the mind. Often what you believe about birth ends up to be what is. The mind is extremely powerful. That is why the scripture that the battle is in the mind is so absolutely germane to smooth birth. God knew when he gave us this insight into ourselves. Much of health and well being reside in the mind. We need to take off our cultural blinders and put on our spiritual glasses to be able to see things God's way. Ponder carefully how God created birth to work. Fears are often based on what has happened to others, but remember almost all complications are nutritional, iatrogenic (doctor caused) or from your own mind. The mind is extremely strong. The bible tells us to watch what we think. Guard you heart and mind always.

Every baby deserves to be nurtured with prayer, nutrition and love, not technology that does not improve outcome. Every motherbaby is meant to birth in privacy and in love encouraged in the way God created our bodies and souls to work and be strengthened. Use the first hours God created after birth to greet, bond with and marvel at your child and God's creation. Let your husband quietly be there to protect and be with you. Satan will not like this turn of events. It will totally foil his plan. Remember the hand that rocks the cradle controls the world

Galatians 1:15 "But when God, who set me apart from birth and called me by his grace." God already has a calling on your baby's life. Because this little one is sacred in God's sight and plan you can trust and believe that your baby is a gift straight from God. Treat your baby with love and respect, always. Above all, your calling is to protect and nurture this little one. Bringing life from your body, the temple of God, into their own being is truly a miracle, and you perform it mom. You are from a long line of women who birthed their babies naturally.

When God brings a baby into your life motherhood becomes your purpose. All of life including pregnancy and birth do come with an instruction manual—the Bible. Remember you are wonderfully made. You were designed by God to carry and give birth to your baby. Choose God's perfect plan for pregnancy and birth. The process can be pure joy with very hard work. For many women it is pure ecstasy. Have a joyful pregnancy and birth and remember *Philippians 4:13* you can do it. "I can do all things through Christ who strengthens me."

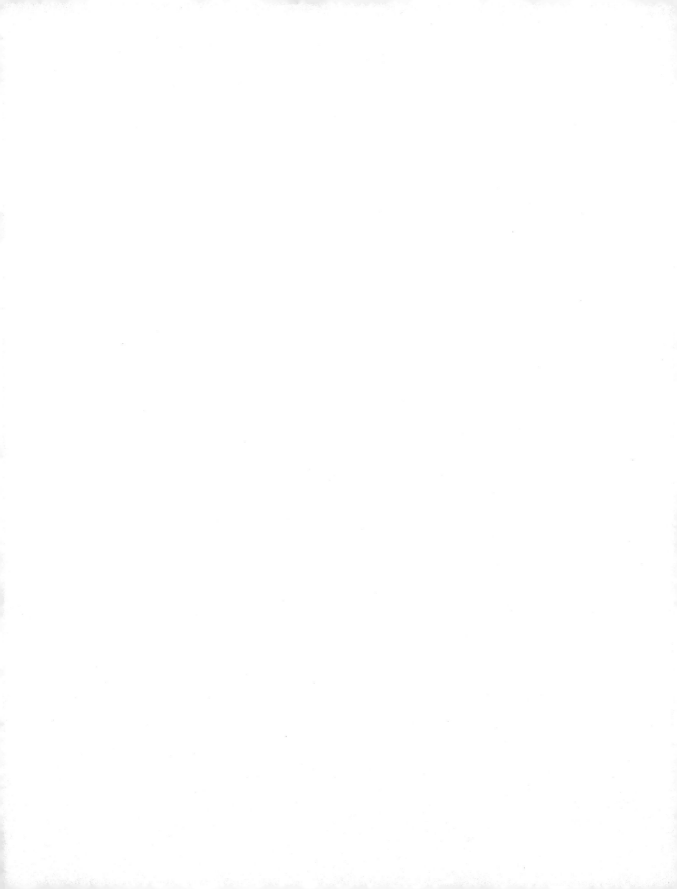

Subject One

Christian Childbirth

Topics:

What is Christian Childbirth?	3
How Faith Affects Labor	7
Biblical Principles for Childbirth	12
Forming Opinions	15
Drawing Conclusions	18
The "Curse" by Kathy Nesper	20

2

What is Christian Childbirth?

Christians are a varied group of individuals throughout the world. Income, family size, political preferences, education or race will not help you identify them. You may not recognize them by the way they dress, the music they listen to or the style of health care they choose. The only factor that distinguishes someone as a Christian is faith in Jesus Christ as the Son of God. Along with this faith, Christians choose to live by basic beliefs from the teachings of Christ and the Bible as a whole. However, the living out of the beliefs can look very different from Christian to Christian.

Being a Christian is not a mandate on your outward appearance, but a manifesto about your heart. There is great freedom in Christ, freedom that stems from the knowledge you cannot earn your way into heaven. Freedom that grows when your realize God does not need the little you have to offer him. Freedom that, when applied by the heart loving God and seeking to do his will, blossoms into a life which demonstrates God's glory to the world around you.

> It is for freedom that Christ has set us free.
> Galatians 5:1

Christian childbirth is not a term to define specific comfort measures, positions or tools for use during labor. Christian childbirth does not require a strictly defined birth place, a preset number of people in attendance or the environment in which a woman gives birth. Christian childbirth cannot be classified by the medical procedures used or the holistic practices participated in. Christian childbirth cannot be recognized by the ease with which a woman gives birth or degree of difficulties she encounters while laboring. Christian childbirth exists when a woman chooses to live out her faith in Christ in labor, and that cannot be identified simply by the actions you see taking place.

> How is living as a Christian different in your daily life?

If you are preparing to have a Christian childbirth, you may be wondering then just what you are supposed to "do." Having a Christian childbirth is no different from being a Christian at work, a Christian at school or a Christian in your day-to-day life. You should be familiar with the basic principles of the Bible to help you determine God's will. In addition, there are basic Christian disciplines you should be practicing to help you fall more and more in love with God. You can even choose to use these disciplines as comfort measures during your labor. However, what that specifically looks like when you live it out is between you and God.

The decision to become a Christian is the decision to live your life for the eternally significant rather than the temporary. It is the decision to imitate Christ and to follow God's will instead of your own. It is a decision that affects every aspect of who you are and what you choose to do. In that way, being Christian will affect how you choose to give birth.

Eternal significance of childbirth

Pregnancy and childbirth are the introduction of a new soul, one of God's children, to this world. You may begin to look at this time in your life with great reverence and remember the impact of everything you do on this new life. Through pregnancy and giving birth you are participating in the creation of a new soul. Eve looked at her newborn Cain and said, "With the help of the LORD I have brought forth a man."

> Genesis 4:1

Pregnancy is a spiritually fertile time in your life. It may be the first time you have questioned who you are, what you believe, and what you want to pass on to your children. It may be the first time you seek God face to face and ask him tough questions. It may be the first time God asks tough questions of you. Focusing on the eternal significance of your relationship to Christ, it becomes apparent that you can use the time of pregnancy to build your faith and mature spiritually.

When you look at it from an eternal perspective, the common concerns of how to give birth, whether to use medication and how long pregnancy lasts are insignificant. Your individual goals for labor seem meaningless except for the goal that labor glorifies God. However in pregnancy, as in the rest of your life, there are things that need to be attended to even though they are not spiritually significant in themselves.

You do need to make decisions about health care for you and your baby. To do this requires you learn as much as possible about the process of normal, healthy pregnancy and birth. You will be making daily lifestyle choices that affect you and your baby. You will need to make decisions about how to handle the labor process. All this requires you learn as much as possible about your options.

As you learn more about the options available, you may begin to discover that what seemed spiritually insignificant is actually an eternal heart issue for you. Learning about options may reveal differences between your plan and God's plan. You may find the preparations expose parts of your heart given to laziness, selfishness, desire for control or pride. You may be challenged to make lifestyle changes, let go of fear or let God be in control. These challenges grow your faith while you begin to make changes.

The choices you make are important to God because they reflect the condition of your heart. This is where the eternally significant meets day to day living, in your life glorifying God. Your daily life is built from the decisions you make, and the decisions you make reveal where your heart is.   Matthew 6:19-20

It all comes down to your heart: Why did you make the decisions you made? Did you do this for you or for God? Decisions you make do matter to God because they expose (not cause) the condition of your heart. God is not interested in phony religion, but in real lives of sacrificial love, kindness, faith and seeking after God.

You cannot turn off your Christianity

You cannot labor separately from the beliefs you hold in your heart. Because of your belief in Christ and God, you enter pregnancy with a set of tools that can help you during labor. For example, Christian faith in God's awesome design naturally gives you trust in the birth process. A Christian who already practices disciplines of prayer and meditation on scripture can use those tools to stay focused and relax during labor.

However, other aspects of Christianity may clash completely with what you thought was true about childbirth. As you study and learn, you will be challenged to test everything you think you know about having a baby against scripture. After your baby is born, you can look back at this time of preparation and see how God used it to mature you.

Your preparation for childbirth can help you grow closer to God. As a Christian, you cannot learn to have faith and trust in the birth process apart from God. You can marvel at his creation, lean on his strength and mature in your faith through this unique time of welcoming your baby. It is nearly unavoidable; the challenges of pregnancy and preparing for birth continually ask you to look into your heart, discover who you are and how that affects what you need. The self-reflection you will do helps to identify your strengths and overcome your weaknesses. In addition, the practice of working through the challenges strengthens your patience, perseverance, contentment and faith.

How Faith Affects Labor

A word like faith has several definitions. In some instances, it is used to mean a religion or the sum of beliefs. Other times it is used to mean a trust or assurance in God or something else. Both of these uses are accurate, and both need to be addressed when discussing faith and labor.

Many people talk about Christianity as their faith, and rightly so. The backbone of Christianity is a trust in the Bible as accurate, God as real and Jesus as deity. With the collective "faith" come some understandings of God you may have that can help in labor.

God created the female body to bear children before the fall. This is why in Genesis 3 God says the work will be increased during childbearing, not that a woman will suddenly have to give birth. His design for giving birth works. *Genesis 3:16*

Because God is good, he meets the needs of his people. This includes their needs during childbearing. *Philippians 4:19*

God is a good creator intending to give hope and a future, not to bring you harm. *Jeremiah 29:11*

A child is a blessing. Never does God call a baby a punishment or anything other than a blessing in the Bible. *Psalm 127:3*

Possessing a faith that includes these points can help to reduce the amount of fear you have about giving birth. This will have a significant effect on your labor. Dr. Grantley Dick-Read concluded years ago that the amount of fear and anxiety a woman has going into labor correlates to the amount of pain she will feel during labor. Women with more fear and tension experience more pain while giving birth. There are physiological reasons for this. The chemicals your body produces in response to fear and stress work to decrease the blood flow to the uterus and begin the process of closing the cervix. This can result in a very painful, long, unproductive labor.

> Q: How have birth horror stories affected you already?

One factor that increases fear are birth "horror" stories. Christians hear the same horror stories that scare many women, but with Christianity, there is a trust in God and the divine creation of our bodies that should make us stop and think, "God did not create a flawed system." Christians also deal with concerns about the "Eve Curse" which some Christians take to mean extensive and unbearable pain for all women giving birth. Christians who believe this expect labor to be excruciating, entering the childbirth experience with more fear and tension, creating the very unbearable experience they expected.

Your overall faith in God as good and wise, loving and caring, can help you go into labor calmer, decreasing the effects of fear on your labor. But not all fear goes away because you have faith in God. There are normal, healthy concerns that motivate you to make good decisions for your health and your baby. It is natural to be nervous about the unknown or even apprehensive about a big job you have to do. This type of fear should drive you to take action, not become a paralyzing fear.

> Psalm 34:4

How you react to concerns is important. If you dwell on fear, trying to avoid labor because of it, you are letting fear control you instead of God. This is a problem. If you try to ignore the fear using a false pride, you are letting your fear control you. The only way to overcome the fears is to acknowledge them to God, and choose to continue to follow his word. This is the second type of faith.

Individual faith, your personal trust in God that allows you to follow his plan is the type of faith that leads ordinary people to do extraordinary things. In Hebrews chapter 11, we see a list of men and women who stepped outside the comfortable and "safe" because they knew God had called them to do something. In these cases faith is not about the absence of fear or concern. Jonathan did not know if he would be successful when he headed off to face the Philistines; Shadrach, Meshach and Abednego did not know they would come out of the furnace alive, Esther did not know the king would not have her killed. In all these cases, faith in God leads people to do what they feared, what could have caused them pain or death, because it was more important for them to obey God than for them to remain comfortable.

1 Samuel 14
Daniel 3
Esther

Gideon and his men were ready to fight when God sent them. Yet God seemingly removed their chances to win by reducing their numbers. In reality, it was never about how many men Gideon had or what types of weapons he could fight with. The battle was always the Lord's, and he could have won it without any army. Still, Gideon had his job to do. God sent him and his men to fight. They had to accept that some of them might not come back from the battle, that some of them could get hurt. It was not just God fighting, and it was not just Gideon's army fighting. It was Gideon and his men following God and using the resources given to them to accomplish the job God gave them. It was faith that moved Gideon to do what needed to be done.

Judges 7:22

Most women worry about possible complications—it is only natural. Genuine complications are rare, but they do happen. It may be helpful to shift the focus from "what might go wrong" to "what I can do." Many women find that activating their imaginations and thought life in a pro-active way, through visualization, affirmations, creative art projects, journaling and intentional relaxation is very helpful.

As Christians, we have the Word of God showing us the way—in taking thoughts captive; to 'think on theses things' according to Philippians 4:8; and the many scriptures that show us how to defeat fear. The Word of God is a treasure trove of promises that we can choose to meditate on rather than ruminate over disaster scenarios. When well-meaning 'prophets of doom' regale you with horror stories, you can go back to the Word of God and choose to speak out what He says in His word. Meditate on His Word and let your soul be filled with His peace.

Julie Bell

God has as much control over childbirth as he does over battle. He could have your baby be born with no effort on your part as easily as he could win a war without an army. But labor will more likely require you to work. You will be acting in faith to follow the plan God set out for you.

Measure of Your Faith

The outcome of your labor is not the measure of your faith. You can not tell how much faith you have by your possessions, your physical blessings, how easy your labor was or any other thing we can see with our eyes. Faith is not determined by the outcome—Paul still had a thorn in his side, Job lost everything he had, Stephen was stoned.

<small>2 Corinthians 12:7-10
Job
Acts 7:59</small>

Faith is measured by what you do, not by what happens because you do it. Faith is shown by the works—by Abraham moving away from his family when God said go; by Jonathan attacking the Philistines because God said go; by Ruth leaving her home to stay with Naomi; by Esther approaching the King. The faith of each of these people would have been just as strong if their stories had ended differently. Would Esther have had less faith if the king had killed her? Would Ruth have had less faith if she had not found a husband? It was the faith that made them do what they did. God determined the outcome.

<small>Genesis 12:4
1 Samuel 14
Ruth
Esther</small>

Faith is based on a trust in God's control and working out his plan, not a hope for a specific outcome. God's plan does not always turn out to be what you wanted. David prayed and fasted for a week because he had faith that God could keep his child alive, but in the end the child died. John the Baptist was following God's plan to prepare the way for the Messiah, yet he was beheaded. Paul asked to have his thorn removed and God told him no. You can have faith in God having the power to do something, and he still may not do it.

<small>2 Samuel 12:15-19
Matthew 14:1-12
Acts 7:59</small>

God does say things happen because we have faith. God never says faith is the only reason things happen. If you consider for a moment the statement, "Cars go when you step on the gas pedal," you can see the statement is 100 percent accurate, but not complete. In addition to stepping on the gas pedal you must make sure there is gas in the car, the car must be turned on and put into the proper gear, all the parts you do not control in the engine need to be in good working order. Yet none of this negates the truth of the statement that cars go when you step on the gas pedal. The gas pedal is simply one part of a greater system that makes the car go. It is the same with our faith—it is only one part of many reasons God works the way he does.

Job's friends had very formulaic ideas of how God worked. To them God was a cause and effect deity that man could control. If you did X, Y would happen. But God's response to Job's friends was, "you have not spoken of me what is right." You cannot use human wisdom to reduce God to simple if-then statements. Human wisdom cannot fathom the divine wisdom and understanding of God. There is no promise of an easy labor if you do this or that. There is no guarantee of a painless childbirth because you trust God. Yet there is the faith that God is good, and his plan is for good, even if we cannot see it.

Job 42:7

Laboring in faith looks like a mother and father doing the hard work that needs to be done, whether it is a two-hour intense labor, a slow 24-hour labor or a surgical birth. It looks like a mother doing her best to follow God's lead and God's plan instead of her own, making decisions not out of fear but out of faith in God's plan. It looks like a family participating with God in bringing about the miracle of a new soul. There is no script for laboring in faith; you simply have to be willing to step outside your comfort zone and follow where God leads you.

Biblical Principles for Pregnancy and Childbirth

Though individual lives are different, and reflect different choices, Christians base decisions on the principles laid down in the Bible. These principles give guidelines, goals and insight into ways to build a closer relationship with God. While the entire Bible is the guide, there are a few principles that weigh heavily on the information presented in this book.

Freedom

1 Corinthians 10:23

"Everything is permissible"—but not everything is beneficial.

Christianity gives great freedom. Christians do not live under the law. With freedom comes responsibility. Although there is no mandate on your decisions, you always have the ability to either honor God or honor yourself. Christ urges Christians to use freedom to love and serve God. What this looks like in your pregnancy and childbirth depends on the places God has called you.

Stewardship

The principle of stewardship, described in the parable of the talents, is making the best use of the things God has given you. Everything belongs to God; it is only loaned to you. Your time, money, skills, possessions, job, home and your education are just some of the examples of things God has given you to use to further his purposes.

Matthew 25:14-30

In pregnancy, God has given you the ability to make decisions that impact your overall health and the health of your baby. Though you are not in control of what happens to you, your decisions will have a large impact on how you are able to handle labor. Stewardship is making choices for pregnancy based on the knowledge that your new baby belongs to God, not you.

Love

This is my command: Love each other.

John 15:17

Biblical love is evidenced by humbling yourself and seeking the good of others first. It is said that Christ took the nature of a servant, coming not to make himself equal with God, but instead choosing to die so others might live. It is this sacrificial love Christians are called to practice. It is not easy, and it is not always comfortable. Serving the needs of your baby first is an example of Biblical love.

Faith

My message and my preaching were not with wise and persuasive words, but with a demonstration of the Spirit's power, so that your faith might not rest on men's wisdom, but on God's power.

1 Corinthians 2:4-5

Throughout the ages humans have relied on technology for strength, power and salvation from the troubles around them. In the Bible, God is clear that it is only through his power that you receive anything. While technology is a tool that can help achieve a goal, it is not the only tool. God has power far beyond your wildest dreams; he is not limited by human understanding of pregnancy and childbirth.

Instinctual Wisdom of God written on your heart

John 14:26 — *But the Counselor, the Holy Spirit, whom the Father will send in my name, will teach you all things and will remind you of everything I have said to you.*

When Christ left this earth, he sent the Holy Spirit to be your counselor. Through the Holy Spirit, God can lead you to the answers you need. Along the way, the Holy Spirit will be leading you, convicting you of places your heart needs to change and interceding for you. The voice can be quiet; you may need to learn to hear it.

Blessings of Children

Psalm 127:3 — *Sons are a heritage from the LORD, children a reward from him.*

Each child is uniquely designed by a loving creator—knit together within the womb to fulfill a purpose already designed by God. Blessings are not always easy. The land of Israel was a blessing, but Moses and the Israelites had to wander in the desert 40 years before they could enter. After entering, they had to fight the people already living there to take possession even though God said he had given the land to them.

Peace

John 14:27 — *Peace I leave with you; my peace I give you. I do not give to you as the world gives. Do not let your hearts be troubled and do not be afraid.*

Jesus has a peace that surpasses understanding. Jesus did not promise to make everything perfect. Instead, in the midst of chaos you can have peace. This peace gives strength in difficult situations. Regardless of the circumstances of your child's birth, you can have peace.

Forming Opinions

Though the Bible gives us standards and principles, there is very little in the way of "Thou Shalt Not" when it comes to giving birth. It is probably no surprise to you that families can read the same Bible and believe they are called to different actions. Listed here are some of the most common debates in Christian childbirth with the Biblical reasoning given from each side.

You will quickly find yourself leaning toward some interpretations and away from others. That is normal. However, the purpose of this section is to challenge yourself to dig deeper. Be willing to explore both sides of each issue, searching the Bible for clear understanding. When you are done, God may have given you a new outlook on a topic you thought you understood, or he may have strengthened your faith in things you already believed.

Is Childbirth Supposed to be Painful?

Yes

Pain in childbirth is a consequence of the first sin. — Genesis 3:16

Paul and Job are both examples to me that God does let bad things happen to good people. God does not prevent all problems, and does not promise to make childbirth easy. — 2 Corinthians 12:7-9

No

Genesis 3:16
Women are not cursed. When labor is painful it is because of the fallen world.

Galatians 3:13
I have been redeemed. I am not under the curse and so do not have to suffer the consequences as they pertained to giving birth.

Matthew 9:22
Matthew 8:16
Jesus did heal those who asked him. I have no reason to expect him to refuse to heal my body if I ask. I can have the easiest and safest childbirth possible by asking Jesus for it.

Should I use a midwife or a doctor?

Midwife

1 Timothy 2:9
1 Corinthians 12:23
I am interested in remaining as modest as allowable during labor. I understand there are parts that need to be exposed, but I do not need to expose them to a man who is not my husband.

Matthew 9:12
I do not mind using doctors when I need them, but pregnancy is not an illness. Instead it is a normal and healthy state for my body to be in. It is not the well who need a doctor, but the sick. A midwife is trained in the normalcy of birth. I can always get the advice or assistance of a doctor if I have a problem.

Genesis 35:17
Exodus 1:17
The Biblical model is for a midwife to be attending the laboring woman. I want to follow that model.

Doctor

Galatians 3:28
I'm not concerned so much about who attends me, as long as I have someone who is willing to work with me to achieve my goals.

Proverbs 15:22
In my area, there are no midwives, or they have to practice illegally. My choice is reduced to hiring a doctor or being alone. I do not feel safe being alone because I do not have any experience with giving birth. I believe my doctor's experience and knowledge make him a valuable part of our birth team.

Should a Christian plan to use pain medication?

Yes

My faith and freedom in Christ allows me to use medication in labor. I have only to answer to God for my decision, and I believe he has given me the freedom to choose to use it.

Romans 14:1-4
Galatians 5:1

I accept the pain medications as a gift from God, and I am thankful that he has made them possible. Why should I be judged by someone else's conscience? Why am I denounced for something I thank God for?

1 Corinthians 10:23-31

No

I have the freedom to choose to use medication; however, I know there are risks involved in its use. I want to use wisdom and discernment to make sure I only resort to medications if they are medically necessary so I do not add risk to the health of my baby or mine. I will not plan to use them because I am afraid. Instead, I'll let God strengthen me.

1 Corinthians 10:23-24
Galatians 5:13
2 Timothy 1:7

I do not think God wants me to rely on current technology to "save me" any more than he wanted the Israelites to rely on the powerful technology of their day. There is nothing wrong with technology, but it cannot take the place of God and I must be sure that my faith is in God, and technology is only a tool I use if necessary.

Psalm 20:7
Isaiah 31:1

It is not easy to love sacrificially, but it is what God calls me to do. I do not expect labor to be a piece of cake, but I am willing to plan for a labor without medication because it is the safest thing for my baby. I can sacrifice my comfort for a few hours.

Ephesians 5:1,2
Romans 12:10-12
1 John 4:9-11
Philippians 2:3-8

Drawing Conclusions
Review of Section One

Christian Childbirth
Write your own definition of Christian childbirth. In a sentence or two, describe what it is and what it is not. Share your definition with a trusted friend who will work with you to help you prepare for a Christian childbirth experience.

Praying for Baby
If you have not already started praying for your baby, this would be a great time to make it a daily habit. In addition to the standard prayers for health, you could be praying for:

Psalm 49:3	**Wisdom**	Your child may learn and gain understanding easily.
Joshua 1:9	**Courage**	You child would be willing to do what is right even when it is hard.
Galatians 5:13	**Servant Heart**	Your child gladly meets the needs of those around her.
Psalm 119	**Love of the Bible**	Your child to desire to learn more about God through the word.
1 Timothy 4:12	**Leadership**	Your child to help others stand firm in faith.
1 Timothy 6:6	**Contentment**	Your child to be satisfied with that which is given to him.
Psalm 16:11	**Joy**	Your child to radiate the glory of God to those around her.
Galatians 5:21-23	**Kindness**	Your child to be gentle and loving at all times.
1 Peter 5:8	**Self-control**	Your child to learn the strength to tell himself, "no."
Romans 5:3-5	**Perseverance**	Your child to continue trying, even when it is difficult.

My Perfect Labor

Take a few minutes to write down some words you want to use to describe your labor experience after it happens. If you have difficulty coming up with ideas, move through the alphabet coming up with a word that starts with each letter, then choose your favorite few words.

After choosing your words, spend some time in prayer asking God to reveal what these words say about you, your upcoming childbirth experience and your expanding family. Answer these questions:

1. Does God agree with the words you have chosen?
2. Are there changes you need to make to help ensure your labor can be defined by those words?
3. Does your family support you in trying to have this type of labor?
4. What do you still need to learn in order to be prepared to have this type of labor?
5. In what ways are you already preparing for this type of labor?

Ten Questions about...
Christian Childbirth

1. In what areas is your faith strong?
2. In what areas is your faith in need of maturing?
3. Where has God been growing you recently?
4. What situations have resulted in the most spiritual growth for you?
5. How do you expect your faith to affect childbirth?
6. How has your faith changed during pregnancy?
7. In what ways have your friends or family supported your faith during this pregnancy or a previous pregnancy?
8. In what areas do you feel you need more support for your faith?
9. How are you incorporating Christian disciplines that bring about spiritual growth into your daily life?
10. How do you know when you have grown spiritually?

The "Curse"

Kathy Nesper
Apple Tree Family Ministries
www.AppleTreeFamily.org

Maybe it was in a sermon, a Bible study, or a casual conversation. Wherever it was, you have probably heard that God cursed women to suffer in childbirth as punishment for Eve's sin.

This belief is widespread, but it misunderstands the message of Genesis 3. We need to take a fresh look to discern God's intent for childbirth.

Genesis 1:22

We know the story well. Eve and husband Adam have been given God's assignment to "be fruitful and multiply and subdue the earth." Only one thing is forbidden, and if they disobey, they will "surely die." They cannot know what death is, but having disobeyed they hide when God calls.

God confronts them, and they confess their fear. God begins to speak, turning first to Satan, in the form of the serpent.

You are cursed... I will put hostility between you and the woman and between your offspring and hers. He will strike your head, and you will strike his heel. (vs. 15)

Consider how God's words must sound to Eve, expecting the punishment of death. God acknowledges her enemy and curses him, taking vengeance on her behalf. He then speaks of her *offspring*. What? Is she to live to have children after all, fatally crushing her deceiver in the end? Hope springs in her heart at the words!

God speaks to her:

I will greatly multiply your sorrow and your conception; in sorrow you will have children... (vs. 16)

With these words, her hope increases. No, it will not be as it could have been. The sorrow she now feels will be a constant part of her life. Eventually death will come for them both, because of what they have done. But there is no curse in God's words. Instead, he makes clear to her enemy and to her that she still has the privilege of participating in God's assignment to be fruitful.

The "Curse"

God turns to her husband:

The ground is cursed because of you; in sorrow you will eat from it all the days of your life... (vs. 17)

The message is the same. The soil is cursed, and he too will experience sorrow and distress in providing for his family. But he still will participate in God's task to cultivate the earth.

God used the same Hebrew word to both of them, only one verse apart. Yet most modern Bible translations say the man will experience "toil" or "labor" while the woman faces "pain" or even "intense pain and suffering." There is no good reason for this difference. The translators have "read into" the passage their belief that birth must bring physical agony.

We cannot know what changed physically with the curse on the ground, what birth would have been like without it. It is indeed one of a woman's most physically intense experiences. But what was God communicating to them—and to us?

In Bible passages that do not refer to childbirth, the Hebrew word spoken to both of them and another spoken to her are most often translated with emotional terms such as "grief "or "sorrow." Those words indeed paint an accurate picture of the uncertainty and struggle of life—*all* of life—in a "fallen" world.

That includes childbirth. We worry, uncertain about its outcome. In the intensity of labor, we struggle to retain control of the overpowering experience. Sometimes, the curse on the earth intrudes with a complication that brings true physical suffering or even loss.

But we are not cursed. God's *love* permits struggles that constantly urge us to surrender to our dependence on him—the dependence Adam and Eve had forgotten.

Those of us who provide emotional support for women in labor know that in a normal birth, the most important thing is *surrender*—to the physical sensations, releasing the tension in the muscles. To the uncontrollable emotions. Surrender to *God* in dependence upon him.

Amazingly, in the wisdom of our loving Creator, surrender also makes the experience more physically comfortable. Bearable. Empowering. "Worth it."

No, it is not as it could have been. But we still have the privilege of fruitfulness. And when we surrender to our Creator in it, our lost wholeness is restored.

Note: Scripture quotations are my own paraphrases, using various sources.

22

Subject Two

Healthy Pregnancy

Topics:

God's Design and Control	25
Stewardship of Good Nutrition	30
Stewardship of Adequate Exercise	36
Spiritually Healthy Pregnancy	42
Drawing Conclusions	48
Making Positive Lifestyle Changes by Christy Callahan	48

God's Design and Control

The changes you experience in pregnancy happen for a reason. Conception begins a series of hormonal changes that allow pregnancy but also cause side effects. It is a beautifully intricate design that allows your body to carry a child with relatively few problems.

Your body begins preparing for pregnancy as soon as your menstrual period has begun. A hormone called follicle-stimulating hormone (FSH) prepares a follicle in one of your ovaries to release a mature egg. About 14 days after your menstrual period begins, your body releases Luteinizing Hormone (Lh) which causes a mature egg to be released into the fallopian tube where it can be fertilized by a sperm.

If the egg is fertilized, the outer covering of the egg, the corpus luteum, grows and begins producing small amounts of progesterone. Progesterone prevents the uterus from contracting to ensure the fertilized egg will not be forced out of the body during a menstrual period. Progesterone also prepares the uterine wall to support the pregnancy by increasing the blood vessels in the walls.

About 10 days after fertilization, the egg begins to develop a connection to the uterine wall which will become the placenta. As the placenta grows, it begins producing estrogen. Estrogen causes growth and changes in your uterus, cervix, vagina and breasts. Estrogen also

> There is a time for everything, and a season for every activity under heaven.
> Ecclesiastes 3:1

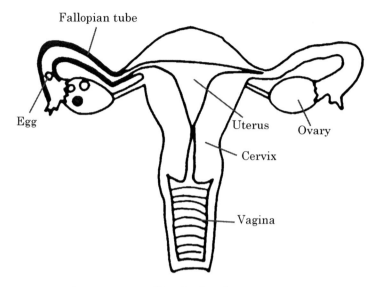

promotes the storage of body fat for extra support during pregnancy. Levels of estrogen increase slowly until about the twelfth week when it begins to increase more rapidly.

The hormone human chorionic gonadotropin (hCG) produced by the immature placenta keeps the corpus luteum producing progesterone until about the twelfth to sexteenth week of pregnancy when hCG levels drop. From the twelfth week on, progesterone is made by the placenta, which continues to increase the amounts of progesterone until after your baby is born.

Your placenta will also begin seceting hPL (human placental lactogen), which allows your baby to be nourished through the sugars and proteins available in your blood. The hormone also stimulates your mammary glands to begin developing. Mammary glands are the only glands that do not mature during puberty. While this happens, your breasts may be sensitive.

While your body undergoes major hormonal changes, your baby spends the first trimester developing every major body system. His major organs are in place, although they will continue to mature. His heart beats, his digestive system moves and absorbs glucose, his bones are hardening and his muscles are developing.

The levels of estrogen and progesterone continue to increase throughout the pregnancy. The increased presence of these hormones causes many changes in your body which help you meet the needs of your baby.

Increased levels of progesterone make your body more sensitive to carbon dioxide in your blood. This is helpful because the carbon dioxide level lets your body know when to take a breath. The increased sensitivity allows you to breathe more frequently, ensuring you have enough oxygen for you and baby. However, as a result of the increased sensitivity, you may feel a shortness of breath from time to time.

Another affect of the increased progesterone is the relaxation of smooth muscle systems in your body. This is helpful because your circulatory system is smooth muscle, and the decreased tone of your blood vessels allows them to carry more blood, accommodating your increased blood volume. However, your digestive tract is also smooth muscle and it becomes relaxed as well, so you may feel more frequent indigestion, heartburn or constipation.

The increased levels of estrogen help your body to support the growth of the uterus by increasing the number of cells in the uterus, the size of the cells and the blood flow to the uterus. The uterine veins enlarge to sixty times their normal size, which allows for adequate drainage of your baby's waste products from the uterine environment.

Estrogen also helps support your baby by increasing the blood volume and increasing the available proteins in your blood so your baby gets all he needs to grow. However, the increased estrogen levels cause a decrease in available gastric acid and pepsin for digestion, so you may have more frequent digestive upsets.

By the end of the second trimester your baby is moving around, spends time sleeping and gets the hiccups. His senses are operational, although they will need maturing. He sucks on his thumb, blinks his eyes and swallows amniotic fluid. If "he" is a "she," her ovaries are formed and already contain all the eggs that will one day become your grandchildren.

As your pregnancy progresses, the placenta produces larger amounts of a hormone called relaxin. Relaxin loosens the joints of your pelvis to ensure it has an adequate stretch to allow your baby an exit. However, relaxin does not just affect the joints of the pelvis, so you may find that you begin to feel wobbly all over as your knees, hips, shoulders and wrists feel loose.

As your baby nears readiness for birth, his brain and placenta begin releasing a series of hormones that cause his body to produce oxytocin which stimulates the uterus. These same hormones cause his adrenal glands to mature so they can produce cortisol, a hormone that stimulates the lungs to finish maturing.

While this is happening, these same hormones increase your estrogen production. As estrogen production increases, it increases the uterine sensitivity to oxytocin, which is being pumped into your blood stream by the baby. You will slowly begin to feel Braxton-Hicks contractions in response to the oxytocin. These contractions help to strengthen the uterine muscle for labor.

Another effect of the increase in estrogen is the increase of prostaglandins. Prostaglandins help to soften or "ripen" the cervix (opening of the uterus) so it will be ready to stretch to allow the baby to pass through. With the increase of uterine activity and the ripening of the cervix, you may find you have completed some of the necessary work of opening the cervix before you actually begin labor.

> "Do I bring to the moment of birth and not give delivery?" says the LORD. "Do I close up the womb when I bring to delivery?" says your God." Isaiah 66:9

As your cervix, uterus and vagina are stimulated and stretched by the contractions and increased prostaglandin levels, your pituitary gland is stimulated to release oxytocin. How your body begins labor is a mystery only God understands, but it seems the increase in prostaglandins and oxytocin start contractions which then increase the levels of prostaglandins and oxytocin further for even more contractions. This cycle continues to build on itself until your baby is born.

There is not a consensus among Christians as to how much control God maintains over the processes of our bodies. There is evidence God is intricately involved in the daily workings of our bodies. There is also evidence that God created a system over which we are able to influence a measure of control. How much control is in God's hands and how much control is in your hands only matters if it makes a difference in the way you view your pregnancy.

Psalm 139:13

Psalm 139:13 says, "For you created my inmost being; you knit me together in my mother's womb." Knitting is a technique for building clothing one stitch at a time. Unlike the seamstress who creates a garment by stitching fabric together, the knitter has touched and directed the creation of every inch of what she has made. The knitter makes the fabric as she stitches it together. God creates the baby and directs the pregnancy from conception to birth.

Your child is on loan to you from God. You are the steward of that which is entrusted to your care. This means you have some control over what happens, but it is not without responsibility. Authority always comes with responsibility. God will hold you accountable for how you have cared for his child, because he does have a stake in the outcome of your pregnancy.

Gift From God

I give thanks to You alone
Who sits on the throne
To loan me this precious gift
And to call it my own.

May I always see, Lord
In every waking hour,
Your majesty and grace
In this delicate flower.

Help me, O God,
To guide and preserve,
This wonderful blessing
To love and to serve.

Doran Richards © 2001

Stewardship of Good Nutrition

At prenatal appointments, you are being assessed for overall health. Your weight is being monitored, your urine is being evaluated, your blood pressure is being measured, your baby's heartbeat is being counted and the height of your fundus (top of the uterus) is being recorded. All these measurements are done in the hopes your caregiver will identify any place you need to improve your health. Yet these measurements are only an overall assessment of your physical state. They do not keep you healthy, and they may not tell you anything is wrong with your health until damage is done.

There is a difference between being healthy and assessing your health. An assessment is no more than looking at what is going on and making decisions based on it. These measurements give you useful information, or they can give you a false reassurance, but they can never make you healthy. To be healthy, you need to regularly act on good decisions.

Q: Has your weight been an area of struggle for you during this pregnancy?

Your weight is an indicator of how much and how fast you are gaining. You can gain weight eating healthy foods or you can gain weight eating junk foods. By eating healthy foods you and your baby have everything you need to stay healthy. By eating junk foods your body must break down your own muscle tissues to provide your growing baby with the proteins and other nutrients he needs. Your health will be different, but you can still show a normal weight gain on the scale. You might not even know damage has been done until you are sick or try to lose weight postpartum. These regular assessments have their place; they can help you identify unexpected problems. But to consider "healthy" to mean the lack of a serious problem is missing the mark.

While you cannot control every aspect of your health, you can have a huge impact on it by eating a healthy diet. Pregnancy increases your body's demands for food and changes your body's needs. After the first trimester of pregnancy you need around 200 extra calories a day, but towards the end of your pregnancy you may need as much as 500 extra calories a day just to be healthy. If you eat too little your body will rely on its own stores of energy and protein (your muscles and tissues) to meet the increasing demand. Even with that your baby will be at a disadvantage. However, if you overeat, your body stores the extra energy as fat which increases health risks during and after pregnancy. So one of the easiest things you can do is to gently increase the amount of food you eat without overeating.

Because you are pregnant, your body needs extra protein to build the baby, nourish the placenta, increase your blood volume and enlarge the uterus. Your body does not have a way to store extra protein; it only keeps the protein it uses and excretes the rest. Your baby cannot be built from your extra fat stores; the fat does not have the amino acids necessary to build body tissues. If you do not eat enough protein everyday, your body will break down your tissues, usually your muscles, to get the building blocks it needs for your baby. If you want to stay healthy, you need to eat enough protein.

All day long we eat either junk or health foods. What are you feeding mama baby? Christians are generally remiss in the area of nutrition. Talking to them about their eating habits parallel talking to them about the behavior of their children or their very souls. It has a "high place" in our lives, almost idolatrous. Even the mere mention of the importance of drinking half your body weight in ounces of water rolls eyes and conjures attitudes. *Carol Gautschi*

Because your blood volume increases in pregnancy, your need for water and salt increase. If you try to limit your water intake to prevent bloating or to minimize bathroom trips, you run the risk of being dehydrated. Water accounts for 75 percent of your baby's weight at birth, and it is also necessary for your body to produce amniotic fluid, which is constantly being remade so it is all new clean water every three hours. Water is essential for every function in your body; not having enough can make you tired, give you headaches, cause you to see stars or decrease your blood pressure (which may already be decreased as your body tries to prepare a larger blood volume).

> On-line nutrition analyzers are an easy way to see if you have areas of deficiency or excess.

Some nutrients are extremely important during pregnancy; for example, folate helps prevent certain birth defects known as neural tube defects. Unfortunately, the most important time for the prevention of neural tube defects is within the first six weeks of gestation, usually before you confirm your pregnancy. Calcium is important during pregnancy since your baby's bones are forming. If you do not have enough calcium in your diet, you may lose calcium from your own bones, which increases your risks for osteoporosis. Iron is used to transport oxygen in the blood, so your increased blood volume means you will need extra iron during pregnancy. During the last trimester, as your baby builds his own blood supply, you will again need more iron. If this is your second pregnancy in a short amount of time, you may find your need for certain nutrients is even higher since pregnancy can deplete some nutrient stores.

What you eat does matter to a healthy pregnancy, but it will also affect your body after your baby is born. If you are not eating enough food during pregnancy, your body is forced to break down its own tissues to make up the difference. Although it would be nice if your body targeted fat for its energy supply, more likely your body will break down both fat and muscle. Breaking down muscle provides your body with what it needs to build your baby and feed your brain—something it cannot get by breaking down fat.

When your body breaks down muscle, you have a few problems. First, your body does not care what muscle it breaks down, so you are just as likely to weaken your heart or uterus as you are your legs or arms. Second, breaking down muscle makes you weaker and causes you to get tired faster. Third, muscle holds your body together, making the normal fat deposits look like soft curves rather than big blobs; without it you will look flabbier. Finally, muscle uses more energy than other body tissues, allowing you to burn calories faster and return to a healthy weight faster.

Important Nutrients		
Nutrient	Why Needed	Good Sources
Protein	• To build your baby, placenta and amniotic fluid • To increase blood volume and maternal tissue growth • Main source of food for brain	Eggs, lean meats, poultry, fish, cheese, legumes
Carbohydrates	• Main source of energy, allows protein to be used for tissue growth	Whole grains, fruits and vegetables, pasta
Fat	• Additional source of energy • Required for baby's brain growth	Lean meats and proteins, eggs, nuts, seeds, olive oil, fish.
Fiber	• Helps move food along the digestive tract to ensure good nutrition	Whole grains, vegetables, legumes
Folate	• Blood formation • Prevention of neural tube defects	Dark leafy green vegetables, dried peas and beans, whole grains, citrus fruits, bananas, cantaloupe
Calcium	• Bone maintenance and baby's bone formation	Dairy products, dark leafy greens, broccoli, dried beans
Iron	• Needed to deliver oxygen to you and baby	Lean red meats, spinach, dried fruits
Vitamin C	• Keeps tissues healthy • Important for iron absorption	Citrus fruits, broccoli, tomatoes, berries, peppers, melons

Though you may expect to cut calories to lose weight quickly after your baby is born, continuing a healthy diet will still to be important. During the early prenatal period your body will go through a process of healing the uterus and returning to its pre-pregnancy chemical balance. If you are not eating a healthy balanced diet, you are more likely to have problems getting your body back to normal. Similarly, the early days with your newborn will be exhausting with frequent demands and short blocks of sleep. If you are not eating healthy, you will be more likely to suffer severe fatigue or illness. This can be even more so if you are recovering from a surgical birth.

If you are breastfeeding, your body's need for excellent nutrition and extra calories will continue. It is estimated the breastfeeding mother needs about 500 additional calories a day to support milk production. Foods with low nutritional quality will not give you the building blocks of good milk, and once again your body will suffer as muscle tissue is broken down. The idea that you can just eat less to safely lose weight was never true. To safely lose weight you will need to eat a high quality diet and get regular exercise. It is the only way to ensure your body burns fat, not muscle.

Healthy Eating Guidelines

See Appendix 1 for menu ideas.

There is no standard menu to follow for a high quality diet. Instead, there are guidelines to use as you select the foods your family enjoys. This gives you the freedom to design your diet around your favorite flavors.

There are two commonly followed recommendations for a healthy pregnancy diet. One is the governmental sources, and the other is from Dr. Tom Brewer, an obstetrician and pioneer in the health of pregnancy (Brewer & Brewer, 1985). The governmental guidelines have almost caught up with the recommendations Dr. Brewer first made to his clients about 50 years ago.

The reason for recommending number of servings per day is to ensure you get the right balance of nutrients. The ranges are given for all adults. Individuals with smaller bodies or who are less active will need fewer calories and so eat according to the lower level of the guidelines.

Food Group	Dr. Brewer	USA	Canada	Australia	UK
Protein	4	2-3	2	1.5	Moderate
Dairy	4	3	2	2	2-3
Fruits and Vegetables	5	5-9	7-8	9-10	5
Grains	4	6-11	6-7	4-6	1/3 of diet
Pregnancy Specific	NA	NA	Add 2-3 servings of any group		NA

As you select your foods, you should aim to eat a minimum of 75 grams of protein a day, drink water to thirst and consume salt to taste. Because these are guidelines and not rigid rules, there is a lot of freedom for your family to select the foods they enjoy and are comfortable with. Whether you abstain from certain foods for health or faith reasons will not matter, you simply substitute with appropriate foods you are willing or able to eat. However, when making your selections you will want to keep the nutrient density in mind.

Nutrient density means how much value a food has compared to the number of calories it contains. Calories are a measure of the energy in food, and a food has calories whether it is mostly protein, mostly carbohydrates or mostly fat. Your body will need a certain amount of calories every day, probably somewhere between 2000 and 2500 but it varies based on your lean body mass and your activity level.

If you are struggling with food aversions, indigestion, heartburn or nausea, you may not be able to eat as many calories as your body needs in a day. If you consume more calories than your body needs, you are overeating. Both over and under eating can damage your health. If you have chosen to eat foods with high levels of calories but low levels of nutrients, you will be undernourished, even if you eat enough calories every day. It is possible to overeat and still be undernourished.

Q: What has been your biggest struggle as you try to eat healthy?

Stewardship of Adequate Exercise

One of the easiest things for a pregnant woman to avoid is exercise. Exercise takes time, it takes work and many days you just do not have the mental energy to get up and move. Most people understand exercise is important because it burns calories, helping you maintain a healthy weight, but you are not trying to lose weight during pregnancy, so why bother?

> Most adults overestimate their activity level.

Activity is important because your health is not singly defined by what you eat. The foods you eat are the energy and the building blocks of your body. The activities you participate in help determine how the energy and building blocks are used. Physical activity can help you stay comfortable during pregnancy, prepare you for a more comfortable childbirth and give you the best chances for returning to your pre-pregnancy health.

God did not design the human body to be sedentary. Instead, the human body is designed in a way that the physical activities you perform every day help maintain your overall health. Physical activity affects your body's physiology, what chemicals are present and how they work. Physical activity also stimulates your body's systems, improving the function of the circulatory and digestive systems, and pumping materials through the lymph system. Physical activity improves the functioning of your body, building stronger bones, muscles and maintaining healthy joints.

Exercise is able to increase endorphin production. Endorphins are the chemicals your body produces to make you feel good, the ones responsible for the "runner's high." In addition, exercise improves your focus and concentration, helping you remain calm and clear in everything you do. Exercise also gives you a physical way to work out tension. These combine to make exercise one of the best ways to reduce stress during pregnancy.

Exercise works to give you more energy in two ways. First, a fit circulatory system is able to deliver 25 percent more oxygen per minute while at rest than an unfit circulatory system. Oxygen is needed by your body to do nearly everything. When your body is able to transport the oxygen properly, you have more energy. Secondly, fit muscles are better able to endure longer periods of moderate work then unfit muscles. This muscular endurance allows you to do things for longer periods of time, hence, more energy.

Overall, exercise will keep you more comfortable during your pregnancy. It will help to improve your mood and your sleep, which significantly impact your comfort. Keeping your muscles strong keeps them able to do the work of supporting your growing baby. This means you are less likely to have backaches and fatigue. Exercise helps keep your digestive system operating properly, reducing the effects of pregnancy constipation. Exercise also helps to maintain your flexibility, the ability to use your muscles throughout their entire range of motion.

If you stay active during pregnancy, you will find your body has increased stamina for labor, which will be a key to your comfort. If you practice some pregnancy specific activities, you will find you have strengthened and improved flexibility in muscles needed for childbirth. This can also work to keep you more comfortable and reduce the stress of labor on your body.

After your baby is born you will find exercise has improved your strength and stamina for carrying your baby around. You will also find a healthy body has the best chances for a speedy recovery from the process of giving birth.

Many mothers are concerned about weight management after their baby is born. They want to know how to return to a pre-pregnancy weight as swiftly and easily as possible. The answer to that question is to stay active during pregnancy. Exercise is not only good for burning calories at the time you perform the activity. The real benefit for weight management comes after the initial calories are burnt.

Aim for 30 minutes of exercise every day.

The stronger muscles you have built exercising regularly are the strong shapely part of your body and support the normal fat deposits you need for good health. You will find your body maintains extra fat for pregnancy and breastfeeding, which is healthy. The key to avoiding flabby and unsightly fat deposits is to firm the muscles under the fat so it can be supported properly. Stronger muscles also improve your body's ability to burn calories. Muscle burns more calories than fat, so you will maintain your weight or lose weight while eating a larger amount of calories.

Types of Activity

There are three types of activity important for your physical health; aerobic training, strengthening and flexibility. Aerobic training is the repetitive movement of large muscle groups that improves your cardiovascular health, increases stamina and burns calories. Strengthening of muscles is done with resistance through a range of motion. The additional weight can be your body weight, handheld weights or a weight machine. Flexibility activities are the stretching done to improve range of motion, prevent soreness and give your muscles a lean, long look.

The easiest aerobic activity to engage in is walking. It is free, can be done anywhere and does not require any special equipment beyond walking shoes and comfortable clothes. If you are new to exercise, start slowly. You may only be able to walk 10 minutes before you feel tired and need a rest. As your body becomes stronger, try to work up to 30-minute walks once or twice a day. If you were active before pregnancy, you may be finding you feel "out of breath" sooner due to your body's increased demand for oxygen. Measure your intensity level by your ability to talk, stopping or slowing down your activity if you are no longer able to carry on a conversation. If you prefer an aerobic class or working out with a video, then choose those types of activities.

Strength and flexibility exercises can be combined in Pilates or yoga style activities. Not only do the exercises use your body weight as resistance to strengthen your muscles, but the stretching done as part of the movements improves your range of motion. There are a wide variety of books, classes and videos that explain various body weight resistance and stretching techniques. You may want to find one specific to pregnancy to avoid stressing your changing body. If you prefer to use weights for resistance, be aware of your changing center of gravity and alter the movements to allow more stability for you (such as using seated movements).

Pregnancy Specific Activities

Kegel exercises are the strengthening of the pelvic floor muscles. The pelvic floor muscle is actually a group of muscles working together to support the weight of your abdominal contents. In the center of the pelvic floor are the openings for your urethra, vagina and anus. The muscle acts as a sphincter, shutting the openings until you physically relax it to allow the contents to exit.

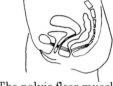

The pelvic floor muscles stretch from the pubic bone to the coccyx bone.

During pregnancy, the pelvic floor is put under extra stress from the weight of your growing uterus. This can cause the muscle to become weak. You can check the strength of your pelvic floor muscle with your index finger. After washing your hands well, insert the finger into the vagina to about the second joint and try to move it against the sides of the vagina. If you have good muscle tone, you should meet resistance in all directions. You should also be able to contract the muscles around your finger.

If your muscle has become weakened, your vagina will feel roomy with thin walls that seem separate from the surrounding structures. Not only does this cause the unintended leaking of urine when you cough, laugh or move suddenly, it also puts you at risk for internal tearing while giving birth. A strong pelvic floor is

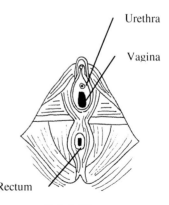

Pelvic Floor

necessary to help your baby's head line up properly in the pelvis. The muscles make your baby flex his chin to his chest so the smallest part of the head comes first, giving you the best chances at effective contractions and even dilation.

To prevent loss of muscle tone and to regain muscle strength, you will need to exercise your pelvic floor muscles. This is done through any number of a variety of contraction-relaxation patterns. The most basic exercise is to contract the pelvic floor and then release. Recommendations vary, so it is best to pay attention to your pelvic floor and do as much exercise as is necessary for you to keep strong tone. This may mean you do ten or twenty every time you use the bathroom, or it may mean you do fifty each night before going to bed. If you do not know how to contract the pelvic floor, it is the same internal contraction used to stop the flow of urine. It is not pulling your legs together tightly.

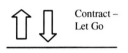

Contract your pelvic floor muscle and let go. Then relax it by bulging the muscle and then release.

During pushing, you will need to relax the pelvic floor to make the opening as large as possible for your baby. This will be the opposite of the muscle contracting you are doing with the rest of your abdomen to push. The relaxation is similar to feeling as if you are bulging the pelvic floor out. Once you know how to contract the pelvic floor, try relaxing it by pushing it beyond the release of the contraction. You may want to practice this on the toilet, as you are likely to release urine during this exercise.

Pelvic Rocking is a strengthening and flexibility activity to help you increase the range of motion of your pelvis. During pregnancy, the changing center of gravity affects your posture. Proper posture involves the abdominal muscles holding the pelvis in the correct alignment. Since the abdominal muscles are under stress, many women mistakenly adjust their posture by pulling their shoulders back. This causes backaches and tightening of muscles that reduce the flexibility in your pelvis. Pelvic rocking exercises will strengthen the abdominal muscles and lengthen the lower back muscles.

During labor, movement of the pelvis will help your baby line up properly. The pelvic inlet is shaped like a circle, but the outlet is shaped like a diamond. To move through, your baby will need to rotate. Pelvic movement during labor helps your baby make the necessary rotations. The more flexibility you maintain, the easier it will be to work with your body by making pelvic movements and adjustments in labor.

In its most basic form, pelvic rocking is the tipping of the pelvis forward (think up towards the abdomen) and returning it to neutral. This can be done on hands and knees, while lying on the floor or while standing. When you become more flexible you can add pelvic circles, figure eights or other "belly dance" style movements to increase your strength and flexibility. Regular, moderate, practice is better at improving flexibility than infrequent, intense workouts.

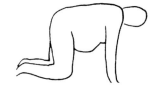

It may be easiest to learn pelvic rocking in a hands and knees position.

Squatting works to improve the flexibility of your legs to allow better positioning for pushing. The best positions for pushing are ones that mimic a squat, however many women in the developed world do not use squatting positions in everyday life. When you do not squat, you lose the flexibility to squat.

You can easily work squatting into your daily routine by using a squatting position to reach objects on low shelves, retrieve items from the floor or talk to a toddler. Real squatting is achieved by keeping your heels on the floor while you bend at the hips and knees. If you are inflexible, this is likely to be difficult at first. Although it will become easier to balance as your flexibility increases, you will need to find a comfortable way to practice.

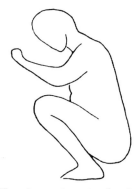

Hanging onto a sturdy piece of furniture or another person can make learning to squat easier.

To support yourself in a squat, you can hold a firm object such as a counter or heavy piece of furniture. If you have a willing partner, you can hold someone's hands while you gently squat. If it is still too much of a stretch, place a thick book under your heels. As you become more flexible, reduce the thickness of the book until you are able to squat with your heels on the floor. Spending time sitting cross-legged on the floor can help you gain the flexibility you need to squat.

Pushing contractions will not last longer than 2 minutes, so you do not need to engage in marathon squatting sessions. Instead, squat when appropriate throughout the day. You will find squatting stretches your lower back to help relieve back-aches. Squatting can also help you to go to the bathroom when you feel constipated, so keep a stool in the bathroom to put your feet up on.

Spiritually Healthy Pregnancy

> 1 Timothy 4:8
> For physical training is of some value, but godliness has value for all things.

Spiritual dry spells. Being stuck in the valley. Feeling far from God. These are all very real experiences for women at any time of life. Sometimes it seems to last forever, and when you break out you realize how much more mature you are and how much you were growing even without knowing it. Other times it comes and goes for weeks and months and you get stuck in a spiritual rut.

It is not a coincidence that times of such heightened spiritual awareness, such as pregnancy and the immediate postpartum, can also become the times women feel the most spiritually empty. With so many new demands on your time and your body, it is easy to find yourself spending shallow or no time with God. When the challenges of a new baby become overwhelming, it is not uncommon for new mothers to wonder what is spiritually wrong with them.

If you are not feeling overwhelmed or struggling to spend time with God, it is still completely normal to feel as if your spiritual needs are not being fed. This can happen even when you continue your normal routine of Bible reading and prayer. It is hard enough to feel as if your efforts to connect to God are not working when you are not dealing with the demands of a pregnancy or a new baby. When you add feeling far from God to the list of stressors, your whole life can feel out of control.

With children, your life is in a constant state of change. Your schedule is never the same from month to month, and time you could count on this week may not be there next week. It can be challenging to stay connected to God when everything in your life is changing every day. The God of the Bible is a God of paradox. To be the greatest you must be the least. The first shall become the last and the last shall be first. The leader must be the servant. And to maintain your spiritual discipline, you must be flexible.

Matthew 19:30
Luke 9:48

You must be disciplined. You must ensure your priorities are in order and that your spend time with God everyday. Through your time with God you will be refreshed and refilled. You are able to lay out your hurts and fears and concerns and allow God to heal your broken heart. God opens your eyes and helps you understand him and his word better. Your can learn spiritual truths without spending time with God, but if you desire to become spiritually mature you must spend time with God. You cannot get stuck on one idea of what spending time with God means so that if you do not have time to devote to it, you just do not spend time with God that day. You need to have several ways to spend time with God ready so when the opportunity arises you can enjoy it.

Spending time with God must be a priority every day. But do not lock yourself into believing spending time with God has to fit the picture in your head or your favorite discipline. Give yourself the flexibility to try other ways to connect with God when needed (or wanted) to ensure you spend time with God every day. This will help keep your relationship fresh, stretch your comfort zones and give you wonderful opportunities to explore other dynamics of God's personality. The point is to discipline yourself to spend time with God everyday, not to make sure you do the same thing with God everyday.

There is a wide variety of ways you can spend time with God. There is amazing variety even within the spiritual disciplines, so you should never be bored and you should never run into the problem of not being able to meet with God. The list is not intended to be all inclusive, please add to it other ways you can spend time with God.

Bible Reading

<small>Psalm 19:8
Matthew 22:29</small>

The Bible is God's Word, and reading it helps you understand who God is and what he requires of you. It also shares the stories of men and women who were learning how to trust and follow God which can teach and inspire you today.

Need Something New?

Read a Bible divided into daily readings; go through an entire book in one sitting; read the Bible as a letter to you; set a specific time every day when you read; set a specific amount of time every day to read; try reading a different version; check all the notes and cross-references; read the Bible out loud; listen to a dramatized reading; record yourself reading the Bible; read the Bible to someone; let someone else read to you.

Scripture Memorization

<small>Psalm 1:2
Psalm 119:99</small>

When you memorize pieces of the Bible, it makes it easier to recall what the Bible says. By meditating on verses, you can gain new insight and are forced to look at your own life in relation to the words of scripture.

Need Something New?

Listen to songs based on scripture passages; keep scriptures posted in places you frequent (bathroom and kitchen); use a verse a day calendar; use a calendar with a verse to memorize each month; memorize some verses with a friend.

Prayer

<small>Psalm 88:2
Luke 11:1-4</small>

Prayer is your direct connection to God. It is not only telling God about your needs, but also listening to God's replies. Through prayer you can lay down your fears, worries, hurts and confusion so God can help you.

Need Something New?

Pray alone or with someone new; pray out loud; write your prayers in a journal; sing your prayers; spend time just listening to God; pray in tongues; use a new prayer posture such as kneeling;, pray scripture; pray at a specific time every day; record the answers to your prayers in a journal; spend time praying specifically to thank, praise or adore God.

Fasting

Fasting is forgoing something with the intent to focus more time and energy on God. The deliberate absence of the item fasted from is a reminder to be with God. Though you may not feel comfortable fasting from food during pregnancy, you can still participate in this discipline by fasting from other activities.

Isaiah 58:3-6
Daniel 9:3

Need Something New?

Fast from a specific food; fast from a frequently visited restaurant; fast from a hobby; fast from the Internet or computer games; fast from cleaning for a day; fast from the telephone; fast from shopping.

Worship

Worship is you looking at God in awe. Although almost anything you do can be done "in worship" of God, worship as a discipline refers to the specific time you set aside to spend time with God and marvel at all he has done.

Psalm 95:6
Psalm 100:2

Need Something New?

Sing and dance while at home; write a song; write a love poem to God; draw a picture for God; buy a new CD to sing along with; try listening to a different style of music.

Service

God calls you to help others out of love. Although it may seem your acts of service are only beneficial to those you assist, God is able to use your acts of service to help you grow and mature.

Psalm 2:11
Ephesians 6:7

Need Something New?

Volunteer at an agency outside your church; start volunteering in your church; practice random acts of kindness; visit a shut-in; go on a short-term mission trip; participate in a fund-raising walk; choose to serve your spouse or children; choose to serve your parents or siblings.

Giving

Proverbs 3:28
Luke 9:12-13

When you give, your money or objects help support physical needs. God says where a person spends her money shows what they value. Giving also helps you to feel free, not controlled by the things you own.

Need Something New?

Break up your regular giving differently such as giving every week or only once a month; give money to a ministry for a specific purpose; give your firstfruits; give ten percent; give to a new charity; give away old clothes or furniture; have a garage sale and donate the money; give used books to the library or a school.

Teaching

Romans 12:7
1 Timothy 4:12

When you teach what you have learned to another person, you are helping to spread the love of God. Although it can be uncomfortable to think of yourself as a teacher, the Bible says we are all adequate to teach and to learn from each other.

Need Something New?

Attend a retreat to learn something new; join a small group to share your stories and learn from others; volunteer to teach a Sunday school class; begin teaching your older children about the Bible; share some of your experiences with a friend or neighbor; help another pregnant woman learn what you have learned; ask someone to disciple you, or disciple someone else.

The placenta is nourished by what you eat and breathe physically. There is another "placenta" called the soul. What you feed on comes into your body-mind-spirit as well.

Carol Gautschi

I have given birth to three beautiful boys, each one of them a wonderful event. However, my second birth was by far the most amazing.

My first delivery was a joyous event—a miracle bringing new life into this world. I had wanted to try to have a natural birth since I had heard it was best for me and my child. Unfortunately, my perfect birth turned into 16 hours on my back with Pitocin, an epidural, a huge episiotomy and my son being pulled out with a vacuum. I was glad to have my son, but felt lied to about giving birth. I did not understand why it was so hard for me.

After becoming pregnant for the second time, I felt God urging me to try a natural birth again. I was so afraid to go through the disappointment and feeling like a failure. I was afraid of the work and how much it would hurt. Everyone I knew was telling me to just plan an epidural because I was too big of a wimp. I prayed desperately to God, asking him to show me what I needed to do.

God answered my prayer in a pushy friend. She continually offered to give my husband and me a crash course in natural birth, and reluctantly we accepted. It was during time with her I began to realize that although a miracle, my first delivery was actually not so wonderful. I had no clue I had choices or that I could affect the way things happened. I just did whatever I was told by my doctor and his team. I learned so much useful information from my friend about nutrition and exercise, about how God had designed my body to give birth and about how my choices were important to God.

I decided I could try again, but I was not going to get my hopes up. Although still a bit nervous in anticipation of more unbearable pain, I tried the things I learned from my friend. I ate healthier, I exercised, I prayed, I stayed home until I was ready to push, and I ate during labor. What a difference!

Imagine 16 hours in the hospital, in pain, on my back, ice chips only. Compare that to being at home, eating when I was hungry, with only 2 hours in the hospital and manageable pain. I gave birth to an 11-pound baby boy without any medication at all; without any episiotomy and no tearing! Who knew I could do it? God did! I went on to give birth to my third son naturally as well.

I am so grateful that God cared enough about my babies and me to answer my prayers in that way. He gave me the information I needed to work with him, and helped me through my labors. I had been a Christian for years but still grew so much from giving birth.

Erin Lowery

Drawing Conclusions
Review of Section Two

Stewardship of Pregnancy

Your pregnancy and the resultant new baby will make many changes in your life. Some changes you may have expected, others may have come as a surprise to you. Take a few minutes to consider the ways your life has changed since becoming pregnant.

Make a diagram similar to the one below. Begin filling in the changes you expect to experience in each of the categories. How will those changes affect your other responsibilities? What can you do now to prepare for these changes?

As you complete this exercise you may find there are responsibilities you can let go. You may also find there are places where you should take on more responsibility. How can you begin making those changes in your life?

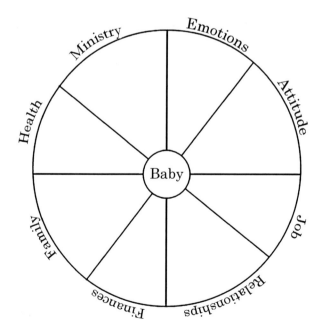

Ten Easy Changes I Can Make

Think about the changes you would like to make and what steps you need to take to accomplish those changes. Select ten things you can start doing today that will help to achieve those positive changes. Write out your list of ten changes, and post it in a place that will make it easily viewed every day.

Exercises I Like

There is no reason for exercise to be boring. Instead, find some activities you really enjoy and work them into your schedule. Take a few minutes to think about the types of exercise you really enjoy. Make a list of activities you can easily participate in on any given week with very little preparation.

Ten Questions about . . .
Lifestyle

1. How does your lifestyle reflect your faith?
2. In what areas does your lifestyle not reflect your faith?
3. How difficult will it be for you to make healthy changes to your lifestyle?
4. What experience have you had with making lifestyle changes?
5. What improves your chances of successfully making changes to your health?
6. What are the areas of most physical concern for you?
7. What can you do to improve your health in those areas?
8. Who can keep you accountable to making healthy lifestyle changes?
9. How does your health affect your spiritual life?
10. Are you satisfied with your current spiritual life?

Making Positive Lifestyle Changes

Christy Callahan
Prenatal Coaching
www.PrenatalCoaching.com

First off, before discussing how to make positive lifestyle changes, I want to encourage you to let go of the need to be perfect. Whew! You can wipe that sweat off your brow and breathe out a sigh of relief. God does not demand perfection, so there is no need to expect perfection of yourself. Lowering the bar sets you free to experience grace as well as the ability to make positive life changes—in God's timing. Now that we got that out of the way, here are a few questions to ponder:

1. What is the most important change you need to make right now?
2. What is it costing you (financially, physically, emotionally, and spiritually) to not make this change?
3. What is your level of commitment to making this change?
4. What steps do you need to take?
5. What kind of support systems need to be in place to move forward?

Let's start with question number one. Be honest with yourself and be willing to take a good look at your life. Something may be staring you straight in the eyes that you have been unwilling to see.

Now that you have faced reality, the next step is to examine how this situation is affecting your life. In other words, take an inventory of the way a particular habit or pattern is negatively impacting your life.

Next, ask yourself how badly you want to change. Sure, you talk on and on about how you want things to be different. Ask yourself: Am I willing to do the hard work it takes to make different choices?

Once you get a feel for your willingness to change, look at specific actions that will bring you closer to your goal. Pick something you can realistically do but have been putting off, perhaps out of fear. Even more importantly, write down what you will do and when you will do it.

Finally, surround yourself with people who will keep you accountable and provide encouragement when things get tough. This means you may decide to let go of friends who make excuses or run you down. You may start to set limits on how you allow others to speak in your presence. The New Living Translation of Proverbs 27:17 says, "As iron sharpens iron, so a friend sharpens a friend." What better time than the present to seek out a group of like-minded persons and/or a life coach who will support you through the ups and downs.

Proverbs 27:12

At the same time that we need boundaries to make changes in our lives, we must also rely on divine grace. When we know deep down that we are OK in God's eyes, we gain a wonderful freedom to be transformed day by day into the likeness of Christ. We read in 2 Corinthians 12:9 (NIV):

2 Corinthians 12:9

"My grace is sufficient for you, [God says,] for my power is made perfect in weakness." Therefore I [Paul] will boast all the more gladly about my weaknesses, so that Christ's power may rest on me.

The same passage in The Message, by Eugene Peterson, goes like this:

[God speaking:] My grace is enough; it's all you need. My strength comes into its own in your weakness. [. . .] I [Paul] just let Christ take over! And so the weaker I get, the stronger I become.

What a relief that we do not have to do it all. God working through us is the One who brings about significant and lasting change. God's grace is all we need.

When you become more gentle and loving with yourself, you gain freedom from self-judgment (trying to determine what is right or wrong about yourself), introspection (obsessively turning your thoughts inward) and unrealistic expectations (thinking you have to do and be too much). You also realize that you no longer need to compare yourself with others, knowing that when you do, you either feel superior (better than others) or inferior (always falling short of your impossible-to-meet standards). This combination of true honesty and God-given grace will propel you to experience new levels of change in your life.

One final note: it is alright to start small when you take action. In fact, Jesus said that if you have faith even as small as a mustard seed you will see mountains move. So do not despise humble beginnings. Just as the little foxes ruin the vineyards in bloom, even one degree of change can alter the course of your life.

Song of Songs 2:15

Subject Three

God's Design for Childbirth

Topics:

Overview of Labor Process	55
How to Measure Progress	58
Before Labor Begins	66
Early Labor	69
Active Labor	73
Transition	76
Pushing Phase	79
Immediate Postpartum	83
Drawing Conclusions	86
Preparation for Labor by Nerida Walker	88

Overview of Pregnancy and Childbirth

God has designed an amazing system for bearing children. You may question God's wisdom in creating a reproductive anatomy that requires such work from the mother to give birth, but looking at the pregnancy as a whole gives a better understanding of the importance of human reproductive design.

When deciding how humans should bear children, God had to create a system that did more than simply allowed the mother to get the baby out. First, there has to be a way to get the baby in, a way for conception to occur. It had to be a way to ensure pregnancy could happen, but self-limit the frequency of pregnancy because human infants need large amounts of care for a relatively long time. God's design of sex for conception prevents random pregnancies. It also provides such an intimate beginning that there is usually a mother and father who have a vested interest in the child conceived.

After the baby is conceived, there has to be a way to protect the baby until he is ready to be born. The baby must have access to nourishment and oxygen to keep him alive and growing, and must be allowed the time to develop the organs and systems necessary to live. However, this must be done in a way that does not

The uterus is designed for the working for creating babies.

damage the health of the mother since any compromise to her health would also endanger the baby.

> Female bodies are a beautiful demonstration of God's creative genius.

Once again God has demonstrated tremendous wisdom by creating women's bodies in a way that the baby does have a safe place to grow and develop. The uterine environment keeps the baby the proper temperature, allows the baby food and oxygen, removes waste products, stretches to accommodate the growth of the baby, and even allows the baby to interact with the parents before birth. As this happens, the mother's body grows and adapts to the new life living inside by increasing the blood supply, increasing the rate at which she eliminates waste products, increasing her lung capacity to allow for more oxygen, slowing down her digestion to allow for more nutrients to be absorbed, and changing her hormone levels to keep everything working properly. All of this happens with relatively few side-effects to the mother.

When it comes to giving birth then, the object is to safely get the baby out of this protected place. God's wisdom shows just as much in the process of birth as it does in pregnancy. In most births, everything happens slowly enough that the mother's body is able to stretch, but not so long that the mother becomes exhausted from the work. The mother's body prepares ahead of time by loosening the pelvis, emptying the bowels and strengthening the uterus so when labor begins the body is ready to work. Once the baby is in position, the mother's body uses the familiar sensation of having to go to the bathroom to signal the mother to begin pushing, and it is the exact same expulsive effort she uses to go to the bathroom.

God has created many ways for adults to bear young, and he could have chosen any way for humans to give birth. However, God understood there was more at stake than the ease with which a child enters this world. The hormonal control that directs the birth process balances the mother's and baby's needs, almost always ensuring the baby is ready to be born.

The main contraction hormone, oxytocin, is a love hormone. It is produced in men and women alike during times of close contact, while eating together and during sexual intimacy. Right before your baby is born, your body will get a surge of oxytocin. This oxytocin surge encourages you to hold and touch your baby. The skin-to-skin contact helps to control your postpartum bleeding and promotes successful breastfeeding. This improves the health of both you and your baby. God's design for birth works not only to have a living mom and baby, but to have healthy and thriving mothers and babies.

Exploring the problems humans would have with other reproductive systems speaks even more to the wisdom of God in the way he created humans to give birth. Take some time to consider why God opted against these seemingly easier reproductive systems for humans.

God's reproductive designs are not random, but intentionally species specific.

- Some plants have a reproductive system that uses wind to pollinate.
- Fish mothers lay large numbers of eggs, then the fish father swims over them to fertilize the eggs.
- Baby birds develop inside eggs that remain in the nest, outside the mother's body.
- Insects lay many eggs that go through distinct larva and pupa stages before becoming an adult.
- Cats and dogs give birth to liters of 4 or more babies at a time.

Measuring Progress in Labor

> Hosea 4:6
> My people are destroyed for lack of knowledge.

There is more than one way to measure anything, just as there is frequently more than one correct answer to a question. A piece of cake can be measured for weight; height, width or depth, volume, density, or calories. These are all quantitative measures, meaning they give value to the question, "How much cake do we have?" You can also measure a cake for taste, flavor and texture, color or the beauty of the icing. These are all qualitative measures, meaning they give value to the qualities of the cake.

In the same way, your blood can be measured in a variety of ways. You can determine amounts of iron, cholesterol, presence of bacteria or T-cells by analyzing the blood. You can also determine blood pressure or the pulse by analyzing the effects of the blood on other body tissues. These are all useful measures and have their purpose. But you would never look at one number and assume it represented your overall health. Although they are somewhat related, you cannot make assumptions about the cholesterol level by measuring blood volume. To get an accurate understanding of your overall health you need to look at all the measurements and how they relate to each other.

It is the same when you measure progress in labor. Focusing on one way to measure does not give you an accurate picture of the overall progress. You need to determine several things and look at how they are related to get an accurate understanding of where you are. The following measures should be used together to determine progress in labor. Understanding how far along in labor you are can help prevent going to the birth place too early (or too late). It can also help your companions find appropriate comfort measures for you.

Cervical Changes

Your cervix is the doughnut shaped opening of the uterus. The word cervix means neck, and most of the time your cervix does look like a neck on your uterus, although it is upside down. Before pregnancy, your cervix was about 2.5 cm (1 inch) long and felt about as firm as the tip of your nose. Pregnancy hormones changed your cervix by lengthening it, softening it and plugging it up with mucus. When your body begins preparing for labor your cervix will change again to allow your baby to pass through into the vagina.

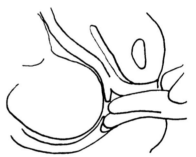

The cervix is the narrow opening at the bottom of the vagina.

Cervical changes can be assessed during labor if your midwife performs a vaginal exam. Your midwife will insert gloved fingers into your vagina to feel the cervix and determine dilation, effacement, station and position. Although care is taken to prevent introducing infection, inserting anything into the vagina does increase the risk of uterine infection. The risk becomes greater if the bag of waters is broken, so many midwives and doctors will minimize the use of cervical checks if the bag of waters has been broken.

Cervical changes are assessed by inserting fingers into the vagina.

Birth is God's time. It can't be rushed or programmed to suit anyone's clock. It is a time to simply be there, respecting the woman's space and the natural rhythms of her body. Think of how time ceases to have relevance when you are caught up in the presence of God worshipping Him or when you are in love and spending time with your beloved.

Time flies by and you barely notice. Birth time is the timing of nature. Who knows when spring will come? Can a budding flower be forced open? Yet, in time, these things unfold. So does birth. I sometimes suggest to my clients that they visit the ocean and see the rhythm of the waves on the shore. That right there teaches you, deep within, so much about the patterns, rhythms and power of labour.

Julie Bell

Dilation

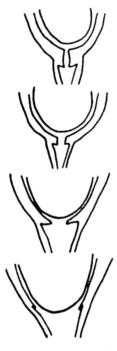

Progression through dilation refers to the cervix opening.

Dilation is the measurement of the opening of the cervix. A closed cervix is given the value of 0, while a completely open cervix is given the value of ten. These roughly approximate centimeters, but there is no ruler used to give the number. Instead, the number is estimated by the midwife, nurse or doctor during an internal vaginal exam.

In general, the further you are dilated, the further you are in labor. Average dilations are given for the different stages of labor, and the baby cannot drop into the birth canal until the cervix is dilated enough to allow the baby's head to pass.

Speed of labor is sometimes assumed by dilation, however, this can be misleading. While the standard assumption is dilation of one centimeter per hour after 4 centimeters, the actual dilation can occur much faster, much slower or a combination of fast and slow. It is not uncommon for a mother to maintain a dilation of 5, 6 or 7 centimeters for a time then dilate completely to ten in a matter of a few contractions. The Guide to Effective Care in Pregnancy and Childbirth gives .5 cm per hour as the bottom range for normal progress in labor. This means when you divide your dilation by the amount of time you have been in active labor, you should have a number that is .5 or higher.

Effacement

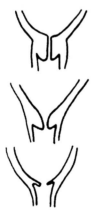

Progression through effacement refers to the cervix thinning.

Effacement is the measurement of the thickness of the cervix. During pregnancy, the cervix is long and thick, acting as a protective barrier for the baby. As labor nears, the cervix softens and begins to react to contractions by stretching around the baby's head. Effacement is measured during an internal vaginal exam and given a percentage value from 0 to 100 based on the midwife, nurse or doctor's assessment. A cervix that is 100 percent effaced is stretched as thin as possible.

Effacement must happen before you can achieve significant dilation. The thinning out of effacement allows the cervix to give way and open. This is similar to the way you cannot open your mouth wide with your lips pushed thickly forward.

Cervical Position

The uterus is anchored to your body by ligaments and the cervix drops into the vagina. Because the vagina, cervix and uterus are all soft tissues, they can be compressed, pulled and generally moved. This allows your cervix to change positions based on signals from your body. For example, when your body is fertile, the cervix gets softer, more open and higher in the vagina. After ovulation the cervix closes, regains its firmness and drops back into its usual position.

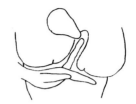

You can feel your cervix on the upper wall of your vagina.

Because of the shape and location of the pelvic structures, your cervix generally points towards your back as it drops into your vagina (posterior position). In order for your baby to have the easiest route out of your body, the cervix will move so it faces more toward your front (anterior position). This generally happens early in labor, and until it happens it may be difficult for your caregiver to measure your dilation and effacement.

Station

Station refers to where your baby is located in relation to the narrowest part of your pelvis. When your baby's head is at the narrowest part of the pelvis, he is said to be at 0 station. Before he reaches the narrowest part he will move between a -4 and -1 station. After moving past the narrowest part, he will move from a +1 to a +4. Plus 4 Station is when your baby is on the perineum, the skin of the vagina.

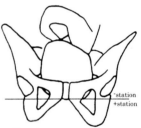

Station measures position relative to the pelvis.

Station is not necessarily related to effacement or dilation, as these can happen before your baby descends well into the pelvis, or your baby can begin to descend before you achieve significant dilation. However, in general, as you progress in dilation your baby will move lower and lower into the pelvis. As your baby moves lower, you may find the pressure on your back during contractions moves lower and lower.

Position

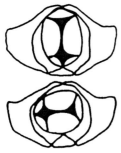

The soft spots on your baby's head let the midwife know what direction he is facing.

Just as a clock assigns a time based on the position of the hands, the position of your baby relative to the pelvis is assigned a value. Because your baby is floating, he has the ability to rotate as if twirling in circles without changing his presentation (head down or buttocks down). Position refers to which direction the back of your baby's head (the occiput) is facing. If the back of your baby's head is facing your back, he is said to be OP or occiput posterior. If the back of his head is facing your front he is said to be OA or occiput anterior. There are also terms for whether your baby is more to the right or more to the left or facing your side. Your baby's position will change during labor. Most babies turn in labor so they are in an OA position because this is the easiest way for the head to move into the pelvis.

When a baby is head down, midwives measure position by feeling the top of the baby's head. Sometimes babies are in positions that make it very easy to tell where the back is because you can feel the spine or back and buttocks through your belly. However it is possible for your baby to turn his head without turning his body. As your baby progresses through the birth canal, the head will rotate to fit through the pelvis, but the body may remain in the same position.

Contraction Timing

Contractions are the tightening of the uterus to open the cervix. The uterus is a muscle and so has the ability to shrink its fibers which causes tightening. This tightening reduces the volume of the inside of the uterus, pushing the baby's head against the cervix and pulling the cervix up around the baby's head. In general contractions will get longer, stronger and happen more frequently as you progress in labor.

To time your contractions, you will look at two things, the frequency (how quickly are the contractions coming) and the duration (how long are the contractions lasting). The frequency is measured from the beginning of one contraction to the beginning of the next. The duration is measured from the beginning of a contraction to the end of the same contraction. Here are some examples:

Begins	Ends	Frequency	Duration
8:45:20	8:46:20	Unknown	60 seconds
8:47:19	8:48:20	119 seconds	61 seconds
8:49:17	8:50:20	118 seconds	62 seconds

For this example, it is appropriate to average the frequency of 2 minutes and the duration of 60 seconds. When you time contractions in labor you will want to adhere to the following guidelines:

Time five or six contractions and then take the average from those contractions.

Only time your contractions if you feel something has changed and you want to verify it with contraction time. Do not time every contraction because it is boring to do and provides useless information.

In general, it is the duration of the contraction, not the frequency that determines how much work is accomplished. Contractions less than 60 seconds long are not really long enough to do much work to open the cervix, even if the contractions are coming every five minutes.

Emotional Markers

Laboring women tend to move through an emotional pattern which varies little from woman to woman. As labor progresses you become more serious; are more inward focused; talk less; want to be disturbed less and slowly let go of the control of labor. These are all normal responses to active labor. As labor progresses further, you may become discouraged; give up; become restless and irritable; feel overwhelmed or trapped and have difficulty relaxing. These are all normal responses to transition.

When using emotional markers it is important to understand who you are. How are you reacting relative to how you reacted an hour or two ago? How has your attitude changed? Some women talk during the entire labor, however the frequency of conversation

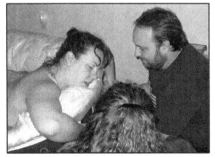

© 2006 Therese Franklin
As labor progresses, women become more serious.

or timing of their comments changes. Other women are quiet by nature and it will be difficult to assess whether there is a decrease in talkativeness.

As you move through labor you will find yourself becoming more focused, using deeper concentration and working more intensely with your contractions. Do not focus on one emotional marker, but use the overall attitude as your guide.

Physical Markers

Just as laboring women progress through emotional markers of labor, they also experience physical markers. The physical markers are caused by the normal hormonal changes during labor. As you move into active labor you will find you move less frequently and more deliberately; lose your appetite; breathe deeper; become sweaty and require effort to work through contractions. As you move into transition you may begin to feel nausea; shaking or trembling; hot and cold flashes; the bag of waters may break and you may begin to have urges to push.

Labor Process

The stages of labor are human-made segments to measure progress, no more, no less.

Labor is a process much like the journey through seasons is a process. The first day of spring may be marked on your calendar, but the weather does not immediately change on that day. Instead, the first day of spring is a guideline used to mark progress through the year. Sometime near that point certain things will begin to happen. You do not necessarily know when or how fast they will happen.

It is the same in labor. In labor, the "stages" are artificial divisions made to help humans understand the progress made. There is a general process labor takes, and certain things begin to happen after other things happen. However, there is no sudden change in feeling or behavior because you reached any particular spot in labor.

As you journey through the stages of labor, it is interesting to note how the spiritual or emotional response at any particular stage is a basic principle of

Christianity. For example, in early labor you will need to exhibit patience. When you are working through first stage labor, you will need to have perseverance and at transition you will discover strength in humility. In his wisdom, God created a physical system for birth that strengthens you spiritually while providing a safe way for your baby to be born.

> To describe a contraction and the sensations therein, I would say that it is your whole boy agreeing to birth your baby. The contraction begins at your shoulders, tingles down through your body as your uterus hugs down on your baby. . .you relax into the intensity amazed at how strong your body is. . . mentally move aside and allow your bottom to release as your lower back and upper legs move into the harmony of this job of birth. As the contraction releases, you breathe deeply and sigh. . .mentally rewarding yourself on a job well done. You are one step closer to your baby.
>
> *MeriBeth Glenn*

Before Labor Begins

Normal Before Labor
Losing mucus plug
Bloody show
Leaking breasts
Irregular contractions
Feeling wobbly
Lightening
Increased mucus

The process of giving birth begins weeks before you feel the contractions that make you catch your breath. Your body and your baby's body will both be preparing for the upcoming event in ways you may not even notice. If you recognize the work before labor begins, it is called pre-labor, false labor, or prodromal labor.

Throughout your pregnancy, your body has been producing a hormone called Corticotropin-releasing hormone (CRH). Near the end of pregnancy, larger amounts of this hormone are being released by the placenta and your baby. CRH does two things. First it signals an increase in estrogen production by the placenta, necessary to prepare your body for labor. Second, it signals your baby's lungs to mature, necessary to prepare your baby for life outside the womb.

The increased estrogen makes your uterus more sensitive to oxytocin, a hormone that causes contractions. Your baby's brain and the placenta respond to the hormones by increasing oxytocin production. As these changes are happening, you may find yourself feeling more frequent and prolonged series of Braxton-Hicks contractions. Generally these contractions are mild and irregular, lasting less than 45 seconds. It is also common for these contractions to stop or slow down if you change your activity. Contractions may stop and start several times as the hormone levels increase.

Higher levels of estrogen also signal an increase in prostaglandin levels. Prostaglandins help soften and efface the cervix to make it ready for the stretching necessary to allow your baby to be born. Prostaglandins stimulate the contractions you have been feeling to become stronger. As your cervix softens, you may find the increased contractions achieve some dilation before labor begins. Some women have enough dilation to release the mucus plug (tissue formed to seal the cervix during pregnancy), and others find the cervix opens enough to begin to see bloody mucus known as bloody show.

At the same time, your body will increase its production of relaxin, a hormone responsible for the relaxation of the ligaments and cartilage of the pelvis. This makes it possible for your pelvis to stretch to accommodate your baby's head. As your pelvis becomes more flexible, the pressure of your baby's head is able to stretch it. You may feel pressure on your pubic bone or notice your baby "dropped" deeper into your pelvis. It is common for dropping (or lightening) to relieve some of the pressure on your lungs or stomach, but increase the pressure on your bladder. Because the relaxin is distributed to your entire body, you may find yourself feeling loose or wobbly in all your joints.

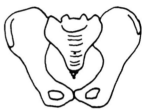

The pelvis has joints on the front and on the sides in back.

Your vagina also prepares to give birth to your baby. The vagina is designed in a way that allows it to open, similar to the way the petals of a flower open. As labor approaches, vaginal tissues become more elastic allowing even more stretch to accommodate the baby. You may find the cervical mucus secreted from your vagina becomes thinner in texture and more abundant.

As labor nears and the placenta ages, it begins to allow larger molecules into your baby's blood. This allows antibodies and immunoglobulins to get to your baby, increasing his protection against disease and illness. Your body also prepares for your baby's birth by producing more colostrum, which you may or may not leak from your breasts. Colostrum is valuable for your baby because it contains your antibodies, which can help prevent your baby from becoming sick.

In addition to the maturation of his lungs, your baby is also preparing for labor by storing iron and fat. The extra iron helps supply baby's needs while breastfeeding. The extra fat helps baby maintain his body temperature, and also helps supply calorie needs until your milk comes in.

> Psalm 119:165
> Great peace have they who love your law, and nothing can make them stumble.

It is common for mothers to become anxious or excited, reacting to every contraction as if it is the start of active labor. It is also common for mothers to become physically and emotionally drained as they go through several cycles of contractions that end without the baby being born. Mothers who are uncomfortable in pregnancy can become impatient for labor to begin, looking for ways to speed the process of labor starting. These physical changes are important to the health of your baby and for your ability to give birth successfully. For that reason, it is important for you to have peace as this process takes place.

> Philippians 4:6-7

Peace throughout pre-labor allows you to remain calm and active regardless of the presence or absence of labor signals. Peace allows you to sleep through mild contractions that come and go for days. Peace lets you go on with your daily activities even though labor may start today.

Peace allows you to live your life until real labor demands your attention. Peace is important when you are frustrated that labor will not start. Peace is important when you are afraid of the upcoming labor.

Peace is not everything being perfect. Peace is being able to do what you know you need to do regardless of what is or is not happening to prepare your body for labor. Peace is trusting you can take a nap and not miss your baby's birth. Peace is being comfortable enough with the process you neither rush it nor avoid it. Peace is knowing this can be a frustrating and exhausting part of pregnancy, but God will give you the strength to get through it. Peace is letting God be in control, and staying willing to do the things you need to do every day.

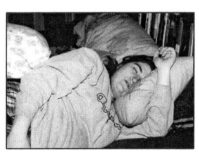
©2002 Jennifer Vanderlaan
You can rest while contractions come and go.

Early Labor

No one knows what it is that finally triggers the start of labor. Progesterone is the dominate hormone throughout most of pregnancy, but near labor estrogen levels rise higher than progesterone. This new hormonal ratio makes the uterus more sensitive to hormones that cause contractions. In addition, the normal Braxton-Hicks contractions increase the production of prostaglandin, which causes more contractions. Eventually, the hormone levels are high enough to start a series of contractions that continue to increase hormone levels which continue to build upon each other in a cycle that eventually ends with your baby in your arms.

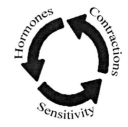

You may not recognize when your Braxton-Hicks contractions become early labor contractions. In all actuality, the difference may only be recognizable with time. In early labor, the contractions will begin to show a regular pattern that increases the length and strength of the contractions. This is not instant, it can take hours or days to move through early labor, with you wondering the whole time if labor has actually started. Generally, the contractions will be 10 minutes apart or less and last less than a minute. Your midwife may consider you in early labor if you are dilated less than 5 centimeters.

Normal Early Labor
Losing mucus plug
Bloody show
Leaking breasts
Increased mucus
Contractions 30-45
   seconds and less than
   10 minutes apart

There are a few physical signs you can use to recognize early labor. Most women will begin labor with a mild diarrhea or digestive cramps. This may be related to the increased levels of prostaglandins, and helps to empty the digestive tract to make room for your baby to be born. Some women also feel cramping or a backache similar to what they experience before a period. This is often accompanied by a feeling of unease, being restless and uncomfortable in every position. Although you may not recognize it until after labor, you may also have a spurt of energy accompanied by an urgency to prepare for baby.

If you have not experienced any bloody show, you may begin to see it at this time. As the cervix begins to dilate and the mucus that closes off the cervix breaks down, the blood-tinged mucus exits your body through the vagina. This will be a pink or bright red blood, not the dark brownish blood you may see after intercourse or a vaginal exam.

It is not a good idea to start timing every contraction as soon as you think they are regular. This leads to a very boring and long time in labor. Instead, time five or six contractions and then wait either several hours or until you can feel a change in the contractions. If after several hours the contractions have not gotten longer, stronger and closer together, you are still in pre-labor.

> **During Real Labor**
> Your contractions will:
> Build in intensity
> Grow closer together
> Grow in length
> Not stop with activity
> Not stop with rest
> Not stop when you eat

There are other tests to determine if this is real labor or pre-labor, such as changing your activity or eating something to see if the contractions stop, but it is not necessary to know at this point. Despite the only thing running through your head being, "Am I in labor?" it may not even be advantageous to know.

Early labor is the longest phase of labor, and generally the contractions are relatively easy to handle. Unfortunately, once a mother has decided she is in labor, it becomes very difficult to ignore the contractions no matter how infrequent or undemanding they are. It is normal for early labor contractions to continue for hours and sometimes days as your body and your baby make final preparations for birth.

We are all familiar with the saying, "A watched pot never boils." In reality, the watched pot does boil, and the watched early labor does progress—they just *seem* to take forever. In the process you miss out on other important pieces of the puzzle. In cooking, you use the time while the water boils to prepare the ingredients to go into the meal. In early labor, you use the time while waiting for

Early Labor

labor to finish a project, catch up on sleep or com[plete] your daily tasks. Continuing your normal routi[ne is] important to making sure your body is able to handl[e the] work of labor because you continue to eat, rest and m[ove.]

Imagine for a moment what labor would be like i[f you] stopped eating, sleeping and doing the normal thing[s you] do during the day because you were in early lab[or. It] might feel really exciting and fun for the first hour. [After] two hours you begin to get bored. After three hour[s you] are hungry, but do not eat because you might be in [labor.] After four hours you are sick of waiting and want to [know] what you can do to make this go faster because you should have been asleep three hours ago but did not go to bed because you were in early labor. By the time you have progressed far enough to be in active labor you are frustrated, overly tired, feel like you've been laboring for hours and just want the whole thing over with—and you've only just begun to feel contractions that hurt.

You will not sleep through the birth of your baby so if you are tired, go to bed. You will do more damage to yourself and your baby by starving yourself than you will do by eating in early labor, so if you are hungry, eat something. Early labor will not move faster if you go to the hospital; in fact, it may slow down or stop, so wait until you cannot ignore the contractions before deciding to get checked.

A good rule of thumb is to be patient, ignoring the contractions until they demand your attention. This is easier said than done, because early labor is often accompanied by excitement and eagerness, especially if this is your first baby. Patience is really a measure of maturity. Children have very little patience; they do not have a full understanding of the passing of time or the things necessary to accomplish whatever it is they are working on. Similarly, children are afraid they may miss something important if they are not paying close attention to, and having their hands all over, whatever has their interest. As an adult, you do have the understanding and skills necessary to be successful at waiting.

True patience is not simply delayed gratification. It is not just waiting to get what you want. Patience is rooted in the understanding of God as sovereign. He is in control

---

Psalm 40:1
I waited patiently for the LORD; he turned to me and heard my cry.

of your labor whether it moves quickly or slowly. Patience is not dependant on your ultimately receiving what you desired. Instead, patience is the calm waiting you exhibit while things are not going the way you desired.

Ephesians 4:2-3

In the Bible we are called to be patient with other believers to maintain unity. This lets us see patience is not simply about waiting for the right circumstances, but about giving God the time he needs to make changes in others and ourselves to accomplish his goal. True patience is giving up control of the clock; everything does not have to be your way right away. Early labor gives you the opportunity to mature spiritually by growing your patience.

Active Labor

When the time is right, your contractions will be strong enough that you no longer question the reality of labor. You will find contractions demand your attention, requiring you to focus your thoughts, breathing or movements to prevent being overwhelmed by the intensity. Generally, active labor contractions last at least a minute and are less than 5 minutes apart. Your midwife will consider you in active labor when you are dilated between 5 and 8 centimeters.

Along with the stronger, longer contractions, you may notice physical changes which can reassure you this is really labor. Most women find their hunger naturally lessens during active labor until they have no appetite. This is a gradual process as labor progresses, starting perhaps with having only a light appetite during early labor to no appetite or even the thought of food causing sudden indigestion.

Many women also find their desire to talk during labor decreases. This is another normal slow progression which may begin with stopping the conversation at the peak of a contraction, then not talking during a contraction, and perhaps even moving to the point of not wanting to talk between contractions. Some women lose their desire to listen to others talking in a similar progression.

You will find it takes more energy to move the further you progress in labor. You may begin by stopping your

---

Normal Active Labor
Strong contractions
Contractions are more than 60 seconds long and 5 minutes apart or less
Decreased hunger
Decreased modesty
Turned inward
Less talking
Less moving

movements at the peak of a contraction, then not wanting to move during a contraction. In active labor you may not want to move even between contractions, though it can be more comfortable to change positions regularly. It is helpful to change your position every half hour to an hour, even if it takes you a few contractions to get into a new comfortable position. You may also find it helpful to rock or sway your hips with contractions, even if the rest of your body wants to be still.

As the intensity of the contractions increases, your body will respond by producing endorphins. Endorphins are feel good hormones responsible for the "runner's high." They are also released by your body during orgasm. Endorphin levels are at their highest level ever during labor, and they have a profound effect on the process.

High levels of endorphins make it possible for you to manage your pain by actually reducing the sensation. In addition, the chemical composition of endorphin causes a unique mental state in which you may appear to be "zoned out" or "in another world."

Endorphins pay a larger role in the process than just pain relief. The high levels of endorphins cause and increase in the hormone prolactin. Increased prolactin levels prepare your breasts to produce milk to nourish your baby. Prolactin is also believed to play a role in the protective "mothering" behavior normal to mothers.

James 1:4
James 5:10-11
To make it through active labor, you will need perseverance. About 17 percent of women give birth with low levels of pain, but most do not. Unfortunately, labor does not end when it gets tough. The initial reaction is to give up, give in or simply want to end labor. You can no more end labor than you can instantly end any other difficult task in your life. The goal is to work with your body appropriately, allowing labor to progress.

Some women lie in bed waiting for the whole thing to be over. Just waiting for labor to be over is not persevering, it is avoiding. It is not good for your body or your baby. Your body will give you signals to let you know what positions are the most comfortable, and usually what is most comfortable for you is also the most helpful for the baby to move through the pelvis. Trying to avoid labor by lying in bed will make you more uncomfortable, and without the help of gravity to move your baby down, can lead to a longer labor.

Some women try to do everything regardless of their body's need for it. Rather than respond to the signals from their bodies, they will try every position for two or three contractions then move on to the next hoping this will speed labor. Using comfort techniques or positions in an attempt to force the labor to move according to your schedule rather than responding to the labor your body needs is not perseverance, it is controlling. While changing positions is good, it should be in response to the signals from your body, not an attempt to force labor to move faster than it should. It also should not come from an expectation that you are "supposed to" be laboring in any particular way. As long as you are comfortable and there is no concern for safety, it is appropriate to continue with a coping technique that works.

Perseverance is accepting the work that must be done, and doing the work you need to do even when it is hard. Perseverance is continuing to do your best, drawing on the strength of God to get you through. To persevere is to continue to do your best even when things do not work out the way you want them to. Perseverance is about not only the physical work, but also the mental focus and taking the time to make wise decisions. It is easiest to persevere when you have someone with you encouraging you to continue.

> Hebrews 10:36
> You need to persevere so that when you have done the will of God, you will receive what he has promised.

Transition

Normal Transition
Strong contractions
Contractions with double peaks and almost no break between them
No modesty
Hot and cold flashes
Shivering or shaking
Nausea
Unable to get comfortable
Feeling panicked or overwhelmed
Giving up

Transition is the time your body is completing dilation and preparing to push your baby out. It is generally very intense with contractions right on top of each other, and sometimes with double peaks. But it is also the shortest part of labor, generally lasting 15 minutes to half an hour. Physiologically, transition serves an important purpose. The increased contractions put tremendous pressure on your cervix. Your body responds to this increasing pressure by increasing the hormone levels.

Stress hormones, which hinder earlier labor, increase naturally during transition. After the relaxing, daydreaming effect of the endorphins, these hormones make you alert and give you new energy. While this is happening in your body, your baby responds by producing hormones that prepare him to breathe. The levels of stress hormones drop quickly after your baby is born.

Oxytocin, the hormone which causes contractions, is significantly increased in response to the stretching of your cervix. As oxytocin increases, the intensity of your contractions increases. These stronger contractions make it possible for your baby to exit your body. In addition, because oxytocin is a love hormone, the high levels cause a feeling of well-being and love that helps you bond with your baby.

The hormonal interplay of transition create a system in which your cervix and vagina stretch and relax, while your contractions increase. In an undisturbed labor, this results in what Dr. Michel Odent calls the Fetal Ejection Reflex. The Fetal Ejection Reflex is a normal, physiological response to labor in which the baby is born quickly and easily. In some cases, midwives say the baby seems to slip right out.

As your body adjusts to the last few centimeters of dilation, just before you begin pushing, the hormone levels are so high you will see undeniable physical signs. Observation of these signs alerts you to the fact that you are in transition.

Some women get hot and cold flashes, cold sweats, nausea or vomiting, shivering or shaking, hiccups, burping and a general inability to feel comfortable in any position. This is the most common time for the bag of waters to break naturally. When you begin to show these signs, it does not matter if you are not dilated to 9 or 10 centimeters, it means you are very close to pushing.

During transition, contractions will be long and close. They may be 90 seconds long and 2 minutes apart, which gives you a 30-second rest time between contractions. The contractions may double peak, or they may seem to be one right after the other without any break. Another physical sign is the inability to relax or be comfortable. A woman who was handling labor well may suddenly find she has no idea what to do and nothing is comfortable any more. At this point, it is the job of your helpers to assist you into various positions in an attempt to find the one that will keep you most comfortable.

Many women find their dilation is not uniform. Rather than dilating a centimeter every hour or two, they will dilate to 4 or 6 or 7 and seem to stop for a time. This does not mean labor has stalled, as long as your contractions continue to get more intense, closer together and longer, simply prepare yourself. Often the body gets ready and then suddenly dilates the rest of the way in a few contractions.

You will also recognize transition by the desire to give up. This is when women claim they can not do it anymore. Most women begin to doubt their ability to go on, and may seem to forget they are in labor to give birth to a baby. This is also the time in labor when most women ask for something to help them with the pain, feeling they just can not go on.

The "giving up" or feeling out of control may be recognized by comments the mother makes. It is not uncommon for a mother to say, "I can't do this," or "I need something." This is not necessarily the mother asking for medication, but for help. She can no longer handle the labor the way she has been, and she needs to do something different.

Transition is the time when you are the most emotionally needy as well. Some women need constant reassurance that they are OK and the baby is fine. This may be due to the overall "giving up" and feeling that you are out of control. Most women will respond well to positive encouragements, and some require no special consideration other than giving them the physical and emotional space to labor.

> Proverbs 3:34
> He mocks proud mockers but gives grace to the humble.

Transition can be the most powerful time of your labor. You will feel the great strength of your muscles contracting. The force of your own muscles will actually stop you in your tracks and many women need to focus to continue breathing. Birth lets you see the raw power God placed inside you. Seeing this power, it can become tempting to worship the creation instead of the Creator, turning giving birth, your body or yourself into an idol. In his great wisdom, God designed transition in a way that although you see the power, you accept your inability to control it. God designed transition in a way that teaches humility.

Humility is not thinking lowly of yourself. Instead, it is the accurate measurement of your strength and limitations. When you get to the point of transition, you will see the power you hold inside. Because of the overwhelming nature of transition, you will also see your need for something outside yourself–your need for God. This very real, very powerful and very raw experience with God is unique to labor. It is not uncommon for women to be more confident, more willing to try new things, less likely to give up and having an overall better attitude about the person God made them to be after experiencing the power of transition.

Second Stage

At some point, the sensation of your contractions will change to a need to push. This can happen suddenly and involuntarily, or can take several contractions to build to a strong urge to push. Most women find their contractions spread out to about 5-minute intervals when they start pushing. Some mothers have a brief time of rest in which they have no strong contractions right before they have the urge to push.

The urge to push is caused by the same nerves that alert you to a full bowel, so it really does feel exactly like you have to go to the bathroom very badly. When the baby is low enough in the pelvis, the pressure of the uterus contracting will push the baby onto the nerves and signal an intense "gotta go" feeling. It may even cause you to push involuntarily, which is completely normal and healthy.

As the contractions push the baby further and further out the cervix, you may need a contraction or two for the uterus to tighten up around the baby and push him down onto the nerves during a contraction. It is normal for you to have between three and five separate urges to push in a contraction. Your job will be to work with your body, pushing when you have the urge.

Pushing, especially for a first time mom, can take an hour or more. It is an exercise in faith, in which the progress you make is unseen. You will push and push and push and still not see any of the baby's head. This is

Normal Second Stage
Contractions space out, have urge to push
Renewed energy
Can take 2 hours or longer
Position Changes can be helpful
Crowning may burn

normal. It is not until the baby is almost born that you begin to see any physical signs of progress. It begins with a small glimpse of the head during contractions that hides again when the pressure of the contraction ends. As the baby moves lower and your vagina stretches, more and more of the baby's head can be seen. Eventually, the baby's head will move beyond your pubic bone and will not be able to slide back in when the contraction ends. At this point, you will begin the crowning.

Your baby's trip through the birth canal is not a straight shot out. Instead, it requires your baby to rotate his head first to one side to get through the pelvis, and then back as he moves under the pubic bone. This rotation and descent happens best when you are upright as much as possible. Positions such as squatting, standing and leaning over something give you the freedom to move your pelvis to help baby navigate the turns, allows the coccyx to be flexed out of the way all

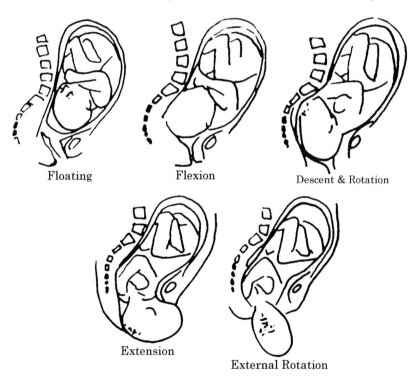

Progress through the Pelvis

while allowing gravity to help the process. Pushing while reclining on your back requires you to push your baby uphill against gravity, prevents pelvic movements and pushes the coccyx bone in the path of the baby. Changing positions is helpful even during pushing, assisting the baby in rotating. As in any stage of labor, select positions based on what is comfortable.

Your baby begins his descent through your pelvis long before you start pushing by bringing his chin to his chest (this is called flexion). By positioning his head in this way, the part of his head with the smallest diameter will move into the pelvis first. Even though heads are somewhat circular, his head will be more oval with a larger and smaller diameter as his head compresses to move through the pelvis.

When he is as far as the ischial spines, his head will begin to rotate so the back of his head is facing your front. In doing this, he is positioning his head so the largest part goes through the largest open area of your pelvis. As you push, he continues to move lower and lower until his head is low enough to slip beneath the pubic arch. At this point, crowning begins to occur. The back of his neck will pivot on your pubic bone allowing his forehead, face and chin to slowly pass over your perineum.

Crowning, the time when the vagina stretches around the widest part of your baby's head, can feel like a burning, tearing or pulling sensation. This is your body's signal to stop pushing and allow the skin to stretch. You may find yourself caught in a small tug-o-war between the urge to push and the burning sensation that says stop pushing. Listen to your body, going slowly, starting and stopping the pushing as needed. Although if feels like it takes forever, it is only a few moments before your body will stretch around the baby's head. If the cord is around the neck, it can be loosened to allow the baby to pass through the cord or slipped over the baby's head before the next contraction.

During crowning your baby's head stretches your perineum.

After his head is out, he will begin to rotate his head again, this time to release his shoulders. The shoulder closest to your pubic bone will be released first. Once the shoulders are released, the rest of his body will slip out.

> Hebrews 11:1
> Now faith is being sure of what we hope for and certain of what we do not see.

It can be difficult to keep faith that your efforts are productive, and you may feel tempted to try to rush the pushing process. But you must remember the system God created works. The slow progress allows your body adequate time to stretch while also allowing your baby adequate time to conform to the confines of your pelvis. Pushing only when you have the urge, and only as strong as your body dictates can help you keep the energy you need for the pushing phase. Directed pushing (where you push through the entire contraction taking breaths at 10-second intervals) may allow the baby to be born faster, but also tires you and decreases the amount of oxygen available to you and your baby. Overly forceful pushing can also hinder the baby's rotation. It is best to push with your body in faith the amount of pushing your body calls for is adequate.

Once the head is out, your baby will rotate again, this time to move the shoulders through the pelvis. When the shoulders are free, it only takes a fraction of a contraction to push the rest of the baby through the canal and into your waiting arms. Your baby may come out with a gush of water that was surrounding him, so be ready to hold someone who feels slippery.

Does it surprise you to know the 'lying on your back, legs in stirrups' position is the WORST position for giving birth? It's bad for the mother and bad for the baby, but the doctor needs you on your back because it makes *his* job easier.

But whose job *should* we make easier? Whose comfort *should* be of concern? There are three very important players in this birth scene: There's the woman in labor, struggling to give birth to a new life, pushing a human being through her pelvic bones. No, we won't worry about her comfort during the process, except to give her some drugs for the pain. There's the baby, who may be oxygen-deprived when the mother lies on her back, causing fetal distress. No, don't worry about the baby, we'll resuscitate if we have to. Then there's the doctor, who is being paid—*well* paid—to catch the baby the mother pushes out. Let's make sure *he's* in a comfortable position!

Sheila Stubbs
Excerpted from *Giving Birth the Easy Way* © 2005

Third Stage

After your baby has been born, the things you do out of love and kindness for your baby will also benefit you. Your immediate interactions with your new baby are not only helpful for him, they help you as well. Allowing your baby to nurse immediately stimulates your body's production of oxytocin, which helps to return the uterus to its normal size. Your baby's gentle kicking on your abdomen while you hold him will also stimulate the uterus to contract and shrink. This shrinking of the uterus causes the placenta to be sloughed off the wall of the uterus, and it will be born without much of a push when you feel pressure. The oxytocin shrinking the uterus also helps to prevent blood loss from the newly opened wound where the placenta was attached to the uterus. It is normal for the placenta to take anywhere from five minutes to half an hour to be born.

Another example of mutual benefit is the skin to skin contact you will have with your baby immediately after he is born. This helps your baby to regulate his heart rate and temperature, helps him to establish a regular breathing pattern, exposes him to the natural bacteria on your skin reducing his risk of illness and soothes him, decreasing the amount of crying.

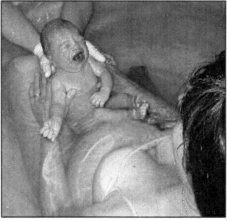

©2006 Joseph Schroer
Immediate skin to skin contact is good for you and your baby.

The skin to skin contact not only helps to build a good breastfeeding relationship. It also helps to maintain your oxytocin levels which continues to help reduce your bleeding and helps to keep you calm and responsive to your baby. Oxytocin is a love hormone responsible in part for human bonding. The immediate skin to skin contact gives you a strong foundation for bonding. The oxytocin can also help to increase your milk production, which further improves breastfeeding success.

There is no rush to cut the cord, as long as it is pulsing your baby is receiving oxygen from the placenta and cutting the cord does not speed up the birth of the placenta. Exposure to the air will begin the process of closing the blood vessels, which will stop the pulsing of the cord. Holding the baby on your abdomen and waiting to cut the cord until it stops pulsing ensures your baby has the proper blood volume.

You may find yourself feeling shaky from the rush of adrenalin. You may find yourself in a bit of disbelief that this really just happened; giving birth is often emotionally charged. You may be excited, nervous, joyful and scared all at the same time. This is normal.

It may take you a few hours to be confident in your mothering skills, but given privacy and patience you should be feeling ready to parent soon. The same is true for fathers. Dads who are given 15 minutes alone with their new babies during the first few hours of life spend significantly more time with them during the first three months than fathers who did not have the opportunity to gain that confidence and bonding. How amazing that simply holding and talking to your newborn is related to successful parenting.

This is the key to kindness, knowing whether we see the result or not. Meeting the needs of others allows God to fulfill our own needs. You do not need to struggle to become a good parent. God has created a system in which meeting your baby's needs helps to make sure your needs are also met.

There's that childhood rhyme "first comes love, then comes marriage, then comes Suzy with a baby carriage . . ." Before I even met my husband, I was reading books on how a Christian woman could work to make her marriage strong. I listened to radio programs on Christian parenting. So why was it that I was pregnant with my second child before I purchased even one book relating the Bible to pregnancy and childbirth?

When I was pregnant with my first child, I had never even heard of the concept of childbirth classes specifically geared toward Christian couples. My husband and I prayed often about the pregnancy, that the baby would be healthy, that the birth would go well. But we never specifically looked to see what the scriptures had to say about childbirth. In Christian circles we are encouraged to apply our faith to all areas of our lives, but I had never been specifically challenged to apply my faith to birth. I am very encouraged to see a growing movement geared toward doing exactly that.

Jennifer Riedy

Drawing Conclusions
Review of Section Three

Ten Questions about...
Giving Birth

1. What do you expect labor to be like?
2. Why have you drawn those conclusions?
3. What do you expect to be the most difficult?
4. Which expectations would you like to change?
5. How do you think you can you change that?
6. What do you need to do to prepare to give birth?
7. What do you want to do to prepare to give birth?
8. Who will help you give birth? How?
9. What concerns do you have about giving birth?
10. Which of your strengths will help you give birth?

Labor Clock

For this exercise assume the average labor is 12 hours long, which is not unreasonable based on many estimates. Using what you know about the length of the stages of labor, estimate how long you might be in each stage of labor. There is a wide range of normal when it comes to time in labor, so there is no right or wrong in this exercise.

Begin with pushing; you could spend 30 minutes or two hours pushing, and either one would be normal. Draw a line at twelve o'clock to indicate the end of your labor, and working backwards from twelve o'clock, put a line at where you might begin pushing.

Transition is intense, but usually no longer than half an hour. Continuing to work backwards count out an amount of time you might spend in transition, and draw a line on the clock to show when it will begin.

Active labor is the time you progress from 4 or 5 centimeters to the time you get to 8 or nine centimeters (when transition begins). You may dilate as slow as half a centimeter an hour or as fast as two centimeters an hour. Estimate an amount of time you could be in active labor, and counting backwards from transition, draw a line to indicate when active labor will start. The rest of the time represents your time in early labor.

Now go back to your clock and answer these questions based on the labor your clock represents:

1. How you might be feeling physically and emotionally:

    2 hours into your labor?

    5 hours into labor?

    9 hours into labor?

    11 hours into labor?

2. What unique challenges does this labor progression pose?

3. When might your contractions demand attention?

4. When should you consider preparing your birth place (going to the hospital or birth center or getting out your home birth supplies)?

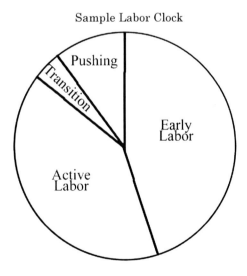

Sample Labor Clock

Preparation for Childbirth

Nerida Walker
Author
God's Plan for Pregnancy
New Life Ministries
www.NewLifeMinistries.com.au

Psalm 127:3
Deuteronomy 28:4

Psalm 139:14

Many women expect birth to be a fearful, painful or negative experience where the whole process is out of their hands. But did you know you do not have to accept the natural course of events; rather you can build your faith and move towards the outcome you desire instead of expecting or experiencing the worst.

Whenever the Bible mentions children it says they are a heritage, an inheritance, or a blessing and a reward from God. Pregnancy and birth is God's designed way to not only populate the earth, but to bring his blessing of children into our lives. The Bible also says that we are 'fearfully and wonderfully made'. God created you to bear children and every part of your reproductive system was created perfectly for this task.

Through my ministry I meet women who are fearful of childbirth, simply because they do not understand the process. I therefore believe it is important for you to get to know the physical changes that happen in your body to deliver a baby. If you understand how your body is going to work, then knowledge can replace fear. You can also begin to prepare and pray more specifically.

The following is a basic outline only and should be read in conjunction with childbirth books. However, it is important to consider the Word of God as you read them and be confident that you do not have to experience pain or complications in labour as may be described.

To prepare for your labour, begin by praying over your body throughout your pregnancy so that your faith can mature, placing it in full submission to the authority and name of Jesus. Once labour has commenced you can continue taking authority by continuing to speak to your body and command it to fulfil its particular function effectively and efficiently as God designed.

I know of babies that have changed position during labour, from breech (bottom first) or posterior (spine against spine) to the correct anterior (face against spine) position. This was simply done by the parents commanding the baby in Jesus' name to move into the correct position for birth.

The first stage is when the cervix thins out and begins to dilate. Transition is when the cervix dilates from 7-10 cm. Take authority and speak to your body, commanding that:

Preparation for Childbirth

- the timing will be appropriate and that you and your family will be comfortable and ready for the birth.
- your body will function perfectly and efficiently as it was designed in order to bring forth this child because you are fearfully and wonderfully made.
- your baby will move into the correct position with its head engaged firmly on the cervix to help with dilation, its face facing the spine, and its back to the stomach wall (anterior position and head down).
- the umbilical cord will be in the correct position, not around the baby's neck, body or shoulders.
- your cervix will efface and dilate efficiently to the full 10cm without any complications.
- your hormones will work efficiently and effectively during pregnancy, labour, delivery and post partum.

During the second stage, the baby is delivered. The mother works with the contractions to push the baby through the birth canal. Take authority and speak to your body, commanding that:

- your bones and ligaments will spread and separate to make room for the baby to pass through.
- your muscles will work effectively and efficiently to push the baby out.
- your vagina and perineum will be elastic and stretch as much as necessary without tearing to accommodate the delivery of the baby and that they will go numb as God designed so there will be no pain as your baby's head crowns.

Third stage is when the afterbirth (placenta, water sac and umbilical cord) is delivered. The placenta separates from the uterine wall and passes through the birth canal. Take authority and speak to your body, commanding that:

- the placenta will completely peel off the uterine wall in one piece.
- your uterus will contract and push the placenta out through the birth canal and then contract (without pain) and return to its original size and heal quickly and efficiently.
- your body will recover quickly after the birth.
- your hormones will get back into balance and begin to release colostrum from your breasts and begin milk production without any blockage or complication.

Be as specific and detailed as you want to be. Any time you start to become tense or afraid, resist the fear and continue to take authority over the situation. And finally in closing, I encourage you to dig into God's Word for a personal revelation for your birth. Faith comes and grows from the Word of God. Faith also enables you to believe what God has said over what your natural circumstances may dictate to you. It is then a matter of acting on what you believe for you to experience a breakthrough. I pray you will experience the joy of giving birth and that not only will you apply these principals to your labour and delivery but to every other area of life as well.

Romans 10:17

90

Subject Four

Birth Planning

Topics:

Birth Planning	93
Should I Write a Birth Plan?	95
Writing a Birth Plan	98
Using your Birth Plan	102
Birth Planning and Guilt	105
Styles of Care	107
Drawing Conclusions	112
Supportive Community by Doran Richards	114

Birth Planning

There is a disconnect between planning and success in the Bible. Nehemiah planned and was able to repair the wall around Jerusalem. Esther had a bit of a plan before approaching the king, but it was hastily devised and built almost solely on prayer. Jonathan had no plan when he approached the Philistines, he simply went because God had said to go and hoped God would give him victory. Gideon made a plan but before that plan could be implemented, God downsized his army. Paul's travel plans were disrupted a few times. Jesus asked if there could be a different plan but willingly submitted when there could not be. Joshua was given the plan battle by battle; Moses was given an overview, and then only told one plague at a time. The wealthy landowner was planning to hoard his wealth by building more storehouses and was destroyed because of his plan.

Book of Nehemiah
Book of Esther

1 Samuel 14
Judges 7

Book of Acts
Matthew 26:39
Book of Joshua
Book of Exodus
Luke 12:13-21

Planning in and of itself is neither godly nor ungodly. Planning is a tool, and like any other tool it can be used to bring glory to God or to satisfy selfish reasons. Planning can be a part of your godly preparations for labor and your stewardship of pregnancy.

Birth planning is not a list of what you want or do not want in labor. A birth plan is not a wish list of preferences for labor. It is the action steps to help you achieve that wish list. Planning is taking action to try to accomplish what you believe to be the best course of action. For example, if after investigating your health and nutrition you realize you should eat more vegetables to be healthy, how will you do that? Or, if you find information that convinces you a cesarean surgery is the best way for your baby to be born, how will you accomplish that with the minimum risk, with the fastest recovery? The wish list is good because it allows discussion about issues, but the wish list is incomplete unless you know how to make it happen.

What things do you think are important for labor?

All planning starts with a goal, something you hope to achieve. You need to take the time to determine what is the most important to you before you can decide how to get there. However, decisions are not made in a vacuum. What seems most important to you will likely be influenced by the opinions and values of those around you. What seems important at any given time may not actually be the most important to God. You should always be considering what God's plan for you may be. In goal setting, you cannot ignore differences that may arise in your plan and God's plan.

It is not a question of the perfect birth plan. The perfect birth plan does not exist. Instead, you need to know the person God made you to be. Know what your strengths are and the places you will need help. Based on your unique makeup, you will find preferences in approach to labor on nearly every option. The point is you cannot look at someone else's list of how to handle labor and adopt it as the "perfect" birth plan. You need to know who you are, what your goals are and what God is calling you to do.

Be sure your planning is preparation out of wisdom, not fear of the worst. You will never be prepared enough to have a plan for every possible complication, but you can be as healthy as possible going into labor so you are less likely to have common problems. You can learn about the various ways to handle common labor challenges so you have a knowledge base to draw from during labor.

Should I Write a Birth Plan?

There are two sides to every issue, and even something as seemingly simple as writing a birth plan can become a complex subject when differing opinions are placed side by side. On the one hand are the professionals who encourage you to become a part of the decision making for labor and birth by writing out your birth plan. On the other hand are the experts who remind you labor cannot be scripted by your birth plan.

There are four key things to recognize about birth plans before you choose to write or not write out your choices for labor. Understanding these things will help you to be a part of the decision making process for giving birth, while allowing you to be flexible enough to handle whatever challenges labor has for you.

You are creating a birth plan whether you write it down or not.

As you learn more about the process of giving birth, you are making plans for the way you would like labor to proceed. It does not matter whether you write your preferences on paper or not because the desire and expectation is already in your heart. Writing your decisions down is a way to help you share those desires and expectations with the rest of your birth team. It is a tool you can use to help the team work together, but it will remain only a tool. Writing a birth plan does not automatically mean you will clearly articulate your goals and desires with your birth team. You will still need to talk with your midwife, discussing your decisions and clarifying the options available to you.

Not committing your choices to paper is not likely to prevent you from being disappointed if you are not able to have the style of birth you would like. It only makes it more difficult to communicate with the strangers who will assist you while in labor such as nurses.

The Process of creating a written birth plan is more powerful than the birth plan itself.

As a finished document, a birth plan is no more than writing on paper. You have no control over how the nurses who receive your plan will respond to your requests. However, during the process of writing the birth plan you have tremendous opportunities to ask questions of your midwife. You will get to know more about her and the way she attends labor; and she will know more about you and the help you will need from her to be comfortable and confident as you labor.

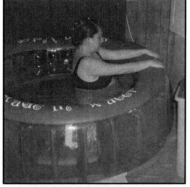
© 2006 Christian Klopka
Options such as water birth, home birth and positions for pushing should be discussed before labor begins.

As you work to make final decisions, you will be sure of your choices and your reasons. In that way, not only are you a stronger labor team, but you are more likely to speak up for the decisions you have made. If you are faced with family members or hospital staff who are not supportive of your decisions, the practice you have had discussing your options will have prepared you to clearly state your reasons and request the support you need.

Birth plans are not necessarily written for the normal, uncomplicated labor.

If every labor followed a specific pattern, there would be very little need for a birth plan. Because every labor is different and you can not know what labor has in store for you before it begins, your birth plan is an additional tool to help you communicate how you have decided to handle both the normal variations of labor and the unexpected situations that may arise.

A written list gives you the opportunity to talk about unexpected situations with your midwife. If you will be in a hospital, it gives hospital staff who do not know you the opportunity to understand what assistance you will need and how they can best support you through a difficult labor.

When a birth plan is fully used, labor generally does not look ideal.

Some mothers have the mistaken idea that when their birth plan is followed, labor will be just like the ideal they imagine. Some women do get to do everything on their birth plan. They get to try every position and pain relief technique, and when complications arise, they get to do every intervention and have a cesarean done they way they wanted. The experience was not the one imagined, however, every action taken followed the birth plan. Other women get to do very little from their birth plan. Labor simply happens too quickly to try all the positions and techniques they had expected to use for comfort. The experience may have been their ideal, but very little from the birth plan was needed.

How much of your birth plan is utilized is dependant on factors you probably do not have control over. But regardless of the circumstances of your labor, your birth plan can help you and those assisting you determine how you will respond to the challenges facing you.

Before you go out and buy some hiking boots for your labor kit, I must mention that walking was what worked for *me*. A while back, I was at a friend's homebirth and she was perfectly content in labor lying on her couch. She looked so relaxed, stretched out on her side, she reminded me of a mother cat contentedly waiting for her litter to be born. "I just hope it's soon," she purred.

Sheila Stubbs
Excerpted from *Giving Birth the Easy Way © 2005*

Writing a Birth Plan

If you choose to prepare a written birth plan, there are two things to think about. The first is your content and the second is your format. The content is the meat of your birth plan, the information about the choices you have made and options you would like. The format is the way in which you present your choices to make them easy to read and understand.

Choosing Your Options

Depending on the caregiver you have hired, the birth place you have chosen and your overall health, you will have a variety of options to choose from. If you are not sure yet what options are available to you, review the list on the opposite page as a start. It is a good tool for beginning conversations with your midwife and to take with you on birth place tours.

Find out what options your midwife is comfortable with, and find out if there are policies at your birth place that might restrict the options you have. If possible, tour more than one birth place so you can see the differences in what they offer. You may also find it helpful to interview a different midwife, since options vary between caregivers.

ONSET OF LABOR
  Spontaneous
  Self-induced
    Walk
    Enema
    Castor Oil
    Nipple Stimulation
    Thumb Sucking
  Medically Induced
    Prostaglandin Gel
    IV Pitocin
    Amniotomy

CLOTHES
  Own clothing
  Hospital Gown

EMPTY BLADDER
  Walk to toilet
  Bedpan
  Catheterization

MONITORING
  None
  Intermittent
  Continuous
  Internal
  Telemetry Unit

PAIN RELIEF
  Epidural/Spinal
    Soon as possible
    When uncomfortable
    At 5 cm
    Only if I ask
  Narcotic
    Definite
    Offer please
    Only if I ask
  Relaxation Techniques
    Vocalization
    Relaxation
    Breathing
    Imagery/Visualization
    Close Eyes
    Focal Point

HYDRATION
  Drinking Fluids
  Popsicles
  Ice Chips
  Suckers/Lolipops
  Heparin Lock
  IV Fluids
  No Liquids

COMFORT MEASURES
  Dim lights
  Music
  TENS Unit
  Heating Pad
  Hot/Cold Packs
  Water
    Shower
    Bathtub
  Massage

COMFORT ITEMS
  Pillow
  Tennis Balls
  Rolling Pin
  Wooden roller
  Lotion/powder

POSITIONS
  Walk
  Lunge
  Sitting in chair
  Sitting on side of bed
  Rock
  Stand
  Pelvic Rock
  Dangle
  Back-to-Back
  Hands & Knees
  Squat
  Leaning over bed

SPEED UP LABOR
  Nipple stimulation
  Position changes
  Break amniotic bag
  Pitocin
  Prolonged pushes
  Episiotomy
  Forceps/Vacuum Extractor

PUSHING
  Spontaneous
  Directed
  Prolonged

PERINEAL CARE
  Massage
  Warm Compresses
  Episiotomy
  Prefer tear to episiotomy

CUTTING CORD
  Partner
  Mother
  Doctor/Midwife
  Wait till pulsing stops

BABY'S WARMTH
  On mother's abdomen
  In warmer
  Warmer if necessary

EYE CARE
  Delayed 1 hour

CESAREAN
  Partner present
  Doula present
  Remain alert
  Infant recover with mother
  Describe events
  Video/Pictures

MEMENTOS
  Footprints
  Video/Pictures

ROOMING IN
  24 hour with mother
  Nursery on request
  Partner rooming in

Once you know what options are available, you can begin to determine which options are the most important to you. There is no right or wrong to this, it is simply a matter of understanding who you are and what you will need to labor normally. Your list may be very different from a friend or relative's list.

Take a written list of your choices to a prenatal appointment so you can discuss them with your midwife. If she has concerns about an option, find out what they are and where she recommends you go to do further study. Complete discussion about your choices is likely to take several visits, so the sooner you start the better able you will be to communicate your needs and desires.

You will need to determine if your choices are realistic. It is possible your health or lack of facilities in your area prevent you from having some options. You should also pay attention to the support you are receiving from your birth team. You are not likely to be successful without their support. It may be necessary to hire a doula, restrict some family members from the labor room or hire a different caregiver to make your choices a reality.

Once you have your options selected, you will need to determine which ones should be listed in the birth plan. Generally, you will want to consider listing the options you have chosen for the environment, interventions, pain relief, management of second stage and immediate postpartum care. You only need to list the options that are important to you. If you do not care what the environment is like, you can skip putting information about that in the birth plan.

Format

The way in which you present your choices will have a huge impact on whether or not the birth plan is read by hospital or birth center staff. Remember to keep your words brief, using bullet points or headings if at all possible, as this is the easiest way to share large amounts of information quickly.

Try to put the most important, highest priority information first so it is most likely to be read. For some women, this will mean a fear of needles may be listed first. For others it may mean a desire to give birth without medication will be listed first. Continue the rest of the information either by topic (such as environment or pain relief) or by the next highest priority.

Keep the written plan to one page. Anything longer than that will take too long to read and the information will not be kept in the memory as strongly. Remember, the point of writing your choices is so that the birth place staff can assist you in meeting your goals. Presenting them with a document that overwhelms them is not likely to be helpful.

Sample Birth Plan

Begin with an introductory paragraph about yourself and who will be with you during labor.

Our Goals

* Goal 1
* Goal 2
* Goal 3

In case of unexpected situations

* Goal 1
* Goal 2
* Goal 3

Newborn Care

* Goal 1
* Goal 2
* Goal 3

Using Your Birth Plan

Whether or not you have chosen to write out your choices, you will need to communicate those choices with your caregivers. This will be done during pregnancy as you prepare to give birth, and while you are in labor.

During Pregnancy

Before labor begins, you will work with your midwife to determine the best ways to handle the expected and unexpected situations that may arise. It is through this discussion you will determine how well you work as a team. If you find you are not a good team, you may want to search for a different midwife.

Some women get nervous when they talk to their midwives. This nervousness is unnecessary. Remember, your midwife is working for you because you hired her. If you are dissatisfied with the quality of work she is doing for you, hire someone else.

If you have a difficult topic to discuss, try not to prejudge your midwife's responses. Listen carefully and contribute to the dialogue. Bring any information you have that supports your choices, and be open to exploring additional sources she may recommend. Take a list of questions with you so you are less likely to forget things. Let your midwife know at the beginning of the appointment that you want to ask a few questions; if she forgets, gently remind her before the appointment is done.

Using Your Birth Plan

When possible take something you have read on the subject with you. Share with your midwife the sources of information you have on the subject and why they have led you to the conclusions you have made. Be sure to let her know that you are interested in her thoughts and opinions of the options in general and in your case specifically. Ask your midwife if she has any literature on the subject, or if she can recommend a book or website to you so you can keep researching the issue.

When asking questions, ask the specific questions you want the answers to. Asking, "How often do you do episiotomies?" will give you the answer, "I only do them when necessary." Instead ask, "How many of your clients need episiotomies?"; "Under what circumstances do you recommend an episiotomy?" or "What techniques do you use to help keep perineal skin intact?"

If your midwife disagrees with your views on a subject, let her know that you will continue to research the subject and want to talk to her about it again at your next appointment. This will give her time to do some more research and gather information so you can work together to make a decision. It also lets her know that this issue is important to you.

> How have you handled discussing difficult topics that have already come up?

It will be your responsibility to decide if and when your differences are too great. If you are unable to receive the type of care you desire from your current midwife, it is time to investigate your other options by interviewing other midwives in your area.

During Labor

Ideally, your birth plan will be read by anyone who assists you during labor. It will help them to understand who you are and what help you would like to feel confident about during labor. Even though your birth plan states how you would like to handle situations, you may still be asked if you would like one option or another. Simply let your caregivers know you would like to continue to follow your birth plan.

There may be times during your labor when your helpers are not sure how you would like to proceed. Other times you may ask for something not listed on your birth plan. At these times it is useful for your labor helper to remind you what it says on the birth plan and ask if you still want to follow what it says.

Regardless of what was written on your birth plan, the staff at your birth place will want your verbal and perhaps written consent for some procedures. This is because of a major push by the obstetrical industry to ensure women are given the right of informed consent before any treatment or procedure is done. Basically, this means you understand what is being done, why it is being done and the risk it entails. Though the idea of informed consent is a good one, its practice has a few flaws.

The first problem is that informed consent does not happen without the right to refuse treatment. Some women feel pressured by caregivers to accept treatments they do not want. In the Listening to Mothers II Survey, 10 percent of the respondents felt they were pressured to have an intervention they did not want. This manipulation can be subtle, such as not being told of other options. It can also be more forceful, such as being told you are a bad mother or do not care about your baby if you decide not to have a procedure.

Another problem is that many women are not given the information they need during labor to ensure true informed consent. During labor you may not be listening to what is said, or have the attention span to listen to all the other options. There may not be time during labor to explain everything you need to know. This makes it very difficult for a laboring mother to give true informed consent.

It has become increasingly important for a woman to do her own research into the options available for handling labor and the birth process. This is not only due to the impossibility of learning everything you need to know during office visits, but also because standards of care and the common interventions vary not only between communities, but also between caregivers. Never underestimate the value of a second opinion.

If something unexpected happens during labor, your birth plan may or may not specifically detail how you would like the situation handled. Remember that in most cases the decision of how to proceed rests on you. You have the right to refuse any intervention, including one your caregivers believe can or will save your life.

Birth Planning and Guilt

Sometimes, caregivers warn women not to make plans for birth so they do not feel guilty or disappointed after the birth. This issue stems from the understanding a natural childbirth is the safest for both the mother and baby, yet so few women seem to give birth naturally, even when they try. The belief is encouraging a woman to give birth without medication sets her up for failure, and then she feels guilty if she does not achieve the goal.

This causes a struggle for your labor helper as well. How do you help a woman give birth without making her feel guilty? How do you motivate a mother to keep going without her feeling like a failure if her labor does not turn out as planned? Mothers need encouragement and support to achieve a normal birth. When the support is not there, the problems and the interventions used to correct them increase. How do you give support without mom ending up feeling like a failure or guilty for the way she labors?

First and foremost you must decide what, exactly, is the goal and whose goal is it? Pay attention to where the desire for a certain outcome is from. You will probably not feel guilty about not achieving someone else's goal, and you should not be expected to anyway.

Whose choices did you use to set your goals for labor?

If you had a goal of giving birth without medication and ended up with interventions or surgery, you will feel some level of loss. The same can be said if you expected to receive an epidural and ended up unable to have one. This is normal and not something that needs to be changed. It hurts to have expectations not be met. There is a disappointment and in some cases even grieving when expectations are unmet.

How do you deal with anger, frustration or hurt?

Disappointment and loss are not the same as guilt. Neither is the anger, frustration or hurt some women feel–especially if the decisions were out of their control–that somehow she was not respected or listened to. Usually, it is not the mother who fails, but a health care system that fails to provide her with the tools or an opportunity to be part of the decision making. How could a mother be expected to be successful with her goals when her choices are not respected?

Guilt is a very unique sensation, because guilt has to do with sin, not loss. Guilt is the prompting of the Holy Spirit as you are gently (or in some cases not so gently) convicted to make changes in the way you think or behave because it currently does not line up with God's desire for you. It is God and God alone whom you must please. You can be sad about the way labor turned out but not feel guilty when you know the decisions you made pleased God. You can be encouraged to work towards your goals and not feel guilt if they are unmet when your decisions in labor are made according to God's plan.

Styles of Care

In planning for your baby's birth, you will need to make decisions about the style of care you would like. You will have the opportunity to have your labor actively or expectantly managed. You will have the opportunity to choose between pharmacological and natural interventions. You will have the opportunity to utilize procedures based in western medical philosophy and eastern medical philosophy.

Medical procedures, regardless of their philosophy or style, are tools and therefore neither good nor bad. Instead, it is the purpose for which you use them that determines whether you are bringing glory to God or turning away from God. Each style of care has strengths and weaknesses. When determining which type of approach to take for your health, you can consider the risks and benefits of every option and select the methods and approaches that make the most sense in your circumstances.

Management

The type of care you receive from your midwifemidwife is determined by her style of labor management. Expectant management of labor assumes the birth process works most of the time, waiting until there is indication of a problem to intervene. Active management of labor assumes that because some women will have problems with labor, it is best to control as much about the process as possible.

The term "active management" for labor was introduced to describe a specific style of care intended to prevent prolonged labor. Included in the original program are strict criteria to diagnose labor, early breaking of the bag of waters, early use of oxytocin and continuous professional support. As active management has caught on, the practice has changed. Usually it is the strict criteria to diagnose labor and the continuous professional support that are left out. Unfortunately, those are also the two factors of the program that show any indication of preventing long labor when used routinely on their own.

Do you tend to favor a specific type of health care?

If your midwife practices with an active management style, she is likely to recommend induction, prefer continuous monitoring with an electronic fetal monitor, use frequent vaginal exams to monitor progress and encourage the use of methods to speed labor to maintain a specific rate of dilation.

The term "expectant management" describes a style of care that is frequently referred to as the "midwifery model." Expectant management accepts that there may be problems, but does not attempt to manage problems until there is evidence to suggest something is outside the bounds of normal. With expectant management, issues such as a long labor may give the midwife cause to watch for other signs of problems, but without other signs the long labor is not considered a problem.

If your midwife practices with an expectant management style, she is likely to be comfortable with waiting for labor to start, waiting for your body to move labor in its time, recommend position or comfort measure changes rather than medical interventions and monitor progress without continuous use of an external fetal monitor.

Interventions

The question of if and when to intervene in the natural course of labor is further confused by the availability of both natural and pharmacological methods to intervene. Most midwives are familiar with a mix of methods, and will recommend the course of action that is most likely to produce the desired result with the least risk.

Some women find the term "natural" gives a false security about the relative risks of some interventions. Even though something is natural, it can still have side effects, cause problems or not work for you. Some herbs can be harmful during pregnancy or interact with other products used during labor.

Other women find pharmacological methods give them a false security about the relative risks of an intervention. Even though something has been formulated in a laboratory, it can still have side effects, cause problems or simply not work for you. Some pharmaceuticals will drastically alter the course of your labor.

> What types of interventions do you use in everyday life?

There is usually more than one way to accomplish the desired effect for your labor. It is important that regardless of the source of an intervention, you carefully consider the risks and the benefits before making assumptions about which is best. In that way, you can be sure the decisions you are making have the best chance of making the changes you want.

Philosophy

Both eastern and western medical philosophies offer a variety of tools for use during labor. You probably have a tendency to prefer one style or another and may have distrust for one philosophy or the other.

Eastern medicine has the advantage of having been practiced for thousands of years. Most of the treatments that have survived the test of time seem to be effective, although scientific efficacy studies are only now beginning to be conducted. There are likely to be treatments that work and treatments that do not, but on the whole, the practices that have continued through centuries have done so because people believe they have helped them.

Western medicine has the advantage of having been scientifically studied, although many practices in western medicine are begun based on theory and later dropped when scientific study finds them to be ineffective or harmful. However, even the most effective treatments do not work for every person. Even when a drug is shown to have the desired chemical effect, it does not always mean the person is "better" for having taken it. Because of the desire western medicine has for isolating individual "parts," treatments are always changing.

Both philosophies have areas in which they can be supported by the Bible, and areas in which they seem to go against the Bible. Like anything else, either style of medicine also carries a risk to carry you away from the truth of God. How dangerous it is to your relationship with God will depend on your strengths and areas of struggle. The biggest struggle for Christians with either philosophy of medicine is the denial of God or his power. If a practice from either style of medicine causes you to start seeing yourself as a god, as if you are in control and you do not need God, recognize that is a problem.

How do you prefer to manage your physical health?

Some Christians feel any style of medicine interferes with their faith in God. They choose instead to use prayer, trusting whatever happens is God's will. Other Christians choose to use medicines of either philosophy only when necessary to avoid becoming entangled in idolatry. Some Christians do not feel a pull toward idolatry when using any medical treatment. What medical treatments tempt you to be pulled to sin will be dependant on your personality, experience, strengths and struggles.

Making Choices

When trying to decide which styles, treatments and options are appropriate for you, ask yourself the following questions.

Does this violate anything I believe as a Christian?

Regardless of how beneficial other people may think something is, if it violates your core beliefs, it is harmful. Though it is sometimes easier to go along than take a stand, you will feel more comfortable if you avoid those options that you feel are wrong. Most caregivers will understand your concerns and desire to honor your culture and beliefs. If you hired a caregiver who continually pushes you to go against what you feel is right, you may need to find someone else.

To what extent is this likely to help or hinder?

Remember, your primary goal is to have a healthy mom and healthy baby. It is easy to see that options which are likely to help you achieve your goal should be used, while those that hinder your goal should be avoided. How you approach the options that neither clearly help nor clearly hinder your goal will depend on your personal style. Some women are willing to try anything that may help as long as it has little to no risk. Other women would rather not spend their energy on something that is not as likely to help regardless of how little risk it carries.

Do I have peace about using this treatment?

If you are feeling the prompting of the Holy Spirit to avoid or use a treatment you should respond accordingly. It feels wonderful when God gives peace about options you wanted all along. However, it is the peace about using an option you would have preferred to avoid that can have the most impact on your choices for labor. Sometimes God's plan is different from yours. If God is trying to direct you somewhere, follow.

Drawing Conclusions
Review of Section Four

No Rules

Just for today, let go of your preconceived ideas about how birth should happen. Instead, think about how you would like to give birth if there were no rules about where you were supposed to be or what was supposed to happen.

Write a story, draw a picture or sing a song about how your birth would be if there were no rules. Share what you have created with someone close to you.

The Perfect Birth

Imagine for a moment that you have the freedom to orchestrate your labor and childbirth experience. You have the unique privilege of completely planning your baby's birth. Ordinarily you have no control over these factors, but just for today, how would it go?

When does labor begin?

How does labor begin?

Where are you when labor begins?

Who is with you when labor begins?

How strong are the contractions?

How quickly does the labor progress?

When do you go to your birth place?

How long do you push?

How long does labor last?

What do you do after your baby is born?

There are some things about childbirth you may have a choice about, depending on the circumstances of your birth. Although you do still have to deal with the circumstances surrounding you when labor begins, you may have control over what happens. For the purpose of this exercise, think of your ideal childbirth, how would it happen?

Who is your primary caregiver?

Where do you labor?

Where do you give birth?

What is available to you at your birth place?

Who is with you for emotional support?

What do you use to manage pain?

What procedures happen?

What procedures do not happen?

What techniques do you use to avoid the procedures that do not happen?

What happens after your baby is born?

Now that you have worked through your ideal childbirth, finish the following statements based on your responses.

My top three priorities for childbirth are:

My ideal birth place is:

My ideal caregiver is:

In childbirth, I want access to:

In childbirth, I want emotional support from:

My first choices for ways to handle childbirth pain are:

Other things that are important to me are:

The Art of Giving Birth

Spend some time looking at photos of women in labor, art depicting birth or birth movies. What questions, thoughts or concerns come up when you see these visual representations of childbirth? What do you see that you like? What do you see that you do not like?

Get out some crayons, paint, chalk, markers or other creative drawing tool. Make a visual representation of the birth you would like to have.

Supportive Community

Doran Richards
Author
Celebration of Pregnancy
Blessing God's Way
www.BlessingGodsWay.com

Are we surrounded by the ones we love and trust during our pregnancies today? Do we call upon women in our communities to help us? Can we see a connection that has been lost? All of this has had an impact on our birthing culture! We are missing a piece of the puzzle for better birth. That missing piece is the support of our community. This includes the friends and family members as well as the church's support. The Association of Labor Assistants and Childbirth Educators (ALACE) have said:

> Only recently in the long story of humanity has the linkage of knowledge and reassurance between generations of birthing women been broken.
>
> Pregnant women today often find themselves without ties to female relatives who can reliably teach them what to expect from childbearing.
>
> Birth has often come to resemble a mechanized, medical emergency. It is no wonder that many first-time mothers' images of birth are filled with fear and pain.

Oh, how sad this is! Would it surprise to you to know that we should not be filled with fear and pain? It is not how we should feel when being used as a vessel of our Almighty King! He is not the Father of fear and chaos and disorder, but instead, the Father of peace that passes all understanding.

Childbirth as a discussion topic has been lumped in with those faux pas of the past that say you should never talk about politics and religion. Childbearing has essentially become part of that silent creed, distressing to say, and our children are not seeing pregnancy and birth as an honorable event in our lives ordained by our heavenly Father! But we can change this. If we make ourselves aware of the problem, we can encourage our young daughters to pursue serving women in their childbearing years by becoming Christian midwives, doulas and childbirth educators.

As women, we are called to serve. Serving our God is first and foremost, then our husbands and families, yes, but also our fellow woman. What a wonderful avenue for our young daughters to be encouraged in! We teach them to sew, cook, clean, study—but what about birth? Teaching our daughters to serve one another can be taught at a very young age. Why not begin as soon as God gives you opportunity to?

The word ancilla means female servant in Latin. Doula means female servant in Greek. I propose that if you venture to ask your neighbor what these two words mean, she would not know.

I found out how unfamiliar the term doula was while in the hospital helping a friend during her birth. The nurse that was marking charts turned to me while inputting some information in their computer and said, "What is your purpose here; are you a nurse or what?" and I replied, "No, I am a doula." She looked at me like I just had offended her, but she wasn't sure . . . and then she asked, "What is that?" I then explained to her that she could put in her computer that it was female servant. I felt it was an opportunity to enlighten someone who genuinely did not know, in essence, what a doula was. Why is this unfamiliar terminology, especially among the birthing realm and church at large?

Consider this quote and compare it to where we find support for childbearing in our culture today:

> Birth was a thoroughly feminine event, managed by a midwife with the assistance of the lying-in woman's female relatives and friends.
> *Childbearing in American Society 1650-1850 by Catherine Scholten*

I propose to you, the reader, to take a moment to ponder this dilemma in our culture. First, it would be great if we could acknowledge that there is indeed a problem or lack of support in our communities. From there we can begin to take steps in changing the tide for this predicament. It will take work and time. We have to pray for the time to do the work together. If we all make an effort to reach out to those around us, serving women in childbearing, we will begin to see a change.

In this article my intent was to show the severity of our downward spiral of support in our own communities—it is there, we cannot deny it. However, I do want to encourage every one of my sisters in Christ that nothing is impossible with him who loves us. His heart would love to see us serving one another . . . Let us pray that he gives us the opportunities to do just that, according to our gifting and callings.

Subject Five

Childbirth Pain

Topics:

Why Pain in Labor?	119
Forces that Affect Pain	126
Fear and Pain	130
Coping with pain	134
Personal Pain Coping Strategies	139
Abnormal Pain in Childbirth	142
How Painful is Labor?	146
Drawing Conclusions	150
More Than Conquerors! by Kelly Townsend	152

Why Pain in Labor?

Speak about giving birth, and chances are the thoughts of those around you go to pain. In our culture pain is an accepted standard of birth, as normal and as expected as the joy of holding your newborn. Before exploring ways to handle the pain in labor, it is helpful to understand more about pain. What is pain? Why do you experience it and how can you affect the pain you feel?

A common Christian teaching says when sin entered the world, so did trials, struggles and pain. However, the belief that life was somehow blissfully work-free before the fall is a misunderstanding of scripture. Genesis 2:15 says, "The LORD God took the man and put him in the Garden of Eden to work it and take care of it." Adam had a job and was responsible for the garden before the fruit was eaten. Sin did not bring work into the world, it only changed it. In Genesis 3:17 the man is told, "Cursed is the ground because of you; through painful toil you will eat of it all the days of your life." It was not that Adam was suddenly to become a farmer; he already was responsible for that work. The fall simply made the work harder.

There is no record of childbearing before the fall; however, God's words to the woman give a glimpse of how her work would also be changed. In Genesis 3:16 the woman is told, "I will greatly increase your pains in childbearing; with pain you will give birth to children." It was not that sin somehow made childbirth work. Sin did not change the nature of birth; only the intensity of the

Genesis 2:15

Genesis 3:17

Genesis 3:16

work for a woman to labor was increased just as the intensity of the work was increased for the man.

It is worth mentioning that the word translated "painful toil" when God spoke to Adam is the same word translated as "pains" when God spoke to Eve. Both words are "etsev" and in almost every other use of estev, except where it describes the birth of Jabez in 1 Chronicles 4:9, the translation is toil or work.

1 Chronicles 4:9

When trying to understand what the increase in work is supposed to be, it is helpful to look to the man, whose work is more widely understood. Genesis 3:17-18 says,

Genesis 3:17-18

> Cursed is the ground because of you; through painful toil you will eat of it all the days of your life. It will produce thorns and thistles for you, and you will eat the plants of the field. By the sweat of your brow you will eat your food.

You may have some idea of the difficulty in growing enough food to support your family. Just like giving birth, it is a lot of work, but it is doable. There are some other similarities between giving birth and gardening that should be made as well.

Birthing and Gardening

The hard work of growing food changes every day. During the planting season, the hard work involves preparing the soil and nurturing the seed to germinate. During the growing season, the hard work involves ensuring the tender shoots have enough water and preventing weeds from choking out the good plants. Harvesting season brings the work of collecting the crops and storing them for later use. The main point here is that the "hard work" that must be done is not a single exertion but a series of efforts in which a variety of labors meet the current situation. If a farmer had to simultaneously sow and reap the work would be overwhelming. God in his wisdom has spread out the "painful toil" to allow all the work of growing to be managed by humans.

While giving birth, a woman's body goes through a process that actually can take two weeks or longer. Just as in growing food, giving birth has "seasons," and each season has its own work for the mother to do. As the body prepares for labor, the mother must ensure she gets adequate rest and nutrition for energy. As the body begins to have contractions, the mother must work through difficult emotions to keep herself calm and relaxed. As the body contracts the uterus to push the baby out, the mother must work with the body to allow this to happen. Every season of giving birth has its own "painful toil," which God in his wisdom has spread out so the work of birthing is manageable to women.

The painful toil necessary to grow a crop in the desert is different from the painful toil necessary to grow a crop in the mountains, which is different from the painful toil necessary to grow a crop in a river floodplain. It is not better or worse to garden in different areas. However, the wise gardener understands the climate and soil and chooses plants that will thrive under the conditions. It is possible to grow plants outside of their native habitat, it just takes more work. In some areas, it does not matter what you grow, certain parts of gardening will always be more painful toil than in other areas. For example, it will always be more work to water plants in a desert. You can be very good at drawing water from a well, but it will always take many trips to the well to water a garden in the desert.

Think about a time you had to complete a difficult task. What made the work harder? What made the work easier?

Women giving birth also have differences about them which make parts of labor easier or more difficult than other women. These differences are neither good nor bad, they are simply differences. A wise mother uses the strengths she has, whatever they may be, to help her complete the work of birthing. Some women try to imitate what has been successful for a friend or relative without paying attention to who God made them to be. Just like growing a plant outside its native habitat, trying to labor using a strength someone else has will make labor more work. However, even using all the strengths they have, some women may still have a very difficult time with some parts of labor.

The painful toil of gardening is lessened by working with the season. In some areas there are winter, spring, summer and fall. Other areas have a wet and a dry season. If you tried to plant a warm weather crop during a snowy winter season, it would take tremendous work to be even mildly successful. A wise gardener works with the seasons so plants have the best chance to thrive with the least amount of attention.

In labor, the work needs to be completed at the proper time as well. If you tried to push during early labor you would quickly exhaust yourself and still need to work through the entire labor to reach the point where pushing is effective. You might begin to believe that you could not give birth because your pushing efforts were fruitless. However, that is no truer than saying you can not grow anything because planting seeds in the winter does not produce a crop. Pushing is a work of labor, but it is only the work for one season of labor.

Purpose of Pain

If some level of pain or discomfort could have been involved in the original work of labor (before God increased the work in response to the eating of the fruit), the next question that should be asked is what purpose would the pain serve? Pain, by its very nature, is a call to action. There are various degrees of discomfort your body can feel, and along the continuum of discomfort to pain you will also see a variety of responses. The gentle, or not so gentle, grumbling of an empty stomach prompts you to find food. The pressure of a full bladder or bowel encourages you to empty your body. The burn of your skin next to something hot causes you to move your body thereby protecting it from further damage. A sore muscle lets you know you worked too hard so you will be gentler the next time. Pain is your body's call to action.

Pain
↓
Endorphins
↓
Prolactin
↓
Breastfeeding Success

Pain has a physiological purpose in childbirth. The increasing intensity of the pain or discomfort increases your body's production of endorphins. Endorphins are natural opiates that are responsible for "runners high." They are also produced during sexual intimacy. Endorphins are at peak levels near the end of labor, helping you manage the pain of the contractions.

What is even more amazing is the endorphins your body is producing in response to the pain of labor are preparing your body to care for your child. The high endorphin levels cause your body to increase prolactin levels. Prolactin is a hormone necessary to breastfeed. Some level of discomfort during labor helps to control the intricate biophysical feedback mechanism of giving birth and mothering.

Another important reason for discomfort or pain during labor is the way you naturally move your body in response to pain. It is very difficult to hold still while in pain, which works just perfectly for labor since movement is necessary for your baby to properly align in your pelvis. Without proper alignment, either you or your baby could suffer damage. Pain serves as a method of protection against a bad birth position.

Pain ↓ Movement ↓ Proper Alignment

It is probably not a surprise to you that humans do a very poor imitation of God. When humans attempt to rewrite the process of labor to remove the pain chemically, it interferes with the delicate balance necessary for a healthy birth. Subtle movements and minute amounts of hormones are directed by the pain you feel. Labor is about more than just forcing the uterus to contract.

The pain and discomfort women feel during childbirth has varying locations, sensations and degrees of intensity. This is due to the differences in mothers' pelvises, babies' positions and sizes, levels of hormones, sensitivity of tissues and mothers' overall health. Each pain or discomfort is a call to a different action. A backache needs a different response than fatigue, which should get a different response from a slow labor. The wise mother listens to her pain to understand what it is calling her to do.

Pain is not only your physical call to action. God uses pain as a call to action to bring his people back to him. In Amos 4 God goes through the "pains" he gave to Israel and their response. Starting at verse 6 it reads,

> "I gave you empty stomachs in every city and lack of bread in every town, yet you have not returned to me," declares the LORD.
>
> "I also withheld rain from you when the harvest was still three months away. I sent rain on one town, but withheld it from another. One field had rain; another had none and dried up. People staggered from town to town for water but did not get enough to drink, yet you have not returned to me," declares the LORD.
>
> "Many times I struck your gardens and vineyards, I struck them with blight and mildew. Locusts devoured your fig and olive trees, yet you have not returned to me," declares the LORD.

Amos 4:6-11

"I sent plagues among you as I did to Egypt. I killed your young men with the sword, along with your captured horses. I filled your nostrils with the stench of your camps, yet you have not returned to me," declares the LORD.

"I overthrew some of you as I overthrew Sodom and Gomorrah. You were like a burning stick snatched from the fire, yet you have not returned to me," declares the LORD.

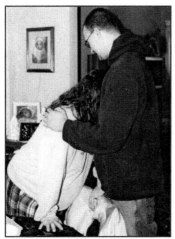
© 2002 Jennifer Vanderlaan
You may have more or less pain than another woman.

God did not send the pains to Israel as punishment, but to cause them to refocus their attention on him. The pain was a reminder, a call to action to serve God. It is possible that some of the discomfort, both physical and emotional, a woman feels in labor is intended by God to keep her focused on God as her provider and source of strength. It is appropriate to respond to labor through prayer, worship and other forms of communion with God.

The idea that pain may have physical and spiritual purposes in labor does not necessarily mean labor should be dreadful. One common belief among Christians is the expectation of a dreadfully painful labor because of the "curse." Another common but conflicting belief is that Christians should not have pain or suffering during labor because we have been redeemed from the curse. Most Christians believe labor lies somewhere in the middle, but you will probably lean to one understanding or the other.

Genesis 29:31
Luke 1:7
1 Samuel 1:1-10
Genesis 18:12

The truth is, there are many variables that go into labor, and the outcomes vary from overwhelming to nearly painless. The amount of pain you feel may be more or less than another Christian, but you cannot compare your Christianity by your labor pain. Expecting every Christian must have the same experience during labor denies the intricacy of God. God works according to his purpose. Even when he answers prayers, the answer comes in his time not ours. Rachael, Elizabeth, Hannah and Sarah all prayed for years to have a child. Their prayers were not suddenly answered because they finally got the words right, or their heart was suddenly right. God opened their wombs because it somehow suited his purpose.

Why Pain in Labor?

Assuming that you will have no problems when you are spiritually right is presumptuous and a lie. As Paul grew closer to God, he did not have less problems, he had more. He did not claim to be more holy, he called himself the chief of sinners. David, a man after God's own heart, still struggled with sin and had trouble raising his children. Being in the center of God's will sent Jonathan into battle with only his armor bearer; made Noah the neighborhood laughing stock as he built a boat in the middle of the desert; caused Moses to leave his home to face off against a powerful king; sent Gideon into battle with only 400 men. Being right with God is no guarantee that life will be easy or labor will be painless.

1 Timothy 1:115

2 Samuel
1 Samuel 14:1
Genesis 6

Exodus 4:18-end
Judges 7

What a Christian can expect, regardless of the amount of discomfort during childbirth, is the peace of God that surpasses understanding. This means in the midst of the storm, with the wind blowing in your face, your hope is not gone, because you know God is protecting you and leading you. The peace is not a perfect labor, but calmness when labor is not perfect. Peace is knowing you cannot make it through labor on your strength, but you do not have to because God will be your strength. Peace is letting go of control, and letting God lead you through labor.

Only God knows to what extent you will need to work during labor. You may give birth painlessly, or you may struggle through many challenges. You are only in control of how you respond to labor. It is how you handle yourself, where you turn for strength, which is important. God will give you the strength to manage whatever labor suits his purpose.

Factors That Affect Pain

There are many forces that will affect the amount of pain or discomfort you feel during labor. Some of them you can control, some of them you can influence and some of them you cannot change.

Physiological Factors

When a woman is laboring, her cervix is stretching. If the cervix is sensitive, this stretching can be a source of pain or discomfort. The same may also be true of the vagina. Some women may be more sensitive than others and may feel more discomfort while stretching.

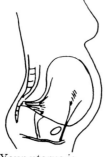

Your uterus is held in place by ligaments.

Along with the cervical stretching, other body parts are manipulated during labor. With each contraction, the uterus is pulling forward, which pushes it against the abdominal wall. At the same time, the ligaments that hold the uterus in place then pull against the woman's back. For some women, especially women who are muscularly tense, there is pain involved in this pushing and pulling.

As the baby descends in the pelvis, the pelvis must stretch to accommodate the baby's head. This stretching puts pressure on nerves and ligaments which can cause discomfort or pain depending on the amount of pressure.

This stretching can also cause a discomfort or pain in the symphisis pubis, the place where the pubic bone connects in the front, which actually opens in labor to make more room for the baby.

There are real physiological reasons why a woman may experience strong physical responses during labor. Certainly the variations in sensitivities among women have some affect on the amount of pain or discomfort they feel. Unfortunately, you cannot control how sensitive your cervix is or how easily your pelvis will stretch.

Physical Factors

Two people can experience the exact same thing differently. For example, playing in water that is deep enough to be over your head can be incredibly fun and exciting if you are a person who is comfortable with your swimming skills and has been trained in ways to move around in water. This experience can be terrifying if you have never learned how to swim. It is all based on the skills you have mastered to handle the situation. Similarly, you can master skills that help you manage labor effectively.

Running a 5K race when you have trained and worked to condition your body can feel fulfilling even though it is a hard workout. Yet, place a woman in the race who does not exercise, and the event becomes overwhelming and the amount of effort she has to exert can make her physically sick. Labor is a tremendously physical work, and asking your body to perform the task without proper conditioning can increase the pain and discomfort you feel.

Getting out of bed in the morning can be easy when you put your things aside and made sure you got to sleep at a reasonable time. However, ask your body to wake up after only two or three hours sleep, and you will most likely experience incredible physical discomfort if you can get your body to wake up at all. Being tired makes anything you do seem more difficult. Adequate rest in the days and weeks leading up to labor gives your body the reserves it needs to function properly.

> It's intense, but it 'feels like' a good, warm, healthy pain—the pain of muscles working really hard, not the pain of awful damage being done. Remember it's a healthy muscle working and it's user-friendly pain.
>
> Put a gun to my head and force me to run for 20 minutes without stopping, I'm dying. I swear I'm dying. It is extremely difficult, excruciatingly painful—but amazingly, I'm not actually dying. I'm simply doing what my body is quite capable of. Under a certain amount of distress! So, it's exertion pain, not trauma pain.
>
> Labour is actually nicer than a forced run. Because you actually get total breaks of pain-free times in between, when you can rest, relax and breathe fresh oxygen and energy in. The only time you might not get these breaks (or not very long breaks) is if you consented to induction for any reason, or sometimes just at the very end when you are in transition.
> *Julie Bell*

Other physical factors can impact your labor as well. For example, if your bladder is full, the pressure of each contraction will be multiplied even though you may not recognize the pressure as the need to use the bathroom. Keeping your bladder empty is a good way to reduce extra pain. Certain positions will affect the amount of pain you feel. For example, staying upright during labor decreases the amount of pain you feel while lying down increases the amount of pain you feel. Staying upright as much as possible can help you have a less painful labor.

Emotional Factors

Although pain is a physical reality, the experience of pain can be influenced by your emotional state. For example, the difference between being physically intimate with your husband as opposed to being raped. In one experience the sensations of touch bring joy and pleasure while in the other they bring fear and pain. In this case the difference is in the trust, the security you feel and your willingness to give yourself to your partner. How much you trust your body to work properly during labor can affect the amount of pain you feel. How willing or unwilling you are to labor can affect the amount of pain you feel.

Several issues can make a woman unwilling to labor. Some women find the issue of modesty and a lack of respect for their modesty to hinder their labor. Other women find that their labor cannot proceed normally until they are in a place where they feel safe. Still other women find they cannot labor with certain people, or without certain people. How you feel about the environment around you will make a big difference in how willing you are to labor and therefore influence the amount of pain you feel.

Some women find they hold back from labor because of a fear of how they will appear. They do not want to be out of control or are concerned they will do something wrong. When you feel "on display," it can be hard to let go and let your body do the work it needs to do to labor. The possibility of expressing pain, not being polite or making noise is very real in labor. If you are not comfortable with these possibilities, it can increase the amount of pain you feel.

<u>**Emotional Issues**</u>
Fear
Trust
Concern
Respect
Modesty

Some women are simply afraid of the pain they expect to feel. They refuse to let go of control because they do not want to be in pain. What they do not understand is this struggle for control actually increases the amount of pain they feel in labor.

Dr. Grantly Dick-Read was the first person to document a connection between fear and pain in childbirth. He observed that the more fear a woman has, the more pain she feels in labor. Dr. Dick-Read taught women how their bodies worked and how to relax in labor to prevent the fear and pain.

Fear can wreak havoc at a spiritual level as well. When you try to hide or ignore your fear, you prevent God from being able to help you with it. It is as if you build a wall to prevent people from seeing your fear, but that wall keeps God out as well. Although you build the wall to protect, it actually hurts by preventing true healing. Do not be afraid to be honest about your fears with God, he is the only one who is able to heal your hurts and fears.

Fear and Pain

Fear of the pain of labor is the driving factor behind most labor preparations. Women prepare because they are afraid of the process, or perhaps of having strong sensations during the process. This is good because it calls women to action, to ready the body and mind and spirit. But this is not good because fear has a negative effect on childbirth.

If you look at the use of term "like a woman in labor" in the Bible, you see a picture of the "pain" and anguish experienced. The physical pain is said to happen because of fear. This may be fear of the expected event, fear of the event being out of your control or fear of anticipated harm or pain. But the verses do not say physical pain in response to a physical cause.

For example, in Psalm 48:6, Isaiah 13:8, Isaiah 21:3 and Jeremiah 4:31 the pain is felt because of the expected event. The fear of what is to come causes the pain. More examples can be read in Jeremiah 6:24, 13:21, 22:23 and 30:6. The Bible equates pain in labor with the fear of the unknown and expectation of loss of control or pain.

What cannot be denied is the universal nature of this fear. Fear of birth is not caused by modern culture any more than the sexualization of breasts is unique to modern culture. Fear of birth and male interest of breasts were accepted enough parts of the ancient Israelites' culture that they were written about in the Bible. Certain aspects of our culture may build upon this fear, but it is not unique to us.

Songs of Songs

Fear and Pain

> Labor is 98% in the head and heart. If women can just get beyond conscious fear–but mostly subconscious fear–they can usually be victorious in natural childbirth. That is why prayer and time spent early on with a loving caregiver is so vital. They have to be able to consistently have someone that genuinely cares they can go to that secret place with; therefore, creating a "safe place" to give birth.
>
> *Carol Gautschi*

You can try to change your environment, hoping it will change your heart. It does not work that way in life, and it will not work that way in childbirth. Fear of labor is a part of the human nature, coming from inside the heart in the same way sin is a part of the human nature. Sin does not happen because this is a fallen world; the sin came first. People sin because it is the nature of the human heart. You are human. In your humanness you have a heart that is drawn to sin in the same way the heart is fearful. No wonder the Bible is so full of commands not to sin and not to be fearful, anxious or worried.

This is neither good nor bad. It is the nature of the human heart—the way God made you and when he created man and woman he said it was good. This is who you are, and God is able to grow and mature you despite the fact that you are drawn to sin and fear.

Dr. Grantley Dick-Read wrote in 1959, "The fear of pain actually produces true pain through the medium of pathological tension" (Dick-Read, 1959). In 1979, a report in Nursing Research found fear or anxiousness was one of the indicators of increased pain during labor (Lederman, Lederman, Wrok & McCann, 1979). In 1980, another report in the Journal of American Psychiatry identified several psychological dimensions that can influence the degree of pain felt during labor (Doering, Entwisle & Quinlan, 1980). These included anxiety and emotional arousal.

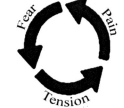
Dr. Grantley Dick-Read's Fear Tension Pain cycle.

During a normal labor, your body responds to the stress by producing stress hormones called catecholamines in normal amounts. Your baby is also producing his own supply of these stress hormones. Normal levels of stress hormones are helpful to labor because they decrease the baby's heart rate so there is less oxygen use. This allows your baby to deal with the normal decrease in oxygen during contractions. In addition, the stress of contractions helps the baby become ready to breathe.

If you are excessively anxious or fearful, your body produces excessive amounts of catecholamines. These "stress" chemicals divert blood away from the uterus to other parts of your body. This gets you set for action, but limits the supply of fresh oxygen for your uterus and your baby.

To understand the full effects of fear on labor, you first need to understand the design of the uterus. Your uterus is a muscle, but unlike other muscles your uterus has muscle fibers that run perpendicular to each other. One set of muscle fibers runs longitudinally from the top of the uterus (fundus) towards the bottom. When these muscle fibers contract, the fundus is pulled down and the cervix is pulled up. This pushes the cervix against the baby's head causing the cervix to open. The other set of muscle fibers run latitudinal, or around, the sides of the uterus and are concentrated near the cervix. When these muscle fibers contract, they pull the sides of the uterus in and close the uterus.

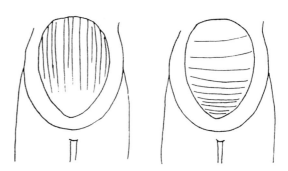

During the normal labor, only the longitudinal fibers will contract so the cervix can open and the baby can be moved out through the cervix. During a dysfunctional labor, fear makes the latitudinal set of muscle fibers contract effectively closing the cervix and preventing the baby from exiting the uterus. The dysfunctional labor caused by fear can result in a long, painful, ineffective labor because the body is working against itself. It is also possible the two sets of muscle fibers contracting could compress the blood vessels in the uterus, restricting oxygen for the muscle and for the baby.

The last resort method to deal with this type of fear is to use medication. However, using medication carries its own set of risks to the health of the baby and the proper functioning of the rest of the labor. Ideally, your fears will be handled before labor begins, giving you and your baby the best chance at a normal, healthy birth.

Fear, by its very nature, is something you experience in anticipation of an event. When the time comes, you are working through whatever happens and the fear is gone because you are doing it. You handle it because you have no choice but to handle it. However, for some women this fear is overpowering and prevents them from allowing their bodies to begin effective labor. It may not be fear of pain. Women report fear of death, fear of being inadequate to give birth and a lack of trust in their doctors or hospitals as reasons for anxiety (Wesson, 1999).

You can do some things to help ensure you are not overcome by the fear of childbirth. First and foremost, do not pretend you have no fear. Trying to hide something about yourself does not work because labor is not controlled by your conscious mind, it is controlled by your sub-conscious mind. You may be able to convince others you are not afraid, but you cannot fool yourself. Secondly, take the fear to the only one who can truly comfort you, God. Be honest about how you feel and let him give you the strength you need.

> See Appendix 2 for an activity to help overcome fear.

Coping With Pain

Giving birth is not like baking a cake where you mix the correct ingredients in the sequential order for the designated amount of time and then bake at a predetermined temperature. There are too many variables to any labor and birth for there to be a one-size-fits-all formula for coping with discomfort.

Labor requires a multi-level approach to manage pain. Most women are not able to rely on one or two comfort measures, but instead use a variety of comfort measures in combination throughout their labor. Positions, relaxation techniques and quick comfort measures are more effective when they are used together.

The Theories

When trying to decide what comfort measures to try, it helps to understand some of the reasons the various techniques work. There are two main theories about managing the pain of labor taught in childbirth education classes. The first is the Gate Control Theory, and the second is the Fear Tension Pain Cycle. An understanding of each will help you find ways to manage your discomfort.

The Gate Control theory is based on the body's having two types of sensory nerves (the nerves that send signals to the brain). These nerves send either pain or pressure signals to the brain at different speeds—but only one signal can be sent at a time. The idea is to stimulate the nerves that send pressure so you block (or close the gate) on the nerves that send pain signals. Ice packs, heat pads, pressure massage and cool moist cloths are all ways to stimulate the pressure nerves and block the pain nerves.

Nerves can become sensitized to a stimulus, so the positive effect of these techniques can be as short as fifteen minutes. This is not a problem because you have lots of activities to choose from, and by the time the next one is exhausted you can go back to the first technique again. These techniques are helpful because they take no previous experience or practice to use them successfully.

The Fear Tension Pain Cycle theory is based on the body's natural response to stress hormones. When the mother is stressed or fearful, her body produces hormones that prepare her body to handle that stress by diverting blood to her arms and legs away from her uterus and shutting down unnecessary functions, like digestion and giving birth, until the danger passes. This shutting down of labor and lack of blood for the uterus causes painful, ineffective contractions that can last for hours. The idea is to stay calm and relaxed, allowing your body to do the work of labor. Relaxation techniques such as visualization, listening to music and choosing a calming environment are all ways to prevent the production of excess stress hormones.

The techniques for staying relaxed take time to learn and prepare for labor. Most require practice to be successful during contractions. When used correctly, these techniques can be very powerful at helping you achieve a deep relaxation. However, you cannot pretend to be relaxed when you are not, and relaxation techniques are no substitute for trust in your body's ability to labor.

Gate Control Theory
Ice Packs
Warm Compresses
Pressure Massage

Fear Tension Pain Theory
Music
Massage
Deep Breathing
Water Immersion
Childbirth Education
Prayer
Companionship

> My grandmother (mum of 5) used to tell us, "Two-thirds of pain is fear." I think that's pretty true for birth. If you build your confidence in your body through knowledge and exercise, and go into birth not too fearful, then you can minimize the release of the stress hormones that make labour more painful. Deep relaxation and regular breathing can help you avoid tensing up, and the better you can manage that, the less painful and more manageable it is. So you can get a "confidence-relaxation-manageable pain" cycle happening instead.
>
> *Julie Bell*

The Research

A few bits of research have considered what is necessary for a woman to cope well with the pain of labor. Contrary to popular belief, coping well with labor does not take a high tolerance for pain. Coping was more closely tied to the interactions with attendants and confidence in ability to labor. This says two important things about giving birth.

1 Corinthians 15:33

First, where you have your baby and who you hire to be with you matters immensely. "Bad company corrupts good character" is true even in labor. If you are surrounded by caregivers who disregard the things you ask for, are offering you medication for the pain and telling you how tired you are going to be it can be very difficult to have a good attitude about the work of labor. On the other hand, being surrounded by caregivers who tell you how well you are doing, respect your decision making ability and patiently allow labor to follow its course, you will be much more inclined to feel successful and cope well with labor. Your birth team will greatly affect your attitude.

©2006 Marcelia Conerly Ambrose
Your ability to cope with labor increases when you are surrounded by supportive help.

More evidence that it is not superhuman strength that gets you through labor is found in the research done on doulas. When a woman has a doula with her in labor, she is less likely to request medication and less likely to need a C-section. She is also less likely to need other interventions. This is not because women who hire doulas are tougher or better at birthing than women who do not. It is because the presence of someone who encourages you and works with you to help you be part of the decision making process changes your attitude about labor. You have more strength because someone else is there to support you. Remember, a cord of three strands is not easily broken.

Ecclesiastes 4:12

Secondly, attitude is important. It is just like anything else in life; if you do not think you can do it, you will give up before you even try. The first painful contraction will be your evidence that you cannot do it and you will begin to panic. Confidence in your ability to handle labor is one of the strongest indicators that you will successfully cope.

Your Body

There are a multitude of tricks and techniques you can use to get through labor. The secret is finding the right ones. You will only know the best ways for you to handle labor if you take the time to really examine who you are as a person.

It does not matter that other women do really well with lots of family and friends. If you always want to be alone when you feel stressed or unwell then you will probably want to be alone for most of labor. It does not matter that other women really enjoy the labor pool. If you do not like being in the tub or a hot tub, you probably will not relax as well in the water.

> What expectations about labor have you formed based on other women's experiences?

It does not matter that walking is one of the best ways to move labor along comfortably. If you have been up all day and you are tired when you start feeling contractions, go to bed. It does not matter that everyone is telling you how to do the breathing patterns for labor. If you prefer to do deep breathing then just breathe.

It does not matter that everyone else thinks classical music is relaxing. If you prefer to listen to rock or jazz then use that music. It does not matter that every hospital labor room has a bed right in the center of it. If you do not want to lie down, do not use it.

It does not matter that everyone else gets tense first in their shoulders. If you get tense, first in your face then ask for a massage of your temples and forehead.

The point is, you need to know who you are and what you need to be successful at using the different comfort measures. You need to understand the signals your body gives you and you need to be familiar enough with the way the comfort measures make your body feel that you know instinctively how to move. It is like the way you sway when you have to wait for a bathroom, or the way you lie just so in your bed. These things are you responding to the small signals your body is sending you, and you already know how to listen. You just need to give yourself permission to respond to what your body is telling you about labor. Start by practicing now in pregnancy.

When your back is sore, do pelvic rocking and try sitting backwards over a chair—which one worked better? When your legs feel heavy, try lying down on your side and sitting with your feet propped up—which one gave you energy faster? When you are tired but cannot sleep, try sleeping on a couch or recliner chair—which position was the most comfortable?

The pushing reflex is the same as the sensation that lets you know you need to use the bathroom. When you feel the need to go to the bathroom, how does your body initially react to that feeling and what hinders you from doing what comes naturally? Can you empty a full bowel better sitting on the toilet or lying on your back? Does it help to have your feet up on a stool simulating a squat?

Get to know your body and the signals it sends. How do you know you are thirsty or hungry? What happens if you do not get food right away? What kind of massage feels the best to you? You are a unique individual created by God for a unique purpose. You are the expert on you, and you are the only one who can tell the rest of your birth team what you will need in labor. You are the only one qualified to interpret your body's normal signals. You will be able to interpret your body's signals in labor too.

Personal Pain Coping Strategies

For most people, childbirth brings to mind painful physical contractions. Although intense physical sensation is part of labor, in reality there is more than physical discomfort and contractions. For some women, the intense emotional and mental work needed to labor causes as much distress as the work of the uterus.

In the Bible, the pain of childbirth and labor are used repeatedly as a metaphor for fear and anguish—not physical pain. Because of the extreme emotional torment happening, the people will look and behave like a woman in labor. What is going on in your head can and will affect what is happening in your body.

During childbirth, women do fear pain. That fear alone could be enough to cause anguish, but it is only the start of what may be going on. When labor is slow to start or seems to take longer than anticipated, fears about how much the body can be trusted begin to grow. If the mother is struggling to make sure she looks in control, not wanting to look bad in labor, it will cause mental anguish during labor. If the mother feels isolated by the experience, because in reality no matter how many people are with the mother she is the only one in labor and the only one feeling the sensations that can quickly turn into emotional pain. When contractions build until there is barely a break between them and the mother sees no end

> References to fear as a woman in childbirth:
> Psalm 48:6; Isaiah 13:8, 21:3; Jeremiah 4:31, 6:24, 13:21, 22:23, 30:6, 48:41, 49:22-24, 50:43; Micah 4:9-10

to labor, she may feel anguish. If the mother is working with labor attendants who are not listening to her or treating her as an object instead of a person, the feelings of helplessness and powerlessness can be enough to cause emotional and mental anguish.

Coping strategies for labor need to cover more than managing backaches and contractions. Real labor coping skills include handling stress, isolation, boredom and fear. To successfully manage labor a mother must be ready to deal with the emotional and mental pain of labor, not just the physical sensations.

You already have more coping ability than you may think. You already have ways you successfully manage physical, mental and emotional pain. Understanding how you naturally cope can help you determine which comfort techniques will work the best for you. Find your strengths and build on them. Learning ways to cope that are outside your natural strengths can be very helpful as well, since it will give you the widest variety of tools to handle whatever happens in labor.

Think about a time you have been very stressed. How did you know you were feeling stressed?

How does your body react to tension?

How can you keep yourself calm if you feel stressed?

How you successfully handle stress and pain will depend on how you are made. Think about who you are and how you naturally cope with pain and stress. Do you:

Focus thoughts inward or find an external focus?

Need to be alone or need companionship?

Seek out silence or seek out conversation?

Desire physical touch or avoid physical stimulations?

Slow down to relax or keep yourself busy?

You will probably find you work best through labor using comfort techniques that fit your answers to the above questions. There is no right or wrong way; it is simply the strengths you have for dealing with stress. Labor does not suddenly change who you are or how you cope. But labor may require you to use more of your strength than you have ever used before.

Personal Pain Coping Strategies

You have already developed your own unique style of coping with pain. Think for a moment about a time you have been in pain. What helped you to manage that pain? What type of environment did you seek out? How much assistance did you desire? What worked to lessen the pain? What worked to help you cope with pain that would not lessen?

Now that you have a good picture of who you are in relationship to stress and pain, use that information to help you find the comfort measures which are most likely to be successful for you. Variations of the most common techniques for labor are listed in the next section. Be careful not to write off a technique before you try it. Some of the techniques are more helpful than you might think.

> One of the things I notice is that labor and pain are always talked about hand in hand. I don't think what I felt could be described as pain. Pain and a urinary tract infection go hand in hand. Pain and cutting yourself while shaving. . .pain and burning yourself on a hot pan. . .pain and diaper rash. . .pain. . .pain. . .pain. But when you say childbirth, I think intensity. I think hard work. I think strength. I think cooperation. I think relaxation. I think joy. I think elation. I think letting go and letting God. But I don't think pain.
>
> *MeriBeth Glen*

Abnormal Pain in Childbirth

In general, your body uses pain as a way to signal a need. Pain occurs when damage or injury is happening and needs your attention. Labor pain is different. There is no damage being done during the normal labor, even if there is pain. Contrary to other pain, when the intensity of labor increases, the labor becomes more productive even if it comes with an increase in pain. In labor, the idea is not to remove the pain, but to get to through it.

In addition to the physical pain is the emotional and mental pain of labor. These have no physical cause but can become the source of physical pain. Your body uses chemical messages to signal needs for change, and the chemical messages of pain or stress can cause a lump in the throat, stress headaches, a queasy stomach or fatigue. In labor, an increase in stress can cause an increase in the amount of physical pain felt.

In labor, how do you know if the amount of pain you feel is not normal? How do you tell the difference between the normal stretching of a cervix and something going wrong? What can you do to make sure you do not have excessive pain during labor?

It may interest you to know that although nearly every woman considers labor to be intense, not all women consider labor to be excruciating. About 17 percent of women claim they had low levels of pain during labor

(Melzack et. al, 1981). There are some characteristics associated with more difficult labors. Some you will have control over and some you do not. For example, if you are a first time mother or are very young, you are more likely to have higher levels of pain during labor. Similarly, if you have a history of menstrual problems or have a history of miscarriage or abortion, you are more likely to have higher levels of pain.

Other characteristics associated with a more painful labor are difficulty accepting the pregnancy or emotional conflict about becoming a mother. Anxiety about labor and fear of being helpless or in pain are also indicators of a more painful labor. Unrealistic expectations or a partner who is indifferent about the baby and labor can further contribute to a more painful labor (Wesson, 1999).

While some of these issues are unable to be changed, many of them are related to your emotional preparedness for labor and mothering and so can be influenced. By working through your fears, educating yourself about the process of labor and communicating effectively with your husband and birth attendants you can improve your chances of having normal or low levels of pain.

It is important to remember, although these factors indicated a greater sensation of pain, they did not indicate problems with giving birth. Removing pain is not associated with birthing more successfully. Even if you know you are more likely to feel more pain, it does not mean you will have problems giving birth. It simply means you will need to rely more on God's strength to cope with what you are feeling.

Increasing Pain in Labor

There are some things within labor that can increase the amount of pain you feel. For example, a full bladder increases the pelvic pain you experience. This can be avoided by emptying the bladder every hour. Another cause of increased pain is the use of a reclining position (lying on the back). For the least painful labor, you should use upright positions such as standing, walking, leaning and sitting. Being dehydrated can also increase the perception of pain. All three of these causes of increased pain will not only make labor harder for you, they also have the potential to slow down the work of labor, making labor longer.

When you are exhausted and discouraged your perception of pain increases. Exhaustion, discouragement and anxiety can all be managed with supportive companions who work with the mother in labor. Sleeping when possible, avoiding arbitrary time lines and allowing yourself to work as your body needs will also help. If your have extreme fear or anxiety, the hormonal response to that fear will increase your pain and decrease the productiveness of your labor. About 20 percent of women fear giving birth, and for 6 percent the fear is extreme. Fears range from the expectation of pain to not trusting caregivers.

If you have a scarred cervix from a previous surgery, it can cause greater pain during labor. Inducing labor can also increase the amount of pain you feel. If your baby is not in an optimal position, it can cause increased pain and a slower labor. Generally, staying as mobile as possible, specifically moving the pelvis will help the baby move into the best position so labor can proceed. If you are feeling excessive pain and the labor is moving slower than anticipated, it may be caused by a hormonal response to fear or poor fetal positioning.

Pain and Labor Problems

In general, as long as what you are doing helps you to cope with labor you are probably fine. If you can not breathe or catch your breath, your partners should breathe with you to help you take deeper breaths. Feeling pain in the back is a normal variation that can be frustrating but is not in itself a sign of danger. Try some different positions to get baby to rotate and take the pressure off your back.

There are two possible danger signs in labor—a contraction that does not go away and pain that remains between contractions. Neither is normal during labor, although back pain between contractions can be normal with some fetal positions.

A contraction that does not go away could indicate a problem with placental separation or hyperstimulation of the uterus. Be sure to let your midwife know right away if this happens. Depending on where the separation occurs you may see blood. Whether you see blood or not a continuous contraction is not normal and should be addressed immediately.

If the contractions are maintaining a pattern but you feel pain between contractions, it may indicate problems with the baby's position which should be resolved so the birth can proceed. By changing positions and staying active, you give the baby every opportunity to get into the best birthing position.

Pushing should not hurt, although it is normal to feel pressure and a burning sensation as your baby is crowning. If pushing does not feel like a relief, or if it hurts to push, your body is probably not ready. Your baby may not be in the right position, or you may have a cervical lip and should hold off pushing until your baby can finish the stretching of the cervix at which time it will feel like a relief to push. Changing positions or walking around may help.

With the exception of placental problems causing continuous contractions, you will not feel any increased pain during a real labor problem. There is no pain that identifies women who will deal with shoulder dystocia or fetal distress. And though you may see signs during labor that indicate a possible problem, the signs are not related to the pain you feel. For more information about problems in labor, see section on Labor Challenges.

> Prior to a mom beginning pushing the contractions usually shift over. They become what some mom's describe as lighter / different and they may stretch out a little. When a mom begins pushing it should feel almost relieving if the cervix is gone. If there is a sharp or intense pain with pushing, particularly right above the pubic bone (this is usually indicative of a cervical lip) I tell her to wait until her body won't let her do anything other than push and it feels better, like a relief instead of intensely painful in one location.
>
> *Brandi Wood*

How Painful is Labor?

There really is no consensus about how much pain you should expect to feel. Even among Christian midwives, doulas and childbirth educators, there is debate about how much labor is supposed to hurt, why it does and how best to prepare for it.

On one side is the knowledge that most women feel pain when giving birth. If they are not expecting to have that pain, they may not take labor preparation seriously. If they do not take the preparation seriously, they will be discouraged by their inability to cope with the pain during labor.

On the other side is the fact that some women have little or no pain during labor. There is no way to predict how much pain a woman will or will not have, but if she lacks the confidence to handle labor, her ability to cope (regardless of the amount of pain she feels) is decreased. Women who expect terrible labors very often have them, so you may be set up for an excruciating labor if you expect the worst.

> Ask five different women to describe what labor feels like. Chances are they will each give you a different description.

The question is further confounded by the simple fact that no one can answer for you what labor pain feels like—whether it is an extremely painful or a painless birth. The baby's position, your overall health, how tired you are, how well supported you are and how well educated you are all play a part in how intensely painful the experience is.

How Painful is Labor?

While most women start with easy contractions and build to strong, frequent contractions, some women start labor with very intense contractions that stay strong throughout labor. Some women never seem to get to the intensely painful contractions. A few women experience irregular patterns where several strong contractions will be followed by a few less intense contractions, which may indicate the baby needs more help to get into a good position. Other women simply take a long time to labor, experiencing whatever levels of pain they have for hours.

Where women feel the strength of contractions and how they describe them is different. Some women say it feels like cramping or aching, others say it feels tight or like pressure. It may feel like a sharp pain or stabbing. The contractions can be felt on the abdomen, back, groin, the sides of the pelvis, on the top of the hips, radiating from the back to front or even starting at the hips and moving down to the legs (Wesson, 1999).

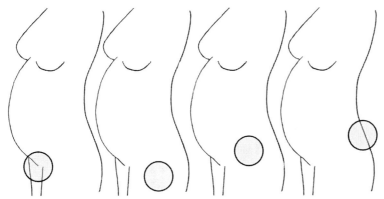

Women report feeling pain, pressure, aching or cramping in different parts of their bodies during labor. You cannot predict what your labor will feel like.

The truth is, unless you have had a baby before (and sometimes even if you have), you cannot really be prepared for what your labor will be like. Which comfort measures will work, or not work, is not something you can know until labor begins. Yet, most childbirth preparation is based on answering the question, "What can I do about the pain?" or more honestly, "How can I get rid of the pain?"

The desire to not be in pain is normal, and for all practical purposes it is very healthy to avoid pain. But if planning for giving birth is based solely on the desire to avoid pain, the focus might be a little off.

If you knew labor did not hurt, what things would you be doing to prepare to give birth? If you knew you were not going to feel pain, what would be your main goal for laboring?

Here is a new paradigm, a new way of thinking about labor. Instead of focusing on the negative aspect of feeling pain, focus on the positive aspect of working with your body to labor efficiently and safely. God created your body to give birth. Instead of trying to "shut off" the experience of labor, plan to turn on to labor so you can understand what your body needs as labor progresses. Let the pain be secondary, if and when it comes you will deal with it. Focus your preparation on finding ways to help labor progress, and the pain will take care of itself.

Stay active, responding to your body's cues to move. Choose upright positions that help you labor effectively, and change your position when your body says it is time. Surround yourself with supportive people who will encourage you and take care of you as you labor. Choose the environment that is most comfortable to you. If your choices are limited then do what is necessary to alter the environment so you can feel safer and more relaxed. Focusing on these things will help your labor to be the most efficient and safe it can be. What is even more interesting, women who labor this way feel less pain and cope better with whatever levels of pain they feel. Changing your focus from avoiding the pain to keeping labor effective not only helps you move through labor as quickly as possible, it also prevents pain.

This really should not be a surprise. God has created our lives in a way that having the correct focus improves life. Think of how your life changes when you get too busy to spend time with God, and how much more you accomplish when you ensure God is a regular part of your schedule. Think of how you can talk yourself out of supporting the church as you struggle to make ends meet, and how the money seems to come in at exactly the right time when you are purposeful about tithing. It is possible labor works in a similar fashion.

How Painful is Labor?

> I have had six pregnancies and four live births. My first was terrible back labor so I would say that that is where I felt it the most. That pain was more overwhelming than anywhere else there was pain.
>
> Second and third births were more natural—no drugs at all, more 'normal,' and I would say the pain was definitely in the pelvic area and also to the right and left of the lower uterus. They were hospital births, and being kept in the bed caused a lot of lower back pain and that felt like a shock type of pain.
>
> I then had my last baby as an unassisted home birth, and all the pain was reduced greatly and was not overwhelming. The place of pain was similar to my second and third birth, but the lower back pain at transition was minimal. The after pains in that birth were "WOW" very intense and worse than the labor.
>
> *Jacinda Montalto*

> I remember labor feeling very intense, pain on my pubic bone and shooting pain in my thighs. All my labors were very fast—4 hours, 2½ hours, and 1½ hours. Because of the quickness, I had a rapid dumping of hormones so I was very shaky and sick to my stomach. On my first son, I pushed the longest—30-40 minutes. He bruised my tailbone so bad that I sat on a "donut" or 4 weeks. His shoulders were also very large.. Pushing the head was not as bad as the shoulders. I remember what a release it was to push.
>
> *Tammy Ryan*

Drawing Conclusions
Review of Section Five

Reaction to Pain

Put an ice cube in a sealed plastic zipper bag. Hold the bag with the ice in your lightly closed fist for sixty seconds. What happens to your body when it begins to be painful? How do you react to the growing pain of the ice?

Give yourself a short break and then try it again, this time working consciously to relax your mind and body while you hold the ice. Did it make a difference?

Letting Go

It is normal to have fears and concerns about giving birth, however, Jesus is clear that we are to cast our burdens of fear and worry onto God.

Schedule at least an hour when you can be undisturbed and alone. Find a quiet, comfortable place to be with God. Pour out your heart until it is empty, being open and honest about all your fears. When you are finished, sit quietly and wait for God to speak to you.

The Bible gives us examples of God having a powerful strong voice, and a gentle, still voice. Stay quietly with him until you can "hear" one of his voices.

Making a plan

Make a list of the procedures or experiences of birth you are feeling afraid about. Include for each fear the worst possible outcome. For example, if one of your fears is needles, your worst outcome might be having a nurse who needs to try several times to insert an IV.

Make a plan for each item on your list. What can you do to try to prevent it from happening? How will you know if it is happening? What can you do if it happens?

Ten Questions about...
Pain

1. What positive experiences have you had with pain?
2. What negative experiences have you had with pain?
3. What expectations do you have for pain during childbirth?
4. How have you come to have these expectations?
5. What techniques do you use to manage physical pain in everyday life?
6. What techniques do you use to manage emotional pain in everyday life?
7. In what ways has pain in your life helped you to grow?
8. How do you expect to respond to pain in labor?
9. What will you do if the pain you feel is less than expected?
10. What will you do if the pain you feel is worse than expected?

Ten Questions about...
Fear

1. What fears arise from previous experiences at birth (as the mother or witness)?
2. What fears arise from your feelings of loneliness or isolation?
3. What fears arise from the understanding you are becoming a mother (again)?
4. What fears arise from the anticipation of the physical process of labor?
5. What fears arise from the anticipation of being "watched" and meeting expectations?
6. What fears arise from the anticipation of being out of control?
7. What fears arise from the expectation of pain associated with labor?
8. What fears arise from the anticipation of breastfeeding?
9. What fears arise from comments made by family or friends?
10. How have you been able to overcome fears in the past?

More Than Conquerors!

Kelly Townsend
Author
Christ Centered Childbirth
Cascade Christian Childbirth
www.ChristianChildbirth.org

Romans 8:35-37

"Who shall separate us from the love of Christ? Shall trouble or hardship or persecution or famine or nakedness or danger or sword? No, in all these things we are more than conquerors through him who loved us."- Romans 8:35-37

As a Christian, we have the benefit of the love of Christ to help us overcome all obstacles in life, including the fear of childbirth! Dear sister, know that the fears you are holding on to are not as big as they might seem, nor do they need to have a grip-hold over you. Each one of us faces the fears of a painful birth, an unwanted outcome, loss of control, echoes of others horror stories, what-ifs', reminders of childhood abuses, needles, and the list goes on. The good news is we can pop the balloon of tormenting scenarios that run through our mind with scripture, a little knowledge, and the blessed assurance of the love of Christ.

First, let us look at the physiology of fear, and how it affects your birth. Each woman faces a measure of fear when approaching the birth of her baby. If she is unable to reconcile those thoughts, she will carry them with her to the day of delivery. During birth, the sympathetic nervous system is triggered by tension in the muscles (furrowing the brow, locking elbows, tightening perineum) and also from thoughts of fear. Just like her heart is affected by being startled (beats faster), so too the uterus can be affected by stress/tension/fear.

The Myometrium, which is the muscle of the uterus, is distinguished into 3 layers. The outer layer contracts to open the cervix and push the baby out. The middle simply supports the blood vessels that are in between the outer and inner layers. And finally, the inner layer contracts and closes the cervix after birth and returns the uterus to the near-original size. However, during times of stress, the inner muscle layer becomes rigid in an effort to stall the birth in order to protect the baby from perceived harm. It fights the productive efforts of the outer layer to protect the baby from a hostile environment on the outside! This can happen in animals as well. A deer in the forest, if she smells a scent of danger, will stop laboring until the danger is gone. Cats will often not complete their labor until they are in a dark confined space and feel safe. This is a protective mechanism built into us just like the pounding heart when we are under stress.

Several things happen during fear in childbirth. First, labor is slowed down because the outer layer has to work twice as long to open that cervix. The process can completely stall and she is diagnosed with "failure to progress," increasing the need for risky medical interventions. Second, the uterus has to work harder to accomplish its work. The muscle layers are opposing themselves, which creates pain. If you try and make a muscle with your arm, and someone tries to extend it and oppose your efforts, your muscle tires quickly and pain soon develops. So too, with the uterus, pain soon develops when the inner layer has been rigid, feeding her fear that labor will be intolerable. The inner layer becomes even more rigid, and the fear-tension-pain cycle has begun. Thirdly, the two muscles working against each other constrict the middle layer where the blood vessels are, cutting off the blood supply to the uterus and placenta. Cesarean sections are often performed due to fetal distress, which may very well have been caused by tension and fear alone.

Conversely, if she is able to relax on her own, if she can overcome her fears, then the inside layer relaxes and the outer layer can be far more efficient. Labor is faster, easier, and safer. However, how many of us can really go into labor with no measure of fear? It is largely impossible to overcome our fears on our own. Praise God that the Christian is able to turn to scripture during these times.

"For there is no fear in love. For perfect love casts out all fear, because fear has to do with torment." — 1 John 4:18

Perfect love. Who can say that they have it? God's love, however, is perfect, and so it is HE who casts out our fear. We must trust that he will cast it out, and he will. Then, if we go in with confidence, peace, and patience, we have a better chance of a less traumatizing experience. Do we have a guarantee of a less painful birth if we are without fear? Certainly not! Many things can and do go differently than we hoped. But the Christian also has the promise of Romans 8:28 that all things happen for good, and that brings peace and understanding in ALL situations. — Romans 8:28

We do not have a lot of control over many aspects of birth. But what we can control is our minds, and Christ, who is the Comforter who comes and comforts us, and takes away our fears, is so essential that we dare not leave him out.

Subject Six

Staying Comfortable

Topics:

Providing Comfort	157
Using Touch During Labor	160
Positions for Labor	167
Movement in Labor	174
Using Water in Labor	177
Relaxation for Labor	183
Comforting Environment	187
Drawing Conclusions	194
Herbs for Labor by Shonda Parker	196

Providing Comfort

Why do women use comfort measures in labor? Quite frankly—because they work.

When trying to determine the best comfort measures to use in labor, you need to look at two things. First, you need to have some sort of concept of what providing comfort means. Secondly, you need to know who you are physically and emotionally to tailor efforts to your individual needs.

> How do you define "comfort"?

The Bible gives wonderful examples of God and his people providing comfort to those who are hurting. These examples give a picture of what is necessary to provide real comfort.

In Genesis, there are two instances of God providing comfort to Hagar. Both times God provided emotional encouragement by acknowledging he was with her. In the second example, God also provided for the physical needs of Hagar and Ishmael by providing water for them. It is interesting to note that in this story God also provided comfort to Abraham by assuring Abraham Ishmael would become a great nation.

> Genesis 16:7-14
> Genesis 21:8-20

In First Kings 19, God is providing comfort to an emotionally drained and frightened Elijah. Elijah is twice told to eat the food God provides, then he is allowed to "see" God is with him by watching him pass by. So here, God again provided comfort by meeting the physical needs and giving encouragement.

> 1 Kings 19

Daniel 6 — In Daniel 6 God comforts Daniel in the den of lions. God once again provides for the physical need by closing the mouths of the lions, and the emotional needs by sending an angel to be with Daniel. The comforting continues throughout the gospels as Jesus meets hurting people. Jesus comforted people by spending time with them, healing their physical bodies and encouraging them.

1 Kings 17
2 Samuel 12 — God's people give examples of how to comfort each other. Elijah's response to the death of the widow's son is to pray with her for God to bring her son back. While David is pleading with God for the life of his child, his household elders stand with him, encouraging him to get up and eat. It was not until the baby died that David responded to their prompting, but when he was ready they served him food.

These examples show two things about providing comfort. First, the comfort should meet the individual's physical needs—it must address any physical hurting they have. Secondly, the emotional needs should not be ignored. Attempts should be made to encourage the person.

Book of Job — Comparing these examples to the story of Job and his friends helps further define comforting. Two things happened with Job's companions that turned their comfort into a source of distress for Job. First, they were uncomfortable with Job's pain and tried to make it go away themselves instead of letting God heal Job. Secondly, they were not really with Job. They did not listen to him enough to hear that Job did not want answers. He wanted to know God was still with him. When they spoke, they used cheap and easy answers to try to end Job's suffering. These answers sound good in books and movies. They are even based in Biblical truth. But when you are really hurting they do not satisfy.

Empty words will never satisfy. They are not comforting, and in the case of Job, they are hurtful. Just the presence of his friends was enough for Job, just to have them there to share his hurt and listen. But many people get uncomfortable with the suffering of others and try to make it go away. This is a disservice to the emotionally hurting people. True healing can only come from God, and every easy answer given only prolongs the sufferer from being with God. The best way to encourage is to be present and to point the individual to God.

Providing comfort in labor should be about meeting the physical needs of the mother. The various positions, pain management techniques and forms of touch intended to lessen her physical pain are helpful forms of comfort. Providing comfort in labor should also be about meeting the emotional needs of the mother by encouraging her—but not with generic answers. In this section you will learn various techniques for both physical and emotional comfort during labor.

> My first baby was posterior. I did feel some contractions in the front, but mostly I felt them as a dull pain that radiated across my lower back, hips and down my thighs. I hesitate to use the word "pain" because, although I was in labor for over 48 hours, it was just not that bad. Exhausting and overwhelming, yes. Painful, not so much. More of a burning sensation.
>
> With my second, I had rather sharp lower abdominal pains. I remember thinking at first that I couldn't be in labor because it hurt too much. Surely I had some sort of intestinal problem instead. In the beginning, labor was a small cramp right in front. Later on, the contractions got "bigger;" that is, I felt them over more area. The sensations became less localized and more generalized. I think it is generally true of labor; as it progresses, it involves more and more of your body, until when you are pushing your whole body is involved.
>
> My third labor was much like the second, but it was longer and less intense.
>
> *Ellen Bauman*

Using Touch During Labor

Your skin is the largest organ in your body. It is sensitive to a variety of touches, able to distinguish pressure from light touch, heat from cold and a painful jab from a relaxing rub. Touch is needed for proper development, and helps to ease pain and discomfort.

<aside>Anointing happens in Mark 6:13; Matthew 26; Mark 14; Luke 7. Washing feet happens in John 13. Crowds surround Jesus in Matthew 8, 9, 17, 20; Mark 1, 8; Luke 5, 22.</aside>

Unlike other comfort measures, touch has the ability to meet both the physical needs of pain relief and the emotional needs of support and reassurance. Biblically, touch is used both to comfort physically and emotionally. Touch is a part of anointing with oil and washing of feet. Blessings were passed on with the father placing a hand on the head of the son. Jesus healed many people with touch, and people crowded around him seeking his touch. In the stories of Elijah and Daniel, angels used physical touch to strengthen and encourage the men.

<aside>Genesis 27
Matthew 28</aside>

The sense of touch is powerful in the stories of the Bible. Isaac knew Jacob by his voice, but because his hand felt like Esau, Isaac believed it was Esau. After Jesus had risen from the dead, the women who met him on the road fell at his feet and touched him. Even today there are those who are able to heal with touch. God created us both physical and spiritual beings, with our physical bodies beautifully intertwined with our spiritual selves. Touch is a powerful way to provide comfort for both the physical and emotional aspects of hurt.

Massage in labor has been shown to reduce the pain and stress of labor. Women who were massaged by a partner for 20 minutes each hour in labor experienced less pain and had shorter labors (Field et.al., 1998). If massage is not possible, more simple forms of touch such as stroking, hugs, holding and rubbing have been effective at helping women through labor (Birch, 1986). Touch is also able to help a mother cope with the feelings of isolation that occur with pain. The laboring mother who is touched feels cared for and has an increased feeling of well-being.

Unfortunately, women giving birth in hospitals are more likely to be touched by machines than humans during childbirth. The increase in routine interventions and procedures, coupled with a culture who seems to have forgotten how to do non-sexual touch creates labor experiences where touch is uncomfortable and clinical. Without actively attempting to use comforting touch in labor, a mother may only be touched to insert an IV or medication, adjust a monitor, take her temperature or blood pressure or to do an internal vaginal exam.

Some women may find they do not like to be touched, preferring instead a personal "space." Other women may not know what types of touch feel best to them. In either case, it is important to the successful use of touch for comfort in labor that touching begin during pregnancy. For touch to be truly comforting in labor, it needs to go beyond the practicing of a skill to meeting the needs of the laboring mother. Some partners may find they are unsure of how to touch the mother, lacking confidence in skills and comfort in the actual touching of another person. Just beginning may be the hardest part. During massage, not only does the mother relax, but the partner giving the massage also becomes more relaxed.

> Describe the types of touch that feel good to you.

When becoming familiar with touch, there are three things to pay attention to. First, are you in a comfortable position? Second, when will touch or massage be helpful and when should it be stopped? Third, what is the best way to touch you? These questions can only be answered by you. For touch to be the most effective, you must have the freedom to say when it is not working or needs to be changed. A mother who feels helpless to change what is happening to her will cope poorly with labor. No one feels cared for or supported when she feels she is ignored.

Position

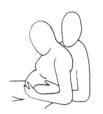

You can use touch in any position. What changes are the parts of your body available to be touched. For example, if you are leaning over a birth ball, it may be easiest for someone to rub your back, legs or head. If you are sitting in a rocking chair, the front of your legs, your hands and your feet become easy places to touch and massage.

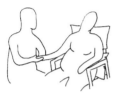

It is not desirable for you to be in one position for longer than 45 minutes, so your labor support will need to be flexible to accommodate your changing positions. You should never be asked to change positions to make it easier for someone to touch or massage you. The rule is everyone else works around the position that is most comfortable for you.

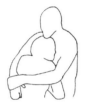

Whatever position you choose, be sure your body is well supported. This becomes especially important when you are using any form of pressure that may cause you to lose your balance. Use pillows, blankets or even furniture to help you be comfortable. For example, if you feel most comfortable in a hands and knees position, consider putting a pillow under you knees and lean your upper body over a chair to support your weight.

Your helpers will want to use good body mechanics to provide a massage that is comfortable for you and them. Proper posture, with a straight back can help prevent lower back pain. Bending should be done at the knees and hips, not lower back. To apply more pressure, your helper should lean in with body weight instead of trying to use arm strength. Kneeling pads can prevent discomfort in your helper's knees, and an asymmetrical kneeling position–with one knee up and one knee down–allows your helper more control with less discomfort.

Timing

Knowing when to touch can be difficult. For example, in the middle of a strong contraction is not the right time to start a massage, but is an appropriate time to hold a hand or to stroke a shoulder. In general, massage should be considered a touch that lasts for several contractions. Your helper will begin the massage in between contractions by placing hands on your body and slowly work up to the full movements. Continue with the massage for fifteen to twenty minutes or until it no longer feels good to you. You may find the pressure you want on some parts of the body increases during contractions and lessens after the contraction has passed.

It is always appropriate to stop any touch when you are no longer helped by it. The nature of labor is constant change. As labor progresses and the baby moves further down the pelvis, the sensations change. A sore spot on your back may migrate downward. Because of this, a touch that felt good an hour ago may not feel good now. Follow your body's cues to be sure what is being done is comforting. Your helpers can watch your face, listen to your sounds and observe your body movements to know you if you are relaxing or pulling away from the touch.

Is the touch helping? If you are not able to communicate with words, your helpers can check your face, body movements and the sounds to determine if the touch is helping.

Be sure to wear loose fitting, comfortable clothing when practicing massage. Your helper should remove any jewelry such as rings, bracelets or necklaces that may touch the skin. Oils, lotions and powders can help hands move smoothly over the skin without causing friction. Some oils contain properties that may help you during labor. Aromas such as lavender are calming while others such as peppermint may help stimulate labor. Be careful the smell of your lotion is not too strong; the sense of smell tends to become more sensitive during labor.

Ticklishness is a sign of nervous tension. Increasing the pressure of your touch and working the areas around the spot can help relax the muscles.

Techniques

The touch techniques you use will depend on several factors. Obviously, some techniques can only be done with a willing helper while others can be done by yourself. If you are coping well with labor, you may only need supportive touch such as holding someone's hand or having someone put a hand on your shoulder. If you are in distress, you may need a more deliberate and firm type of touch.

Comfort touch is not intended to alleviate pain, but instead to reassure you. A hand placed lightly on your body lets you know you are not alone. It can be helpful when you do not want firm pressure. Even if you do not want to be touched, you may find holding someone's hand to be comforting. If holding hands is too much touch, you may prefer resting your hand on a helper's arm or hand.

You might find comforting touch works well when combined with another activity. For example, holding hands gently while praying or having a helper brush your hair. You may also enjoy a "pat on the back" or to be anointed with oil. Gentle snuggling and kisses from your husband also count as comforting touches.

Pressure touch, or pressure massage, is helpful at alleviating back and hip pain during labor. In the same way putting pressure on your temples or the back of your head can help lessen a headache, using pressure during labor can help lessen pain. Pressure is created by pushing a thumb, knuckles, a small firm ball or other appropriate tool, into painful spots on your lower back or hips. To be effective, the pressure must be firm, but not enough to hurt.

Double hip squeeze

The double hip squeeze is a pressure technique a helper can do. Your helper stands behind you and presses on your hips as if trying to push the bones together. The proper position can be achieved by placing hands on the sides of your hips with the thumbs resting along the top ridge of your hip bones. Your helper will push the hips in toward an imaginary spot in the middle of your back with a gentle upward pressure. The double hip squeeze takes a lot of upper arm strength, so helpers may need to take a rest after a few contractions. The same effect can be created while you are sitting if your helper will put a palm on each of your knees and lean forward to gently press your knees straight back into your hips.

You do not have to use the double hip squeeze; any back pressure can be helpful. As your baby's head moves down, he is stretching your pelvis. Using pressure on your back puts the pelvic bones back in place, lessening the discomfort of stretching. Ask a helper to press on your lower back, to the left or right of your spine, until you find the most comfortable spot. If no helper is available, you can try to create the pressure yourself by leaning your back on a wall with a small firm ball placed in a comfortable spot on your low back.

Many people instinctively squeeze their hands in response to pain. Although pressure on the palms can help someone cope with pain, in labor you want your body to stay as relaxed as possible. If having pressure on your palms helps you deal with pain, you can ask a helper to squeeze your palms between a thumb and forefinger to create the same effect. If no helper is available, gripping a small hair comb in your fingers allows you to gently close your hand to increase the pressure. You can also try squeezing the fleshy part between your thumb and first finger with the thumb and first finger of the other hand.

Holding and object like a comb can allow you to put pressure on your hands without adding extra tension.

Other places on your body may respond well to pressure. Some women find gentle circular pressure on their upper backs and shoulders helps them maintain relaxation and cope better with pain. Other women find having pressure applied to the bottoms of their feet helps them let go of extra tension.

Effleurage is a flowing touch or skimming over the body. The effleurage touch is performed with the palm and fingers moving in a rhythmic and smooth glide over the body. When done lightly it promotes relaxation, encourages sleep and can diminish pain. When done with a deeper pressure it can help to relax tense muscles. Try skimming your hands over your belly in a circular motion, either one large circle or two smaller circles (one for each hand).

Effleurage

Kneading touch is performed with both hands together in alternate movements that simulate "wringing" the muscle. Keep the thumbs close to the fingers and push in alternate directions with each hand. This type of touch is best used on fleshy parts of the body when you want to relax tense muscles, work out some pain and be re-energized. Kneading can be done slow or fast, deep or light as necessary to be comfortable for you. You can even use kneading touch on yourself. Be sure you are comfortably positioned in a way that you will not lose your balance, and begin kneading your upper legs or feet.

Guiding Touch is touch which helps you know how to move. In guiding touch, a helper will use his hands to help you understand what to do with your body. For example, placing hands on the sides of your hips or back to gently rock you side to side during contractions can be a comfortable reminder to rock your hips. A hand on the shoulder can help you recognize tension in your upper back so you can release it. Some women practice a form of guiding touch during pregnancy so the touch of a helper becomes a signal to relax. This technique, called touch relaxation, can be difficult to master and requires much practice to use successfully.

Stroking touch is helpful on long pieces of body such as arms, legs and back. Place your hand near the top and gently rub to the end. Use as much pressure as needed, but not so much that it hurts. Move slowly when stroking, it is not the same as rubbing. Generally, stroking should be done in one direction or in a circle. Going up and down at the same spot can be irritating.

You can use stroking touch on yourself by stroking your belly or leg. Or you could ask a helper to touch you in this way. Stroking can be done in many positions, even with you walking. If your helper walks with an arm around your shoulders, he could gently stroke that arm down your back. When you are stopped for a contraction, he can support you from behind while gently stroking down your arms, resting his hands gently on yours when he reaches the end.

Positions for Labor

One of the most interesting connections between heart and body in the Bible is the way posture is related to attitude. When the Israelites were disobedient to God, he referred to them as stiff-necked. When Joshua was met by the Commander of the Lord's Army, he fell face down in awe and worship of God. Bowing down, from a gentle leaning forward to the extreme face to the ground that Joshua did, is a way to show your submission to God.

Exoduc 33:3-5
Joshua 5:14

How you hold your body can say a lot about what is going on in your heart. Humans communicate fear, anger, pride and dislike all with the way the body is held. Think about the subtle ways your body changes just in response to thinking about different emotions. What parts of the body are involved, what muscles are tightened when you are trying to stop what is happening to you and what muscles are relaxed when you are enjoying yourself?

This non-verbal communication does more than express your inner feelings. Your body structure is formed by muscle connected to bone. As the muscles contract and relax, the bones move in response, shifting their position in relation to each other. Unknowingly shifting your body in response to fear can hinder your labor. Understanding how to shift the positions of your bones can help you stay comfortable and labor more effectively.

Your Pelvis

Your pelvis is the center stage for childbirth. During labor your pelvis stretches to accommodate your baby, and your baby twists and turns to navigate through the pelvis. Being familiar with how your pelvis moves will help you be prepared to work with your baby during labor.

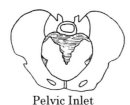
Pelvic Inlet

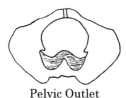
Pelvic Outlet

The internal pelvic structure is similar to a funnel; it starts out wide but narrows near the pubic bone. It is not one solid bone, there are joints that loosen and expand during labor to make more room for your baby. If you put your hands on your hips, you can feel your illiac bones. You can follow the rim of these bones down the front to your pubic bone, which is very low between your legs. The symphisis pubis is the connective tissue between the two halves of the pubic bone that allows it to stretch during labor.

With your hands back up on your illiac bones, you can follow the rim down towards the back to your sacrum (the base of your backbone). The iliac bones are connected to the sacrum in a way that allows them to expand and also to pivot and tilt, making more room for baby. When your torso is bent forward, such as when you squat or kneel, the sacrum tilts in a way that opens the pelvic outlet wider. When your torso is leaning backwards, such as when you are reclining, the sacrum tilts in a way that closes the pelvic outlet reducing the room for baby.

Your goal in labor is to choose positions that promote the expansion of the pelvis. This gives the baby the most room possible to turn and find the way through the pelvic funnel.

Upright Positions

When you keep your body upright during labor, you allow gravity to increase the intensity of the contractions naturally. Interestingly, many women find that being upright also makes them more comfortable during contractions, increasing their ability to cope. When you add pelvic movement such as swaying your hips or walking with an upright position, you create the optimum environment for your baby to navigate through the pelvis.

There are a wide variety of positions which qualify as upright. Early in labor when you have more energy and the contractions demand little of your attention, walking may be very easy and comfortable. As you move into a more active labor or have been laboring for a while, you may find yourself more comfortable leaning on a wall or support person, swaying your hips or slow dancing through contractions. If you want to stay upright, but are getting tired, you might try leaning over a chair or counter, or letting your labor partners support your weight as they hold you up during contractions.

Upright positions not only allow your body to work the most effectively, but also they allow your mind and heart to labor most effectively. Being upright helps you feel healthy, strong and confident. Upright positions make it easy to respond to the cues your body is sending, helping you to feel more successful at working with your labor. Remember, though, to keep your body loose, not stiff, in upright positions. Allow your companions to help support your weight if necessary, and use a wall or chair to lean on during contractions when needed.

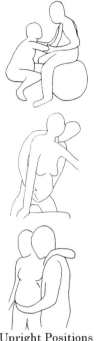
Upright Positions

Kneeling Positions

When you kneel on hands an knees during labor, you take pressure off your pelvic floor. Removing the pull of gravity may help your baby to rotate and can help relieve pressure on your lower back. One of the greatest benefits of kneeling positions is your ability to maintain movement of your hips while you rest. Kneeling positions are associated with prayer and the humility of submitting yourself to God's will. Using kneeling positions may help you let go of the control of your labor and focus on what you can do to work with God.

Kneeling on hands and knees can become tiring very quickly in labor. You might find kneeling so you lean over a chair, birth ball, side of a tub or over a bed allows you to relax your upper body and removes some of the weight your lower body has to support. Some objects, such as a birth ball or rocking chair, allow you to rest in a kneeling position while maintaining mobility.

A unique aspect of kneeling is your ability to kneel in a way that puts your head lower than your hips. This

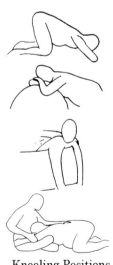
Kneeling Positions

reversing of gravity can be helpful if your baby seems unable to rotate into a better position. Gravity may pull your baby down towards the top of the uterus and off your pelvic bones to make just enough room for baby to move.

Sitting Positions

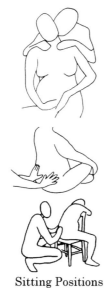

Sitting Positions

When you sit, you are able to maintain an upright position while you rest your legs. You can sit in a chair or even cross-legged on the floor. Using a rocking chair or birth ball to sit on gives you the ability to maintain pelvic movement while you rest. Some women find they prefer to sit backwards on a chair, resting their upper body on a pillow propped against the back of the chair. This allows complete rest for you and gives your labor partners full access to your lower back for massage.

One of the more unusual but comfortable sitting positions is to sit backwards on your toilet, resting your head on a pillow on the tank. Sitting in this way removes upward pressure on your pelvic floor. The coolness of the porcelain is comfortable as your body heats up during labor. Sitting on the toilet may help you feel more comfortable if your bag of waters is leaking, allowing the water to fall into the toilet instead of being held next to your body.

Reclining Positions

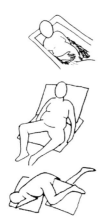

Reclining Positions

When labor is overwhelming or has been active for a long time, you may find a reclining position gives you the ability to rest and relax your entire body. While reclining positions can be helpful at some points in labor, they remove your ability to move your pelvis and the effect of gravity, which can lead to a longer or less effective labor. For that reason, reclining positions should only be used when necessary and for only a short while.

While reclining, use pillows to prop your body to remove the stress from every muscle. If you choose to lie down, lie on your side with pillows under your upper leg, under any unsupported parts of your belly and under your head and arms if that feels comfortable to you.

Some women feel more comfortable if they lean back on their husbands, or have their husbands beside them while they recline in labor. Reclining with someone makes the experience of reclining more relaxing and less like you are sick or helpless. Some women find reclining positions make them feel vulnerable or childlike, putting themselves in a position that makes everyone look down on them.

The one reclining position to avoid is lying on your back. In this position your sacrum will be tilted in a way that makes the pelvic opening smaller, your baby's weight will be pressing on your sacrum and your uterus will have to push against gravity to contract. Not only is it ineffective to labor on your back, women rate lying on their back as the most uncomfortable position to labor in. How beautiful that God has created us in a way that makes the most effective labor positions also the most comfortable.

Positioning with a Hospital Bed

If you decide to labor in a hospital, you can use the adjustable bed to assist you in using a variety of positions for labor.

Put the side bars up and raise the bed as high as necessary to allow you to hold onto the bar for a supported squat.

Place a birth ball on the end of the bed, then raise the bed to a height that allows you to comfortably lean onto the ball while standing.

Position the head of the bed so it is almost vertical, then kneel on the soft part of the bed while supporting your upper body by the head of the bed in a supported hands and knees position.

Raise the bed as high as possible while a labor helper sits on the side. Position yourself between his legs with your arms supported by his upper thighs for a supported dangle.

Choosing Positions

The positions you choose to labor in should be selected based first on what is the most comfortable for you. It is your body, and you are the only person receiving signals

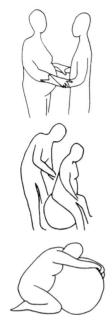

As labor progresses, you may prefer positions that allow you to rest more of your body.

from your baby about what he needs to be born. Learn to pay attention to that still, small voice that lets you know when your body needs to move and how it needs to move.

Use upright positions as much as possible, either standing or sitting. This helps ensure your labor is the most effective. During labor you will want to change your position at least every hour to be sure you are giving your baby opportunity to move and navigate through your pelvis. This change can be small, such as moving from sitting on the floor to sitting on a birth ball; or it can be larger such as moving from walking to kneeling over a chair.

Though you should change position regularly, remember to pay attention to your body. The point is not to force labor to move more quickly than it should. Instead, the point is to work with your body to allow it to labor as effectively as possible.

Some women experience a fear of changing position in labor. They believe it will hurt to change positions, or they do not have the strength to move. Changing positions should feel good, giving you the opportunity to shift your weight and adjust pressure points. Changing positions also allows you to respond to the changes in baby's position, helping relieve some of the internal pressure. Allow your labor partners to help you as you try new positions by supporting your weight or guiding you safely in position changes through contractions. It may take you two or three tries to find the next right position, but you will find it.

Pushing Positions

The most efficient pushing positions are squatting positions. When you squat, the outlet of your pelvis is expanded, the coccyx bone is tilted out of the way of your baby and your perineal skin has the greatest probability of remaining intact during crowning.

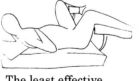

The least effective pushing position is lying on your back.

Overall, upright positions such as squatting reduce the length of the second stage of labor while decreasing the chance you will experience severe pain. Upright positions also decrease the likelihood your baby will have abnormal heart tones during the second stage. There are a variety of ways to stay upright while pushing.

Positions for Labor

If you are flexible enough, you can simply squat on the floor over a clean blanket or towel. Most women in developed countries are not accustomed to squatting and will find squat positions more comfortable with some form of support. You can support yourself in a squat with any stable object, such as a counter, railing or even another person. In the hospital, beds are equipped with bars that allow you to squat on the bed, or on the floor if you lower the bed enough to reach the bar while squatting.

You may prefer using a birth stool to remain upright for pushing. A birth stool is a horseshoe shaped low stool that supports your weight in an almost squat position. The opening in the center provides room for your baby to be born.

Dangling is an upright position that allows your weight to be supported by someone else. You can "dangle" by wrapping your hands around your helpers shoulders and neck, while your helper supports under your arms. Another version of the dangle is for your helper to sit on a counter or high bed so you can rest your arms on his legs and let your weight go.

If upright positions are not comfortable for a time during pushing, you can try some positions that are gravity neutral, which means you are not working with or against gravity. Hands and knees position is gravity neutral and very comfortable for women who have persistant backaches during labor. Another gravity neutral position is lying on your side.

The most common pushing positions in hospitals are lying on the back or semi-reclining. According to the Listening to Mothers II Survey, almost six out of ten women who give birth vaginally in the United States pushed while lying on their backs. Another three out of ten used a semi-reclining position.

There are very real disadvantages to pushing while lying on your back. For example, while lying on your back the weight of your body and your baby press on the coccyx and prevents the small end of your tailbone from flexing out of the way for your baby. While lying on your back you are pushing your baby uphill, against the pull of gravity. This may be a major reason why women who push while lying on their backs are more likely to have vacuum extraction to assist pushing.

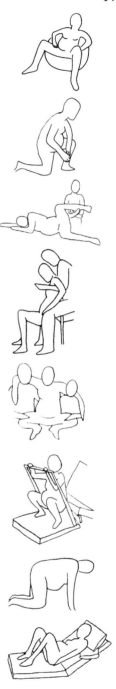

Pushing Positions

Movement in Labor

One of the goals of normal labor is to keep the momentum of the labor going. You want the contractions to continue to strengthen while the cervix continues to dilate so your baby can be born. One of the best ways to maintain that momentum is to keep moving.

Movement in labor does two things. First, it keeps your pelvis moving allowing your baby to find the easiest way through. It is not a straight shot through the pelvis, your baby must twist and turn several times to navigate what equates to an oval on one end and a diamond on the other. Movement helps by keeping the pelvis adjusting around the baby so he can find the best position. This can keep labor progressing as efficiently as possible. The second thing movement does is reduce the amount of pain you feel.

The types of movement most helpful are swaying and rocking that move the hips. This means you will be moving your legs and torso. Some of these movements will come easily to you; others may seem very strange or require practice. Unless you are a dancer, chances are you have not spent much time gaining control of your pelvis. Practicing these moves during pregnancy can help you feel more comfortable now and be useful in labor.

Walking

You do not need to do anything special to move during labor; just walking will help to adjust your baby in your pelvis. If you feel up to it, and baby seems to need help getting into a good position, walk up and down stairs. Some women swear by walking up two stairs at a time to help turn their babies who are putting pressure on their backs.

Rocking

Rocking your hips back and forth or side to side is the easiest pelvic movement to control. It can be done while standing, kneeling or leaning over something. You can even do it while sitting on a birth ball. If you have good control you can do some pelvic rocking while sitting in a chair or lying on your side, although it may be harder to learn this way. You may find rocking your torso or moving your legs is easier than rocking your pelvis when you are in a sitting position.

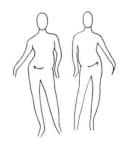

Swaying

Swaying is a side to side hip rocking that includes your whole body. It can help you feel loose and relaxed as you slowly walk or lean over. Some women really enjoy swaying during labor because it feels like slow dancing, especially when you are supported by a husband who sways with you.

Pelvic Circles

If you can rock your pelvis from side to side and back and forth you can do a pelvic circle. While standing, begin by rocking your pelvis to one side, then bringing it forward, over to the other side and then pushing it out behind you. Continue the circular motion for several revolutions as long as it feels good. Once you can control the motion, you can do it while kneeling on hands and knees, sitting on a ball or any other position that gives you freedom of movement.

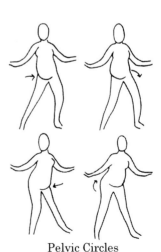

Pelvic Circles

Figure Eights

The most challenging pelvic movement is the figure eight. Similar to pelvic circles, the figure eight requires you to use all four directions of your pelvic movement, but instead of circling you move as if you were drawing the number '8' with your tailbone. While standing, begin by rocking your pelvis to one side, circle to the front and then push your pelvis straight to the back. Circle around to the other side and over to the front, then push your pelvis straight back again. Continue the movement alternating sides.

Hip Circles

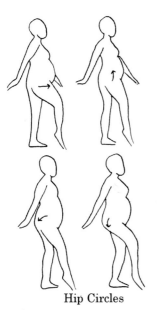

Hip Circles

If you cannot walk, you can alternate hip circles while leaning over a counter or onto a wall to simulate the pelvic movements of walking. While leaning over an object, try to bring only one hip up as high as it will go, circle it around to the back and then down as low as it will go before circling around to the front and up to the top again.

Hip Eights

Hip eights require less full body movement than a figure eight and move your pelvis in an asymmetrical way, but it can be difficult to learn. Choose one side to begin with, and bring your hip as far forward as it will come. Circle your hip up and to the middle, then drop it straight down as low as it will go. Circle around to the other side and back up to the top where you will drop it straight down again. Continue the movement as long as it is comfortable.

Practice these pelvic movements as often as possible to gain full control over your pelvis. In labor, choose the movement that feels the most comfortable at the time. What feels comfortable will change as your baby moves further into your pelvis and you become more tired, so do not be afraid to try a different movement that might not have felt right earlier. If you like, practice your pelvic floor exercises at the same time you practice your pelvic movements. Try contracting the pelvic floor muscle and hold it for five, ten or fifteen pelvic circles depending on how fast you go.

Using Water in Labor

Water is widely available, highly versatile and can be extremely effective at helping you stay comfortable during labor. The question to ask is not if you will use water in labor, but how you will use water during labor. You can shower, relax in a bath, use warm or cool compresses, mist yourself with cool water, place ice on your back and of course—drink it.

Laboring in Water

During labor, you may have the option to use a tub or shower. Either is fine depending on your preferences. Both can be warm and relaxing, helping you to let go of tension. Both can provide you with a change of scenery which can help you overcome some of the fatigue and monotony during labor. Both the shower and tub provide you with a variety of positions to labor in, expanding your repertoire of comfortable positions.

Most women think of soaking in a tub as a relaxing activity. The association with relaxation can help you let go when you submerge yourself. A tub has the added benefit of buoyancy, which means the water helps disperse your weight so it takes some of the pressure off your body. The warm water on your skin feels comforting by itself, and if jets are available they can be used to add a massage feeling to the tub.

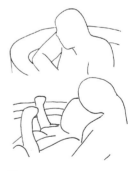

You can use many positions while laboring in water.

The steady noise of a shower can be comforting while it drowns out the rest of the world, helping you to relax and let labor take its course. A shower has the added benefit of being able to position the streams of water on your lower back or belly for a massage. The streams of water can be aimed at your breasts to help stimulate stronger contractions. Showers also encourage you to stay upright, which may help labor progress.

Only 6 percent of the respondents from Listening to Mothers II survey reported using immersion in a tub or pool during labor. This is unfortunate since nine out of ten mothers who used it found it at least somewhat helpful which is the same number who found epidural at least somewhat helpful. Almost half said it was very helpful for managing labor. Only 4 percent reported using the shower, but of those who did nearly eight out of ten found it at least somewhat helpful. If you are interested in laboring in water, here are some things to think about:

1. Your decision to use the shower or tub may be based on what is available at your birth place. If you have the option between the two, choose the one which appeals to you most. Do you prefer showers or do you feel more comfortable in a warm tub? Both have tremendous benefits during labor, and if you decide it is not working as well as you liked, you can always try something different.

2. Keep the water warm but not hot. Some midwives recommend having the water at or just above body temperature. If you are home without a thermometer, simply select water that feels comfortably warm. Closing the door to the room will help keep the heat in, avoiding the problem of having warm water and a cold body out of the water.

3. Consider how much privacy you will or will not have, and what you can do to be more comfortable in that situation. If you will be at home you may be comfortable in the tub naked. Some women feel exposed being naked in a tub with helpers around. If modesty will be an issue for you, wear a piece of clothing such as a tank top or sports bra. You can also use a warm, wet hand towel to place over your breasts. This will keep you covered and keep your body warm.

4. Make sure the tub you use is deep enough to completely cover your belly. If your tub will not do that, rent or purchase one that will. You can find labor tub rentals on the Internet, and the doula or midwife you rent from can give you instructions on the best use. Some mothers purchase a blow-up toddler pool with large enough sides. Some midwives prefer large plastic troughs or crates, which have the dual benefit of firm sides and an oval shape.

5. Do not forget position changes; they can still work to keep you comfortable in the tub or shower. If you are in the tub for longer than half an hour, be sure to rotate your body so you are in a different position. Alternately, you can think of water as one of your positions, rotating between walking, kneeling and the shower or tub.

6. Use props such as shower chairs, low plastic stools, or other items to help you find the most comfortable position. Make sure what you choose can hold your weight.

Giving Birth in Water

If you find the water is very relaxing and comfortable, you do not have to get out of the tub to give birth. Water birth is a gentle way for your baby to enter the world. You will continue to have the benefits of the comfort of the water, and many midwives find there is less risk of perineal tearing as your baby is born.

If you would like a water birth, find a birth attendant who is comfortable catching a baby underwater. Not every attendant is familiar with the way things will look underwater or the research about the safety of underwater birth. Rather than trying to convince a doctor or midwife who is skeptical, find someone else who has been trained to attend water births.

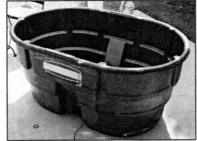
© 2007 Lori Luyten

> Midwife Lori Luyten finds a plastic trough works great for water labor and birth. The firm sides and oval shape give support for a variety of positions. Because it is plastic, it is lightweight and portable and will not break, rip or pop while in use. She simply covers the trough with a heavy plastic liner before filling to keep clean-up easier. Towels placed under the plastic can help create cushioning for comfort.

Giving birth underwater helps you meet the goal of a comfortable and safe birth—it is not the goal in itself. If you do not like being in the water, get out and try something else. Some mothers who plan to give birth underwater give birth on land for a variety of reasons—either they ended up feeling more comfortable out of the water, felt better pushing out of the water or they did not have time to get in the tub. You cannot know before labor begins what will feel the best for you when you are pushing, so be open to trying many positions both in and out of the tub.

Will a tub or shower be available at your birth place?

Staying hydrated

Of course you will need to stay hydrated, so make sure you drink enough water. Taking a sip between each contraction can help. You could suck on ice chips which can also give you a place to focus during contractions. Juice or a sports drink can be available if you want them, or you can just drink plain water. You can add lemon or other flavors if you enjoy flavored water.

What types of drinks appeal to you?

Some women prefer to drink tea or a broth so they accomplish more than just hydrating themselves. Some teas, such as red raspberry leaf, are especially good during labor because of the way they help strengthen the uterus. Broth can give you some added calories for extra energy without making you feel full. Some midwives have special recipes for labor drinks.

Just be sure with all the drinking you will be doing to empty your bladder at least once an hour. There will be many sensations coming from your pelvis, and you may not be able to tell that a full bladder is the reason the contractions are getting so much harder to handle. Avoid the added discomfort of a full bladder by going to the bathroom often.

Using Ice

Because water freezes so easily and can hold the cold for extended amounts of time, it makes perfect cold compresses. You can use the traditional ice pack, or put ice water in a hot water bottle. The coldness of the ice pack can help to remove the pain of the lower back. Be aware the cold therapy may only work for 15-20 minutes at a time. This means you will cycle through cold compresses and other comfort tools coming back to the cold after an hour or so.

You can make your own ice pack by freezing a plastic water bottle two thirds of the way full of water. Take it out of the freezer, fill any remaining space with water and put the cap back on. Using a water bottle as a massage tool, have a partner roll it around on your lower back. Use as much pressure as necessary. When the ice is nearly gone, you can drink the cold water.

> What ways do you use to cool yourself when you feel too warm?

You can also put a few ice cubes in a zippered freezer bag. Be sure it is sealed tight and wrap it with a hand towel. You can use the ice pack to put pressure on the lower back. You can also use some crushed ice wrapped in a cloth to do a pressure massage on the skin between your thumb and forefinger during contractions.

If you are feeling hot and sticky during labor, you may find cool cloths on your face or neck comforting. Have a helper put some ice in a bowl and fill the bowl with water. Completely soak a washcloth, small hand towel or bandana and then wring it out. You can wrap it loosely around your neck, or have someone use it to cool your face. Another way to keep cool at a hot labor is to put ice water in a spray bottle that has a mist setting. Spray your face and neck as needed.

Using Warm Water

Early in labor, you may enjoy soaking your feet in warm water. This can help you relax and can be especially helpful if your goal is to get some sleep before contractions demand your attention. You may enjoy having someone massage your feet with lotion or oils as you soak them.

> What ways do you use warm water to relax?

Just as ice water makes cool compresses, hot water will make warm compresses. Wet a thick wash cloth and wring it out. You can then have a companion hold it while using pressure on your back. You can roll it up and place it under your belly to provide comfort to your pubic bone. Some women find using a warm cloth to wash their faces is helpful. While pushing, your midwife may use warm compresses to help support your perineum.

Sterile Water Injections

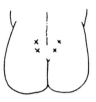

If you experience back pain during labor, you may choose injections of sterile water to help you overcome that pain. Injecting 4 papules of sterile water directly under the skin significantly decreases or removes the back pain without any negative side effects.

Mothers who have tried this technique say the injections feel like a bee sting for about a minute, then the pain disappears. Because there is discomfort during the injections, some midwives recommend you not use this technique unless you are no longer able to handle the back pain. Some midwives administer the injections during a contraction so you would be less likely to notice the sting.

Water in the Bible

One of the added benefits of using water for labor is how the water can remind you to focus on God. There are a variety of references to water in the Bible, and depending on your circumstances any of them might be helpful as you labor. Let the water draw your focus back onto the power of God and the Holy Spirit. There is no right or wrong here; choose the uses that are most meaningful to where you are in life.

Matthew 3:13-17

Exodus 30:17-21

Is God teaching you to lay down your life? Then think of the waters of baptism which give us a picture of death and resurrection. Is God preparing you for the next stage of life? Then meditate on the ceremonial washing of the priests which must be done before they can move on to the next step of worship.

Exodus 7:14-24
John 2:1-11
Zechaiah 14:8
Jon 4:10
Exodus 14
Joshua 3

Has God blessed you beyond your wildest dreams? Then meditate on the water miracles. God turned water into blood as part of the ten plagues used to free the Israelites. Jesus turned water into wine. Are you learning to follow God's lead and letting him perform miracles in your life? Then meditate on the parting of the Red Sea and the Jordon river.

All these references of water from scripture are applicable to all parts of life, including giving birth. In this way, the water you use in labor not only gives you physical comfort, but spiritual comfort as well.

Relaxation for Labor

For many women, relaxation holds the key to coping well with labor. Staying calm and relaxed helps prevent the fear tension pain cycle (important for preventing pain) and can help you to stay confident (important for coping with labor). The relaxation that is beneficial in labor is not just plopping on the couch to watch a movie. The art of relaxation takes time and practice to master for successful use.

When talking about relaxation for labor, it is helpful to differentiate between the physical relaxation and the emotional/spiritual relaxation. Because humans are both physical and spiritual beings, how you feel about what is happening has as much effect on your labor experience as the physical process of labor. To be effective, you must learn to relax your body, mind and spirit.

The techniques in this section can help you keep your muscles relaxed, focus your thoughts and give you the appearance of being calm. However, these techniques are not a substitute for faith in God or his creation. No matter how well you learn to control your breathing, if you lack the faith or have been struggling to trust God, it will affect your labor. The most successful use of these techniques is in combination with the faith you have already strengthened before labor begins.

The biggest trick to labor relaxation is learning what type is most useful for you. Some women are highly distractible and find the mental techniques difficult to learn, but very beneficial during labor. Other women

> What type of relaxation is the most difficult for you?

experience stress and tension first in their backs or shoulders and need to work to learn ways to master relaxation of specific body parts. Understanding who you are and what parts of your body are in the most need of help to relax will help you be more effective at coping with labor.

Abdominal Breathing

The first relaxation technique to learn is abdominal breathing, using your diaphragm to breathe instead of your chest. Abdominal breathing uses less energy while bringing in more oxygen than chest breathing. The slower, deliberate movements and attention needed to breathe abdominally can help to calm you down and regain focus. In pregnancy and labor every breath you take must fill the needs of two lives, not just one, making abdominal breathing the optimal way to meet the need.

To learn abdominal breathing, place yourself in a comfortable position. If a helper will be assisting you, make sure you are positioned to allow your belly to be seen. Begin by taking a deep breath in and out, paying attention to the way your body moves with your breath. As you inhale, you want your stomach to become larger or rise, exhaling will cause your stomach to look smaller or return to normal. If your shoulders rise and fall, you are using your chest muscles. Placing a hand on your belly may make it easier to focus your energy properly.

It may take considerable effort to breathe abdominally when you first learn. Many women unknowingly train themselves not to breathe abdominally to keep their stomach looking as small as possible, and this can be hard to unlearn. Take your time, starting with 30 seconds and build up to longer amounts of time. Eventually, you should find yourself easily taking deep abdominal breaths throughout the day.

> Genesis 2:7
> Revelation 11:11
> Isaiah 57:16
> Ezekiel 37:4-10
> John 20:22

In the Bible, breathing and breath are synonymous with life. Breath is also related to the Holy Spirit and the spirit of humans. Human life is dependent on breathing, though you may live a week without food or a few days without water, you can only live a few minutes without a breath. Abdominal breathing is an exercise that can be used as active prayer during labor, focusing not only on the process, but the significance of the breath of life.

Meditation

Once you have mastered abdominal breathing, you can incorporate meditation into your relaxation. God calls his people to meditate on his Word. Among the wonderful benefits of meditation is the way it stretches your concentration. During labor, it can be easy to be distracted. The art of meditation helps prevent you from being distracted, keeping your attention focused on the work you are doing. Meditation can also be used as a form of prayer during labor, reminding you of the presence and strength of God

A list of verses for meditation can be found in Appendix 8.

Depending on how God created your mind, you may find you think in audible words or pictures. If you think in audible words, you can meditate by reciting phrases, verses or songs to yourself slowly, focusing on each word. If you think in pictures, you can visualize what is happening during a passage of scripture or focus on the work of your body during labor.

The simplest way to add meditation would be to use abdominal breathing as a focal point to meditate on the Holy Spirit. The Holy Spirit is called our counselor, praying for us when we have not words. Meditate on the scriptures that describe the breath of life. Allow the rhythm of your breathing to guide you through thoughts or mental images of the Spirit with you, strengthening you and interceding for you during labor.

John 16:7
Romans 8:26

Once you gain the concentration needed to begin meditating, you can create a repertoire of meditative thoughts or images for labor. Choose verses or phrases that are calming, strengthening and encouraging for you. Learn to pray as you meditate, preventing yourself from being "stuck." The idea of meditation is not to be mindless, but to be mindful, focusing your mental energy on understanding. As you pray over and meditate on your focus, the image or thought may begin to change as God begins to speak to you.

Some women find meditating on their bodies and the work they are doing to be helpful. Phrases such as "open," or visualizing the stretching and opening going on inside can help you stay connected to the work each contraction is doing. Other women will use meditation to imagine themselves somewhere else such as in a garden, on a beach or sitting at Jesus' feet. They either distract themselves from the pressure of contractions or build the contraction into their mental image–such as by imagining contractions as waves of the ocean. If this type of meditation works well for you, you may try imagining yourself in a boat with Jesus tossed about by the waves.

As labor progresses, it can become more and more difficult to be successful at meditation. It can be helpful to write out verses you personally find encouraging and having them available when labor demands too much attention for you to remember the verses you chose. If it becomes too much work to focus on a thought, try listening to music, focusing on the words or notes. You might also try focusing on someone who is speaking or reading to you.

Write the verses you find most helpful on note cards for easy reference during labor.

Physical Relaxation

While other techniques keep your mind focused during labor, physical relaxation is designed to keep your body loose and limp. If you are not familiar with the difference between your body tensed and relaxed, try tensing one muscle, such as your upper thigh, and then releasing it. If necessary, tense and relax every muscle in your body one at a time to learn what it feels like to relax. Once you learn the feeling, you will not need to tense and release before relaxing.

To begin, learn to relax your body one muscle or muscle group at a time. Start with your feet and move up the body. After you are able to relax every muscle, go back and try again but this time keeping the relaxation as you move up the body. For example, you will relax your feet and ankles and while they are still relaxed move up the calves. If you notice any part of your body has become tense after it was relaxed, go back and start again.

After you are able to keep the whole body relaxed, begin training yourself to relax the whole body at one time. Some women are very successful with using a touch or word cue to help remind them to relax completely. The idea is to condition yourself to respond to the touch or word by relaxing. A similar idea is to teach yourself to relax the part of your body being touched.

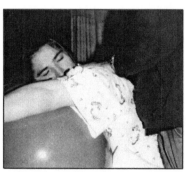
©2002 Jennifer Vanderlaan
Comfortable positions and backrubs can help keep you physically relaxed in labor.

Comforting Environment

You can have peace in any situation and any environment. This is because the environment does not determine the spirit; the Spirit is in control of the environment. But that does not change the fact that humans are sensory beings. You can have peace in the lion's den, but the lion's den is not a peaceful place.

You see, hear, taste, touch and smell your world every minute of your life. As a sensory being, the environment plays a role in determining how comfortable and relaxed you are. You use the information collected by your senses to help understand what is happening and how to react to it. It is an amazing system God created which gives you the ability to avoid many forms of danger. In labor, your senses can either help you or hinder you.

If you give birth at home, everything surrounding you will be familiar and comforting. You know the sounds and smells of your home. You know the touch of your favorite blanket and the sight of your things. This sensory input helps you to feel comfortable and relaxed, safe.

If you give birth in a hospital, everything surrounding you will be new and unfamiliar. Your senses will be gathering information constantly. The smells and sounds of the hospital are not comforting, they are distracting. Though many hospitals have decorated their birth rooms with pretty wallpaper, you will still see medical equipment instead of the comforts of home. All this sensory input can make you feel tense or stressed, hindering your labor.

How much work it takes for you to feel comfortable with birth depends on who you are and where you give birth. God has made each of us unique, and you are the only one who knows how distracting sights, sounds or smells are to you. Therefore, you are the only one who knows which of the environmental comfort techniques are right for your labor.

What are the unique challenges at the birth place you have chosen?

Sight

Your home is probably a comforting sight to you. There are times in life when clutter from life may overtake some of your living space, causing frustration or distress. Focus on making sure you have one room in which you can relax and allow labor to happen rather than trying to redesign your entire home in your last month of pregnancy.

If you want to be surrounded by familiar sights in the hospital or birth center, select a few important things to take with you. You might want a favorite pillow or a picture of loved ones. You may want flowers or something else that looks pretty. It all depends on who you are.

The medical equipment at a hospital can be distracting. Most times the bed is right in the middle of the room with the monitoring equipment right beside it. This blocks your walkway and gives you an unsightly view. The good news is the beds and equipment are on wheels. Ask your nurse to help you push them out of the way, you can always move them back if you decide you want or need them later.

Closing your eyes may help you focus on prayer or meditation.

Regardless of where the birth takes place, some mothers find they do best if they close their eyes during contractions. A great way to labor is in a semi-sleep state in which your eyes are closed and you seem to be focusing somewhere other than the room you are in. If you are really having a difficult time shutting out the busy sights of a labor room, you could try closing your eyes or having a companion place a cloth over your eyes to obstruct your view for a few contractions.

If you find it easier to keep your eyes open, but want somewhere to focus, you can prepare focus objects. Set out a baby blanket or a piece of clothing as a reminder for why you are working so hard. Write out a few verses you find particularly helpful and place them around the room. Let your older children draw pictures that you can look at while in labor. The idea is to select things that are meaningful to you and will help you to feel comfortable.

Sound

Hospitals are busy places with lots of sounds going on. Closing the door to the room you are using will help cut out most of the hallway chatter and intercom talk that goes on at the nursing station. If you decide to use medical equipment that makes noise, ask to have the volume turned down as low as possible to keep distractions to a minimum.

Sometimes your home might be louder than you like. If you are comfortable with the normal sounds of daily life in your home, fine. If you think you might be distracted by the normal sounds of your home, then plan a way to keep the children quiet; television and radio off; telephone from ringing; dog from barking; and any other noise that may become irritating during active labor.

Music is a great way to block other sounds wherever you labor. Some women make a CD or two just for listening to in labor. Select the music that helps you relax, not the music other people tell you is right for relaxing. One woman, a skilled classical musician, said classical music was too complicated to listen to in labor. Instead, she chose folk tunes. Another woman worked at a spa, so to listen to the standard relaxation music made her feel as if she was at work. Instead, she chose rock music. Select your labor music based on your preferences.

If you prefer quieter sounds, you could listen to a book on CD or have someone read to you. Some mothers prefer the white noise of a fan or noise machine. Having someone talk to you can be equally reassuring. If the room you are using has windows that open, see if the sounds of the wind or the birds helps you feel more at ease.

When labor becomes very intense, many mothers make their own noise by moaning. This can be a helpful way to let out excess tension and help you to cope with contractions. Try to avoid screaming sounds, as these can trigger fear and stress. Moaning sounds are made from a relaxed throat, while screaming sounds are made from a tense throat and jaw. If you find your tone becoming more of a scream, just open your mouth wide to help you move into a deeper moan sound. You may find just breathing heavy gives you enough background noise.

What will you need to feel comfortable making your own noise?

Smell

While your home smells just right to you, hospitals have a unique cleaning product smell. Even the pillows and sheets smell funny. You can work around this by bringing a few things from home. Bring your favorite pillow. It will smell like home and you can use it to help yourself stay comfortable in almost every position. Keeping your own clothes on can help keep familiar smells near your body as well.

Some women enjoy using aromatherapy oils during labor. Choose a scent that makes you feel comfortable and find a way to incorporate it into the room you are using. You might place a few drops into a bath or a bowl of cool water you will use for compresses. You might scent a tissue and leave it near you. You could add a drop of lavender to a bowl of cool water you are using to make cool compresses for your face, neck or lower back.

How sensitive are you to smells?

Be aware of how smells affect you. Most women find their sense of smell is heightened during pregnancy and heightened even more during labor. Lotions that smelled good before may be nauseating in active labor. Choose lotions or massage oils that are odorless or have very little scent so they do not overpower you. You might also want to avoid products that have food smells. Most women loose their appetite during labor, and the smell of food could make you feel sick to your stomach. If you are particularly sensitive to smell, it might be a good idea to select a few scented items so you are prepared in case you do not tolerate one of them well in labor.

Taste

You may be hungry in early labor. If you are, be sure to eat light foods you enjoy. Most women lose their desire for food during active labor but will still need to stay hydrated. If the taste of unfamiliar waters makes it difficult for you to drink, be sure to bring along plenty of your favorite bottled water. You could just fill water bottles with water from your home if you prefer that taste.

> What policies at your birth place may limit your food choices?

Some women feel better in labor if they drink something other than water. Be aware that as you progress in labor, you may prefer to have your drink watered down more and more as your sense of taste increases and the flavor feels stronger. If you want a warm drink, think tea or broth. If you want a cool drink, think juice.

Another common taste technique for labor is to suck on hard candies or eat frozen grapes. This gives you a bit of sugar for energy and surrounds you with a flavor and scent you enjoy without overfilling your stomach. You may also like licking honey off a spoon or sucking on a popsicle for the same reason. You may find brushing your teeth or rinsing with mouthwash helps your mouth taste more comfortable.

Touch

Your sense of touch is not just about what you put your fingers on, but what touches your body. In labor this will not only be the furniture you sit on and clothes you wear, but also the hands and any equipment that comes in contact with your skin.

> Mix three drops each aniseed, nutmeg and peppermint with eight drops of lavender into two ounces of oil to make a massage oil that can help ease labor pain while helping labor progress.

Choose a comfortable T-shirt or nightgown to wear in labor. You can purchase something specific for the event, knowing you will just throw it away if necessary. If you get any blood on the gown, you can wash it out with stain remover or peroxide.

You may prefer your favorite pillow and blanket, which will feel especially good if you labor in an unfamiliar and uncomfortable hospital bed or choose positions on the floor or a chair. Some women buy a soft pair of socks or slip on sandals for walking around in. Stroking a velvety blanket or stuffed toy can give you a tactile stimulation that helps you focus.

You should know your skin well. Pay attention to how much lotion or oil you will need to be comfortable during a backrub or having your feet massaged. Think also about how your body feels in enclosed buildings with air conditioning. Would you feel better if you had a fan or opened a window? Change the room temperature if necessary. Generally women prefer it cooler during labor because of the body heat generated.

Think also about the medical equipment available to you at a hospital and how much it will take to feel comfortable if you use it. If you have an external monitor belted to your belly or an IV in your arm, how much is that likely to distract you during labor? Will using a different position, such as sitting in a rocking chair or standing near the equipment, help make you more comfortable?

Favorite Labour Aide:

Juice of a lemon or lime
Active Manuka Honey
Glucose powder
1-2 calcium tablets
Pinch of sea salt
Pinch of baking soda
Add water until it tastes right
Lovely to sip on icy cold throughout labour.

Julie Bell

Meditations on the Holy Spirit

The following questions are given to help you begin meditating—focusing your thoughts on a topic—about the Holy Spirit. You can meditate on these topics whether your thoughts are mostly sounds, images or feelings.

Filled with the Spirit

"When Elizabeth heard Mary's greeting, the baby leaped in her womb, and Elizabeth was filled with the Holy Spirit." What does it feel like to be filled with the Holy Spirit? Can you recall the way your body feels? Is it light or heavy? Do you feel more alive, more alert, more peaceful? If you have never felt the presence of the Holy Spirit, what do you imagine Elizabeth felt like? How did she know she was filled with the Holy Spirit?   Luke 1:41

Led by the Spirit

"Jesus, full of the Holy Spirit, returned from the Jordan and was led by the Spirit in the desert, where for forty days he was tempted by the devil." Have you ever been led by the Spirit? How do you know it is the Spirit? How do you respond when you are being led by the Spirit? Can you sense the leading in others? How different do you feel when you follow the Spirit compared to when you choose not to follow the Spirit?   Luke 4:1

Baptized by the Spirit

"For John baptized with water, but in a few days you will be baptized with the Holy Spirit." Baptism brings to mind very clear images of immersion in water. But what comes to mind when you think of baptism with the Spirit? What are you immersed in? What surrounds you? You know what it feels like to be immersed in water, what does it feel like to be immersed in the Holy Spirit?   Acts 1:5

Power of the Spirit

"May the God of hope fill you with all joy and peace as you trust in him, so that you may overflow with hope by the power of the Holy Spirit." The Holy Spirit has the power to fill you with hope. What other powers does the Holy Spirit have? What does it feel like when your hope is overflowing? What does it take to be filled with joy and peace?   Romans 15:13

Drawing Conclusions
Review of Section Six

Staying Comfortable

Spend some time trying each of the different comfort measures discussed in this section. Make notes about how successful each of the comfort measures are for you, and when you might find them helpful during labor.

	Early Labor	Active Labor	Pushing	At Home	At Hospital	With helpers	While Alone
Touch							
Massage							
Pressure							
Upright Positions							
Kneeling Positions							
Sitting Positions							
Reclining Positions							
Movement							
Tub or Shower							
Ice or Warm Water							
Relaxation							
Abdominal Breathing							
Meditation							
Physical Relaxation							
Closing Eyes							
Music/Sound							
Aromatherapy							
Cool Drinks							
Hard Candies							

Labor Stories

You can learn a lot from a labor story. Take some time to find two or three stories from a book, website or even a friend. After reading the stories, ask yourself the following questions:

- How were comfort measures used successfully?
- What other comfort measures might have been helpful?
- Which comfort measures did not work in this labor?

In Your Birth Bag

How might you use the following items to stay comfortable during labor? What other items could you use for comfort?

Birth ball
Hot sock
Massage oil and Massage tools
Cold pack
Gloves
Relaxing CDs or tapes
Portable tape player
Aromatherapy oil
Pool Noodle
Fan
Washcloths (for cool or heat)
Tennis Balls
Pictures for focus
Toothbrush and toothpaste
Sweater
Complete change of clothes
Book to read
Kneeling pad
Lip balm
Headache medicine
Water bottle or juice boxes

Herbs for Labor

Shonda Parker
Author
Naturally Healthy Pregnancy
Naturally Healthy
www.NaturallyHealthy.org

The best preparation for staying comfortable in labor is to arrive at the appointed time well nourished, well rested, adequately hydrated, and strong, emotionally and spiritually. A whole foods diet will ensure the well nourished part. Raising the head of the bed in the last couple of months, nesting with plenty of pillows, and having delightful back, hip, and foot rubs will ensure the well rested part. Drinking a minimum of 2 quarts of water daily will ensure adequate hydration. Resisting the urge to time every contraction in the last four weeks of pregnancy to see if this is it and surrendering to the fact that God appointed the day of your baby's birth, the how of your baby's birth, and most of all that his grace grants you the freedom to rejoice in his design of your body that was built from the beginning of time to birth babies should imbue you with strength of spirit. Embracing labor for what it is—the work of your body to bring forth your baby—allows us to have joy in the midst of the unknown.

Labor is not unknown to God. He has been birthing babies for over six thousand years. He has a plan just for the birth of your child. He promises it will be good for you. Life is God's specialty. He speaks, and a world leaps into order. He breathes, and life draws deeply of its own first breath. He touches, and what is topsy-turvy, upside-down rights itself and comes into alignment. He created you, part by part, cell by cell; He has entered you and knows you. He has a vested interest in you and will not let real harm come to you.

Preparing the Uterus

The most well-known and reliable of herbs known to help a woman prepare for labor and birth is red raspberry leaf, Rubus idaeus. Mills and Bone in *Principles and*

Practice of Phytotherapy suggest both red raspberry leaf and squaw vine, Mitchella repens, to be taken continuously throughout the pregnancy beginning in the second trimester. Additionally, they recommend the use of red raspberry leaf during labor, up to six 5ml doses in a day.

Prepare for Endurance During Labor:

Siberian ginseng, Eleutherococcus senticosus, has been studied to ascertain whether it truly improves endurance and increases energy, and the results were positive. Ginseng is not an herb that works well with as-needed use. To use during a long labor, mom needs to begin supplementation in the last four weeks of pregnancy. Choosing this support is not planning for labor fatigue; labor is work and Siberian ginseng is indicated for this work regardless. Dosage: 2-3 grams daily during labor.

Relaxing During Labor

Relaxation during labor is one of the main factors influencing the perception of and outcome of the birth. A relaxed mother generally, though not always, opens, or dilates, quicker than a tense and fearful mother. Submitting oneself to the process of birth is "the work" of labor. There is no "secret" to relaxation—relaxation is a process of allowing the tension held in the body's muscles to leave.

What Mom Can Do

1. Eat lightly and drink regularly during labor to avoid hunger which makes it harder to relax.
2. Practice relaxing on a daily basis during pregnancy so the act will be natural and happen readily during labor.
3. A soothing lavender bath can be very helpful for promoting relaxation.
4. If mom is tense and having difficulty relaxing, a combination of ginger, Zingiber officinale, and black haw, Viburnum prunifolium, or cramp bark, Viburnum opulus, may be given to relax mom and allow labor to proceed. Dosage: 20-30 drops of tincture or ¼-½ tsp tinctract.

Excerpted with permission from *Naturally Healthy Pregnancy* © 2008.

Subject Seven

Options for Labor

Topics:

How and Why	201
Birth Place and Attendant	211
Routine Hospital Procedures	221
Induction Options	227
Pain Management Options	236
Newborn Care	248
From Decision to Reality	258
Making Decisions in Labor	263
Drawing Conclusions	272
Home Birth by Marlene Waechter	274

How and Why

Giving birth involves making many decisions. You probably have a wide variety of options available to you. You may even have several options that can accomplish the same thing. Your job is to make the best decision, wisely choosing the options you will use.

When faced with a decision, there are two important components to the solution you choose. One component is the physical—how to proceed—and the other is the reason why you chose to proceed that way. A wise decision will be one in which the how and the why both reflect what you are trying to accomplish.

How to Proceed

How to proceed is important because everything you choose in labor will affect your labor in some way. Everything from medications to positions to birth place will have a direct effect on the way your labor continues. Some options can speed up labor, some can slow labor down, some can help change the baby's position, and others can hinder baby's movement. When selecting how to proceed, be certain you are making choices that have a greater chance of affecting your labor in a way you would like.

How is important because there are risks to every option you have. The risks may be minimal or substantial but they are risks. You will need to determine when the risks of an option are outweighed by its benefits, and when the benefits are not worth the risk.

How is important because some decisions you make during labor change the other options available to you during labor. Choosing a home birth limits your available pain relieving medications. Choosing pain medications for labor can limit your mobility and ability to use positioning to move the baby. Choosing a C-section before labor begins limits your opportunity to try for a vaginal birth. While these limits are neither good nor bad on their own, you probably already have ideas of what limits you are and are not comfortable with. You should be aware of how your decisions can affect the other options available to you before you make them.

> What ideas do you already have about how you would like to labor?

How you choose to proceed is important, but how you proceed is temporary. It is only a reflection of the current circumstances and if the situation changes you can sometimes select a different way to proceed. In fact, it is basically a given in labor that comfort measures should be rotated because your needs will change during labor. What was a good way to handle a backache an hour ago may no longer be effective, so it becomes necessary to try a variety of strategies.

How to proceed is temporary because it is based on the tools, information and resources available to you at that time. When you look back later with more information, you may think a different option would have been a better choice. But that does not mean you did not make the best decision you could at the time with the resources available to you.

> Can you think of a time you made a decision, only to decide later that a different decision would have been better?

Why to Proceed

Mostly, *how* is temporary because God is not as interested with how you proceed as he is with your heart. Your heart is the reason why you choose an option in labor or any part of life. Two people may choose to do the same thing, but one can be honoring God while the other is sinning. Why? Because it is possible to look the same on the outside but have completely different hearts. It is possible to eat a piece of cake in thanksgiving to God for the joy of a friend's birthday, and it is possible to eat a piece of cake in selfish gluttony. The eating of cake is neither good nor bad, but when indulging in gluttony it becomes sin.

> 1 Chronicles 28:9
> Luke 16:15

Why to proceed in a particular way demonstrates your heart, your purpose and what you are serving. It is a reflection of where your heart is. Are you making your decisions out of fear? Are you making your decisions out of pride or envy? Are you making your decisions out of love, peace, faith, joy, kindness, gentleness, goodness, thankfulness, self-control and patience?

Mark 7:20-23

Why is the expression of sacrificial love regardless of the *how*. One woman may choose a particular option because it is best for the health of her baby while another woman chooses a different option for the same reason. *Why* is not a knee-jerk reaction to the circumstances or the situation around you. *Why* is the unwavering faith in God regardless of the chaos you may encounter. *Why* comes from the heart, and it is the heart that will be judged.

Making Wise Decisions

As you consider your options and make decisions in labor, remember both the how and the why. Make decisions based on a heart that is serving God, desiring to honor him while at the same time affecting your labor in the best way with the least amount of risk. You may find you select the same options as a friend or relative, or you may find you use completely different options during your baby's birth. Either way is fine. There is no one "wise decision" for childbirth every family must make.

After learning about the options available to you and making your selections on how to proceed, make another list based on the verses in Philippians 4:8; Galatians 5:22-24; or 2 Peter 1:5-7. This second list should be a list of godly reasons to make decisions. Return to the list of options available to you to see which fit naturally within these motives.

Godly Reasons
Admirable
Excellent
Faithfulness
Gentleness
Godliness
Goodness
Joy
Kindness
Knowledge
Lovely
Noble
Patience
Peace
Perseverance
Praiseworthy
Pure
Right
Self-Control
True

Stewardship of Childbirth

Continuing the Biblical principle of stewardship, the responsibility to make the best decisions possible with the gifts God has given, it is in the considering options and choosing the best available that pleases the master. In the parable of the talents, it was the servants who considered the many ways to care for the master's money who pleased the master, not the one who hid his money in fear of losing it. The master was not angry the servant had not doubled his money. The master scolded him, saying he would have been better to put the money in a bank earning interest than to bury it. He was angry with the servant's apparent inability or unwillingness to accurately consider his options.

Matthew 25:14-30

Many of the decisions that affect how you handle childbirth will be made before labor ever begins. Your choice of health care provider, birth place and attendants will have a strong impact on the process of your labor. However, labor is hardly ever "textbook." Most families must make some decisions about how to proceed or what to choose next during labor. It is in all these decisions the principle of stewardship becomes important to childbirth.

Your midwife can be a great source of information in labor, as can your doula. They have a large amount of knowledge and experience with childbirth. They can give you ideas, suggestions and even opinions about what the best way to proceed will be. However, their advice will always remain suggestions and opinions, not directives or orders. As a parent, it is your responsibility to make decisions about your health and the health of your child. It is your responsibility to be a good steward of the materials available to you. The people you hire to serve you in labor remain in the position of consultant, assessing situations and giving you information when you need it.

Ideally, you will work with your health care provider and attendants as a team. For this to happen, you must hire attendants whose opinion you trust. If you do not feel comfortable with the suggestions and opinions your health care provider shares at prenatal visits, you will not suddenly feel comfortable with her because you are in labor. Instead, you will find yourself unable to work effectively with the person you are paying to be your strongest ally for childbirth.

There are no right or wrong answers for what makes a good attendant in labor. It takes a person whose knowledge, experience, philosophies and opinions about childbirth you trust. If the midwife you hired is not that person, fire her and find someone else. You may be sorry you stayed with an attendant you do not feel comfortable with, but you will never be sorry you found a caregiver you can trust.

Even with the perfect caregiver, the responsibility for decision making is yours. The Coalition for Improving Maternity Services (CIMS) Mother Friendly Birth Initiative states every woman should (CIMS, 1996):

Receive accurate and up-to-date information about the benefits and risks of all procedures, drugs, and tests suggested for use during pregnancy, birth, and the postpartum period, with the rights to informed consent and informed refusal;

Receive support for making informed choices about what is best for her and her baby based on her individual values and beliefs.

Informed consent means no procedures or interventions happen "to you" in labor. Instead, you have chosen to use these interventions because you understand what is happening in your labor, and you understand how the intervention or procedure can affect the labor process. Informed refusal means that with the same information, you have chosen not to use an intervention or procedure which was recommended to you. Informed consent does not exist without the option for an informed refusal.

The following are questions you can work through with your health care provider or other birth attendants when making decisions about labor. You will not be able to get a full understanding of the answers to these questions between contractions. For that reason, it is important to prepare before labor by learning as much as you can about the options available to you and how they may affect your labor. Once you have the background knowledge, the process of considering your options in labor will become easier.

What is being suggested and why?

It may seem elementary, but to make a good decision you need to understand what exactly is being suggested. Doing something to "move things along" could mean changing to upright positions, using synthetic oxytocin, using a cervical cream, or it might mean breaking the bag of waters. Scheduling an induction might mean any one of three different medications. Which option or options is your caregiver thinking about? In the same way, "something for the pain." could mean changing positions, using a systemic medication or having an epidural or spinal block. You cannot make a wise decision without knowing exactly what you are deciding to do or not do.

In the same way, you need to understand why the suggestion is being made. Is there concern for the safety of your baby, or does the caregiver think you want things to change? There will likely be a big difference in your attitude about suggested changes made for convenience and suggested changes made for the safety of your baby, and you have a right to know which type of suggestion is being made.

What do you hope will be accomplished?

Although you may think the answer to this question is obvious, it is not always. There is usually more than one way to accomplish something, and choosing between two or more methods can mean you need to understand what part of the process could use some help.

For example, if you thought labor was taking too long and wanted to move things along, you could try several different ways. Using a synthetic oxytocin may speed labor if it can strengthen contractions. Using a prostaglandin gel may speed labor by ripening the cervix and increasing uterine sensitivity to oxytocin. Oxytocin will not ripen the cervix, so although it may "speed labor," it is not the best choice if your cervix is not quite ripe enough yet.

What will you do if it does not work?

With every option is the possibility that you will not achieve the results you wanted. Not every woman goes into labor quickly with synthetic oxytocin; not every woman has adequate pain relief with an epidural or a systemic medication; not every baby turns vertex from positioning or an external version. The success rates vary with different options, and you need to be prepared for what options will or will not be available after you have tried something and it did not work. For example, if you use artificial rupture of the membranes to attempt to speed labor, your options for waiting for labor to speed up on its own become limited.

What are the risks and benefits?

Every position, medication, procedure and other intervention has its own set of risks and benefits. You will most often choose the option whose benefits outweigh the risks. This means you will rely on less invasive options when labor is moving along normally and move to higher risk ways to change labor only if the benefits of using the procedure outweigh the risks of using it.

What other options are available?

There are many ways to accomplish everything in childbirth; you never have just one option. At the bare minimum you almost always have the option to wait and do nothing. Understanding all the ways you can try to change labor will help you make the best decision.

What are the risks and benefits of the other options?

Once you know what other options are available, you can begin weighing the risks and benefits of all possibilities. This allows you to choose the option with the best likelihood of producing the results you want with the least amount of risk. Sometimes it will mean going with the first thing suggested, other times it will mean going with a different option.

When do you need to decide?

In emergencies, you will make decisions quickly. However, birth emergencies are rare. You will usually have time to decide how you would like to proceed, or to try less risky options before attempting something with more side effects.

Other People and Your Decisions

It is possible to make a decision that other people think is wrong. It is also possible that someone who disagrees with you will treat you poorly because of your decision. Sometimes you catch a medical caregiver, family member or friend on a bad day, or you do not communicate well with each other. When this happens, remember these few things:

Treat her with love and respect. She may be annoying you, but she is still a child of God. Besides, you will get further working with her than working against her.

Acknowledge his concern then share additional information you may have and ask for any more information from him if necessary. When you both have the same information you still may not agree, but at least you will understand where each other is coming from.

Clarify the decision you have made and why. It is possible you have placed greater emphasis on aspects of the decision less familiar or less important to her.

Hold him accountable for how he behaves. Call a bully a bully. Let him know you do not appreciate the way you are treated, give a specific example and ask him to stop. This is exactly what adults expect children to do, but rarely will adults behave this way themselves.

If the behavior continues, either limit the contact if it is a family member or fire the caregiver. No one, including hospital staff, has the right to be with you in labor without your permission. If you really have trouble working with a hospital caregiver, ask to see the head nurse and share the problem with her. She will assign someone else to assist you.

Discerning Between Options

One of the key ingredients in good decision making during labor is understanding the possible outcomes and consequences of the decisions you make. Your decisions are not only going to affect the next few contractions, but the next few hours and days. In some cases it can affect you for months or years. For example, it generally takes longer to heal from an episiotomy than a tear. Another example is that women who hire a doula not only experience less pain during labor but also have healthier babies, are more satisfied with their partners and happier with the birth experience.

The first decisions you make will lay the foundation for the other choices you have—much like building a house. Where you give birth and who attends you will determine what other options are available. It is much more difficult to come back and make changes to the plan after the foundation has been set. For that reason, it is important to research the birth attendant and birth locations available to you. All other decisions will be built upon that foundation.

Knowledge of the various options is not enough. You must have the wisdom and understanding to use them effectively at your birth. Knowledge means simply knowing the facts, no more and no less. But wisdom knows how to apply those facts. Wisdom knows how to handle facts that seem contradictory. Wisdom can balance the benefits and the risks to make a good decision for both mother and baby.

Each of the technologies offered during labor can provide great benefits. But at the same time, they can each have great risks. It is because of these risks you are careful to determine when and if a technology should be used. In the normal labor, adding a technology adds risks. Sometimes that risk is added without significant benefit; sometimes the benefits obviously outweigh the risks.

As the parent, it is your responsibility and right to decide which technologies are a part of your child's birth. You will make decisions based on what you see happening, advice and options from your midwife and your knowledge of the technology available. Before you are treated with a medical option, you will be asked to give informed consent.

As you build your knowledge of the technologies available, pay attention to these three things:

- Are there other ways to get the same result?
- How is this technology likely to affect your labor?
- What ways can you make the use of this technology safer if you decide to use it?

The following pages list the pros and cons of a variety of technologies available in labor. There are three problems with this listing.

1. Although each of these is an option in labor, it should not imply that they are in any way equal. Labor is not a buffet where you can take the technology you like and leave the rest with no questions asked. Some of the options placed before you can have a dramatic

impact on your ability to labor–which can be very good or very bad. Some of the options placed before you are tied together, rarely being used one without the other. Other options will negate each other so if you choose one you cannot have the other. Some of the options are still a normal part of labor in many areas, despite research showing it is either not helpful or may be harmful. As you make your choices, be sure you understand the decisions you are making.

2. The list is long, and includes many things you may not have access to where you live. You will need to decide how strongly God wants you to pursue options that are not currently available in your area.

3. These options in and of themselves are neither good nor bad. They are simply technologies that can be used to help ensure a safe birth for both mother and baby. However, each of these technologies also carries a risk. Because there is risk, there are good and bad uses of these technologies in as much as a good use helps to reduce the overall risk to mother and baby while a bad use would increase the overall risk.

Birth Place and Attendants

Where you give birth and who attends you are very closely tied together. In general, you have three choices for birth attendant and three choices for birth place. For all practical purposes, when you choose your birth attendant, you choose your birth place and vice versa. This is because most birth attendants only care for clients in one type of setting—either a hospital, birth center or home.

There are some basic generalities you can use to help determine which type of care provider is right for your pregnancy, but these are generalities. The way a midwife or doctor practices is dependant on many more factors than the letters after her name. Be sure to interview any birth attendant before hiring her. During the interview you will begin to discover if she is the right attendant for you.

Midwife

Midwives are the safest choice for normal, healthy mothers, and recent research suggests they may even be the safest choice for mothers who have certain risk factors (MacDorman et.al., 1998). A midwife is an expert on pregnancy and childbirth as it normally occurs and its wide range of healthy variations.

Midwives are trained to treat the whole woman, which means they are as concerned about how you are feeling emotionally as how you are feeling physically. Prenatal visits with a midwife are longer than with a physician. Midwives work with you to answer any questions and ensure you feel confident as you prepare to give birth. When the big day arrives, a midwife will remain with you throughout labor, helping you cope physically and emotionally with the work you are doing.

There are two tracks for midwifery education; both require extensive study and time spent learning from other midwives. The first track is to enter directly into midwifery, becoming a Direct Entry Midwife (DEM) or Certified Professional Midwife (CPM). The second is to train as a nurse and then enter into the field of midwifery, becoming a Certified Nurse Midwife (CNM).

> How can you learn about midwifery in your community?

Depending on the laws where you live and her training, a midwife may be able to attend you at home, in a free-standing birth center or a hospital. Both CPMs and CNMs assist women who wish to give birth in a birth center. In most areas, it is the CNMs who attend women who wish to give birth in a hospital. A CNM has the ability to order all the same birth technologies as a doctor, meaning you can have an epidural or other pain relieving medication if you wish. However, unlike a doctor, a CNM is very likely to be familiar with non-medical pain relieving strategies and alternative birth options such as water birth.

While CNMs have the advantage of working within a hospital environment, they have the disadvantage of having to work within the hospital authority structure. Depending on the laws where you live, a CNM working in a hospital may be required to follow an obstetrician's orders regarding your care. Although your midwife may desire to provide care in the midwifery model, the hospital environment may not allow her to. This makes it important to be familiar with the policy and attitude of your CNM's doctor back-up and the hospital she works in.

CPMs tend to assist women who wish to give birth at home. A CPM is able to provide prenatal care including assisting you with the basic prenatal health tests. During the labor a CPM brings to the birth equipment which may or may not include some of the technologies available in the hospital such as artificial oxytocin, IV, oxygen, nitrous oxide and suturing equipment.

In most communities CPMs are required to have a physician as backup for their practice. However, unlike the CNMs who must work directly with physicians in determining your care, CPMs are more likely to be able to direct your care according to the midwifery model.

Family Doctor

If you have a family doctor, you will probably be able to receive prenatal services and birth attendance through that office. Family doctors can be a great choice because generally you will already be familiar with your doctor, and your doctor will already know your family. If you choose your family doctor, you will most likely be giving birth in a local hospital. If anything unusual happens in your pregnancy, your family doctor will refer you to a specialist for additional care but will probably stay involved and may attend the labor depending on your circumstances.

Obstetrician

An obstetrician (OB) is a surgeon trained in the pathology of a woman's reproductive system. Training for the OB centers around what can go wrong and how to use medical technology to improve a bad situation. This is very beneficial for the small number of pregnancies that require obstetrical care. However, when caring for normal, healthy pregnancies, OBs have higher intervention rates without any improvement of outcomes for mothers and babies (MacDorman et.al., 1998).

Most OBs do not stay with you in labor; they either stop in or get telephone updates from the nurses and come only when they are needed to perform an intervention or to catch your baby. This hands-off approach means an OB is not likely to offer you help in coping with labor beyond providing you access to medication. Be sure to interview potential OBs to determine if their style of care meets your expectations.

Support during Childbirth

One of the easiest things you can do to improve the safety, effectiveness and comfort of your labor is to hire a professional labor assistant, also known as a doula. The word doula is a Greek word that means servant. True to the origin of the name, a doula acts as a servant to the family either through labor, the first few weeks post partum, or both.

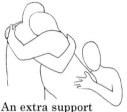

An extra support person increases your comfort options.

Doulas do not perform any clinical tasks, they do not do vaginal exams or check your baby's heart rate. A doula is different from a midwife because a doula is there only for the physical and emotional comfort of the family. This means she may be helping you change position, walking with you, rubbing your back, talking to you or helping your family learn how to do these things effectively. And unlike the staff at a hospital, a doula does not go off the clock at the end of the shift. A doula will stay with you until you give birth.

The research on the effects of doulas is overwhelming. The results are consistent despite the differences in hospital routines, risk factors for the mother and presence of friends and family at the labor. When a doula is present, the mother is less likely to request pain medications, less likely to have a cesarean or operative vaginal birth, and she is less likely to find labor was worse than she expected. Mothers are less likely to feel tense during labor and less likely to feel negatively about the birth experience. Babies whose mothers use doulas have a decreased risk of a five-minute Apgar score below seven, an indicator a baby may be having problems (Klaus, Kennell & Klaus, 1993).

To achieve these great results, the support a mother receives during labor must be continuous. That means she is never left alone. But at the same time, the person in attendance must be providing supportive care activities, either physical or emotional. Physical support could mean a massage, helping the mother walk, holding her hand or putting cool washcloths on her face. Emotional support could be making eye contact, helping her understand the procedures being used, praising and encouraging her or providing information.

Many mothers invite close friends and family to the birth expecting them to provide physical and emotional support. It is important to communicate clearly about the level of support you expect, especially since loved ones may just want to be present for the experience and not participate in the work. There is no research on the support a husband provides or even about the expectations women have of them. However, one study found the women who received continuous support from midwives received more physical and emotional support from their husbands, and the husbands were more satisfied with the experience. Female family members who attended a short doula training were able to provide some of the benefits of a professional doula (Campbell, Scott, Klaus & Falk, 2007).

Many families plan a birth at the hospital expecting the nurse or midwife to support them during labor. Unfortunately, the reality of working in a hospital prevents even the most caring staff members from supporting families as much as they want. Only about ten percent of a nurse's time is able to be spent on supportive activities (Enken et al., 2000). Depending on the type of practice your midwife has, she may be required to attend to several laboring women at one time, preventing her from giving you the support you expected. The only way to have continuous support in the hospital is to hire a doula.

If you plan to give birth at home, your midwife will provide you with continuous support. Midwives who attend home births have the freedom to attend to only one client at a time, focusing on you until they are sure you and your new baby are healthy and comfortable. The continuous presence of a midwife may contribute to the outstanding outcomes of home birth. Women who plan to give birth at home have significantly fewer interventions, with similar outcomes (Johnson & Daviss, 2005).

If you would like to hire a doula to attend you in labor, be sure to interview potential candidates before signing a contract. The doula will be with you at one of your most vulnerable times, so you will want to be sure you hire someone you are completely comfortable with. Personality differences may matter more than her training or experience.

Unassisted Birth

> Unassisted birth refers to families who plan for birth without an attendant, not families that unexpectedly give birth alone.

A small percentage of families choose to give birth at home without an attendant. This is commonly referred to as unassisted childbirth. Families who choose an unassisted birth take total responsibility for the birth of their child. Their inherent trust in their body's ability to give birth leads some of them to forego all maternity care.

Most families who plan an unassisted birth have normal healthy babies. An unassisted birth is planned and prepared for by the family who has learned what they need to feel comfortable in a potentially dangerous situation. Unassisted birth families also have a back-up plan to get help if it is necessary.

In practice, unassisted birth is as unlike the couples who do not make it to the hospital as it is the couples who do. Families who choose this type of labor do so out of faith, and their lack of fear allows them to have some of the most remarkable labors you may ever hear about. In addition, an unassisted birth requires by nature only the family with no additional helpers. This creates an intimate environment for welcoming a new child.

Some home birth midwives allow families to have an almost unassisted birth. The midwife works with the expectant mother to offer advice and get to know her. Then during labor, the midwife maintains a hushed presence allowing her to ensure safety without disturbing the family. When it comes time for the birth, the midwife instructs the family on how to catch the baby, assists with immediate care of the mother and ensures the baby is healthy.

Home Birth

Families choose to give birth at home because it gives them control over what is happening to them during labor. Labor is allowed to progress at its own pace without unnecessary intervention. Home birth also prevents disrupting other children or the routines of the household. Home birth gives families the option to include whomever they desire for support and prevents being cared for by strangers.

Statistically, home is the safest place for normal healthy mothers to have their babies. Midwives who provide home birth care have the lowest rates of interventions, including the lowest rate of cesarean surgery of any maternity care provider (Fraser et al., 2000). In addition, mothers who give birth at home are less likely to suffer a birth related injury and are least likely to have an infection.

> In areas where home birth is not integrated into the health care system, there may be increased risk for mothers and babies choosing to give birth at home.

In some areas, access to home birth is limited by practitioners who choose not to attend home births. Providing home birth services is demanding, requiring twenty-four-hour on call services with very little pay. It is hard on families, especially if the midwife is practicing alone. Because of this, many midwives who could do home birth services choose to work in groups that provide birth center or hospital birth services.

In other areas, laws prevent direct entry midwives from attending home births. In the United States, a midwife who legally provided home birth services in one state may be forced out of practice if she moves to another state because there is no nationally accepted standard for direct entry midwifery. Some midwives choose to continue providing services in areas where they have little or no legal protection, however, depending on the political climate it can be difficult to find them.

Home birth requires the most preparation on the part of the family. In addition to regular preparation for birth, families who choose home birth will be given a list of supplies to have available during labor and birth. Most families find the cost of the supplies to be minimal. In some areas, insurance will not cover the costs of home birth services, so be sure to check your insurance to find out what is available.

Some home birth midwives will travel with nitrous oxide for pain relief, but for the most part families who choose home birth commit to laboring without chemical pain relief. Yet, far from wallowing in agony, mothers who give birth at home marvel in the experience. Giving birth at home is so different from giving birth in a hospital that even though it can hurt very much, women do not need pain medication to handle it. Very few home birth clients transfer to the hospital to use pain medication.

Home birth may be for you if you:
- Have access to a home birth attendant you are comfortable with
- Are willing to do extra preparations
- Desire not to disrupt your family
- Feel most comfortable at home
- Are willing to labor without medication
- Desire the least amount of intervention during birth

Birth Center

Birth centers are a relatively new phenomenon. They offer an in-between point for families that do not need the services of a hospital but are not sure they want to stay home for birth. Because they are designed specifically for laboring but with all the comforts of home, some midwives consider an out of hospital birth center to be the best of both worlds.

Families who choose to use a birth center enjoy the freedom and comfort available, while finding reassurance in the presence of emergency equipment. At a birth center, you will receive continuous support, be encouraged to use positions and movement to keep labor normal and eat and drink as necessary. Depending on your birth center, you may also be able to use some types of pain medication. The length of stay after giving birth at a birth center is usually measured in hours, not days.

In addition to the very low rates of complications and interventions, birth centers also offer families the opportunity to stay together during labor. Many birth centers allow children to participate in the birth. Birth centers provide the large tubs and other props that make good labor positions possible, which some families do not have access to in their homes. Giving birth at a birth center is more affordable than a hospital.

Community birth centers are also a great way for midwives to maintain home birth style care while working as a group. Birth centers often give families a place for prenatal health care, childbirth classes and new parent support groups. Unfortunately in the United States, many birth centers are not able to afford the rising malpractice insurance rates and so are closing their doors.

A birth center may be for you if you:
- Have access to a community birth center
- Are willing to travel during labor
- Desire to keep your family with you
- Feel most comfortable out of your home
- Are willing to labor without medication
- Desire to use the labor equipment

Hospital

Many, if not most, hospitals provide maternity services. Hospitals are designed to monitor high-risk labors, provide pain medication and perform surgery. Some hospitals do offer tubs, showers, birth balls and other equipment to assist you in having a normal labor.

Care in a hospital is different from care in a birth center or at home. In most hospitals, the labor is monitored by a machine, not a person. Hospitals are not able to provide continuous support, even in places where they have one on one nursing. Because of the nature of their work, hospitals require several people you do not know to attend to your needs.

Despite their drawbacks, hospitals are popular places to give birth. Four million women gave birth in United States hospitals in 2005. Delivery was the second most common reason for discharge from US hospitals, beat only slightly by heart disease. Childbirth was the reason one out of five women were hospitalized, and obstetrical procedures accounted for one out of every four hospital procedures performed on a female. Cesarean surgery was performed more frequently than any other surgery for any reason (Centers for Disease Control and Prevention, 2007).

Some women choose to give birth in a hospital because they feel safest where there is medical equipment. Unfortunately, women who plan to have a vaginal birth in a hospital are more likely to have a cesarean surgery than women who plan to give birth at a birth center or at home. They are also most likely to have artificial oxytocin, pain medication, be restricted in their movement, be left alone, have an episiotomy and suffer illness or injury after birth (Goer, 1999).

Some women give birth in a hospital because they choose to have an epidural or a cesarean surgery. A hospital is the only place to have either one. Some women give birth in a hospital because the midwife they have chosen only provides services in a hospital. Other women find they have no option other than a hospital for birth.

Understanding the importance of a woman's feeling comfortable where she gives birth, many hospitals have created elaborate birthing suites that provide room to walk, tubs or showers for laboring in, beds that can be used in a wide variety of positions and decorated in a way that hides the medical equipment. Despite the change in environment, the rates of interventions have continued to increase during hospital births, demonstrating that it is not the wallpaper that creates a good birth atmosphere.

A hospital may be for you if you:

- Know cesarean surgery is the safest choice for you and your baby
- Have chosen to use pain medication with labor
- Have chosen to work with a midwife who only provides services in a hospital
- Are not comfortable with the options of home or birth center
- Have decided a medical induction is safest for your baby
- Have reason to believe you are at a higher risk for problems during labor

Routine Hospital Procedures

There are a variety of procedures which have become routine during in-hospital birth care. Any procedure can be helpful in certain circumstances, but when something is done on every woman regardless of indication, the potential for causing harm rises. Of the six commonly routine hospital procedures, only one is regarded as beneficial by *A guide to effective care in pregnancy and childbirth.*

Although you have the right to refuse any procedure, you are likely to have a difficult time refusing any of these hospital care standards. If you plan to give birth in a hospital, you will want to work very closely with your midwife to understand which procedures she will or will not require of you.

Is It Safe?

As you consider the options available to you, a question on many of the options is probably, "Is this safe?" Unfortunately, that is a question that is too subjective to answer across the board for all labors and all options.

Whether something is safe or unsafe is an assumption made by the person reading the research based on the results. For example, if the percentage of people who had trouble with a cold medicine is below a certain number, it is generally considered "safe" even though there are a percentage of people who will have problems with it.

Further complicating decisions is the understanding that not all medical research is designed to follow the scientific processes. Much of our body of knowledge comes from observational research intended to explore what is possible, not examine the risks of procedures.

Your situation can change how safe or unsafe a certain option is. For example, chemotherapy is generally not safe and the average healthy person is well advised not to undergo this treatment. However, if you have cancer, chemotherapy may very well be "safer" than not having chemotherapy because it can decrease the risks of cancer and may be able to eliminate it. If you know you have certain health problems, pay attention to how they can affect the safety of the options you are considering.

Finally, a good experience does not change the risks. It may change your perception of the risks or your assumptions about the risks, but it does not change the fact that they exist. You can know there are risks and still decide to use an option. Your goal is to find the options that provide you with the least harmful risks. The question is, are you willing to feel safe with the level of risk?

What safety concerns do you have about birth options?

Something can be safe and still have risks. Safe is only going to be defined by you and can only be defined after you have learned as much as you can about whatever you are considering. Your midwife's, best friend's or mother's definition of safe may not be the same as yours. The following information is based on the recommendations found in *A guide to effective care in pregnancy and childbirth.*

Eating and Drinking in Labor

Depending on where you live, giving birth in a hospital may mean accepting a restrictive policy preventing you from eating or drinking. If you move to the hospital environment late enough in labor that you no longer desire food, this may not be an issue. However, if you do want to eat, being denied food can be unpleasant and lead to poor progress in labor.

Withholding food was believed to prevent the risk of aspiration of the stomach contents in case general anesthesia was needed for surgery. Most women undergoing surgical birth receive epidural or spinal anesthesia, so the risk of aspiration is very low. In addition, withholding food does not ensure the stomach is empty but can result in dehydration and ketosis. When food is withheld, the stomach contents increase in acidity, increasing the risk of damaging airways and putting women at the greatest risk for aspiration.

There is no published data on the nutritional needs of laboring women; however, it may be similar to women undergoing athletic activity. The alternatives to drinking and eating during labor are often ice chips and an IV. However, the current practice of IV fluids does not provide a source of energy for the laboring mother and does not do any better job of hydrating during normal labor than allowing the mother to drink water or juice would do.

Intravenous Fluids

Intravenous (IV) fluids can be helpful if you are suffering from dehydration and are required for administration of some medications during labor. In the recent past, having an IV was a normal part of having a baby to prevent dehydration caused by the withholding of food and drink. However, studies are beginning to find there are risks to IVs that do not exist when a mother stays hydrated by drinking water.

Having an IV decreases your mobility and can be uncomfortable. Yet, the biggest problem with IV fluids is the increased risk of fluid overload for both you and your baby. When glucose solutions are used, the baby's blood chemistry changes with a decreased pH and increased insulin production. *A guide to effective care in pregnancy and childbirth* recommends avoiding these hazards by allowing women to eat and drink during labor.

Episiotomy

An episiotomy is a cut to the perineal skin (skin between the vagina and anus). It was once believed performing an episiotomy improved outcomes for mothers by decreasing the risk of tearing and improving healing.

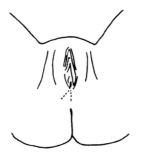

An episiotomy may be cut straight towards the rectum or off to the side.

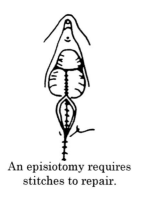

An episiotomy requires stitches to repair.

However, research shows routine episiotomy does not improve outcomes; instead, it increases the risk of a deeper tear and increases the healing time for the mother. There is no evidence episiotomy improves outcomes for babies or prevents incontinence for mothers.

If the idea is to prevent trauma to the perineum, routine episiotomy is not the answer. An episiotomy cuts through skin and muscle, the equivalent of a second degree tear, one hundred percent of the time. Midwives have tried both hands on support, holding the perineal skin, and hands off support to prevent adding pressure. There appears to be no difference in outcomes. There is very little research on perineal massage; however, in one small study women who used massage during labor had fewer third or fourth degree tears. Many midwives find women who give birth underwater have less perineal tears, as do women who use upright pushing positions.

Though routine episiotomy shows no benefit, restricted episiotomy does result in less risk of perineal trauma, fewer complications and less need for suturing. However, the difficult part is ensuring your caregiver is one who understands the difference between a helpful episiotomy and a harmful episiotomy.

Electronic Fetal Monitoring

There are three ways to monitor your baby's heart rate during labor. One is to use a fetoscope intermittently. The second is to use a hand-held doptone. The third way is to use an electronic fetal monitor which can be used continuously throughout labor.

When the electronic fetal monitor was first introduced, it was heralded as a great advancement for the safety of babies. The expectation was the instant information could help identify problems sooner and babies could be saved by cesarean surgery. Its use was adopted and now ninety-nine percent of women giving birth in the United States use electronic fetal monitors during labor.

Unfortunately, electronic fetal monitoring has not proven to be as effective as the medical community had hoped. When mothers are monitored continuously with electronic fetal monitors instead of using a fetoscope intermittently, both cesarean surgery and operative vaginal delivery rates are higher without any improvement in the health of their babies. There is no evidence monitoring with an electronic fetal monitor helps prevent death of babies, decreases risk of admission to special care nurseries or improves the health of babies.

In addition to increasing your risk of cesarean surgery, electronic fetal monitors limit your mobility. When an internal electronic fetal monitor is used, your risk for infection increases. Although some women find the rhythmic swishing of the monitor reassuring, others find the apparatus uncomfortable and have increased anxiety each time the heartbeat is "lost" because they changed positions.

Another problem with electronic fetal monitors is their tendency to reduce your quality of care. When a labor is monitored by intermittent auscultation with a fetoscope, you see the nurse or midwife every fifteen minutes. When an electronic fetal monitor is used, the nurse or midwife checks the monitor—not you. Sometimes the monitor can be read from the nursing station, meaning you may not be attended to for an hour or more.

If you will be giving birth in a hospital, your midwife may have the ability to use intermittent monitoring (listening for one minute every fifteen minutes) instead of continuous electronic fetal monitoring. Different hospitals within your community may have different policies about electronic fetal monitoring. Discuss the options with your midwife before labor begins so you can make any necessary adjustments to your birth plan.

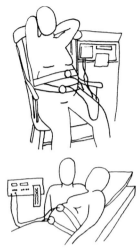

You can choose an upright position while being monitored.

Cervical Checks

Most women find the cervical checks during labor uncomfortable or painful. Cervical checks increase your risk for infection and increase the risk your bag of waters will accidentally be broken. Because of this, they should be limited to as few as possible.

The biggest value of cervical checks is their ability to let you know what is going on in the uterus. If you have been progressing in labor but your cervical changes are minimal, you may be dealing with a poorly positioned baby. Knowing this information, you can begin to use positions and techniques to help your baby move into a better birth position so you can continue to birth normally.

Cervical checks become a problem when they are done often, such as once an hour. Although the generally accepted rate of dilation is one centimeter per hour, it is an average taken over a length of time, not a requirement that each hour produce another centimeter. Checking the cervix can alert you to potential problems, but too frequent cervical checking gives the appearance of problems where none exists.

Hospital Gowns

One of the first things you will be asked to do in the hospital is to put on one of the hospital gowns. Although there is no physical risk to wearing one, there can be emotional risks. Hospital gowns are uncomfortable, unflattering and can leave you feeling like a sick patient instead of the strong, confident laboring mother you need to be.

The hospital cannot refuse to allow you to wear your own clothing. If you think you will be more comfortable in something from home, select clothing that gives you ease of movement. You will also want to consider how easy it will be for your midwife to listen to your baby's heart, how easy it will be for you to push or have your cervix checked and how easy it will be to breastfeed.

Long, flowing skirts can easily be pulled up to push or for checks but also allow lots of movement without leaving you feeling exposed. Button-up tops can be easily opened for nursing or to listen to your baby. Sports bras can provide easy access for any medical need while maintaining your modesty.

Induction Options

Near the end of your pregnancy, you may be asked to consider artificially starting labor. This process, called induction, is "one of the most dramatic ways of intervening in the natural process of pregnancy and childbirth" (Enkin et al, 2000). While there is much research about which methods of inducing labor work the best, there is very little research on when it is appropriate to induce.

Choosing to induce

The decision to induce is not always a simple one. Choosing to induce means making several assumptions.

First, it must be assumed your baby is developed sufficiently enough to be born safely. This is generally done by estimated gestational age and checking the lungs for maturity. However, you must remember the maturing of the lungs is not the only late pregnancy changes happening to your baby. During the last few weeks and days your baby increases fat stores to help regulate body temperature, begins gaining immunity as the placenta allows larger molecules to pass and stores larger volumes of iron.

Secondly, it must be assumed your body is ready to labor. The last few weeks of pregnancy are times of great hormonal adjustment in your body. These hormonal changes prepare the cervix to stretch, prepare the uterus to contract in response to hormones and prepare your pelvis to stretch and open. If your body is not ready to labor, the induction process will be lengthy, uncomfortable and unproductive.

Third, it is assumed you or your baby would be in better health if your baby were born. The standard list of reasons given for induction includes high blood pressure, diabetes, broken bag of waters, big baby, prolonged pregnancy and baby not thriving. Each of these variations of labor is covered in the labor challenges section, and you are encouraged to learn about each one.

Finally, it is assumed the process of induction is safer than allowing pregnancy to continue. Whether this is true or not must be determined on a case-by-case basis. Not all induction methods carry the same risks, and neither do all reasons for considering induction. Regardless of the method of induction chosen, you can be sure of the following:

1. Induction can be a very slow process, especially if your cervix is not ripe. Think in terms of days, not hours. Fatigue and discouragement are common when induction takes longer than anticipated.

2. The methods used to induce can cause contractions that are too strong for your baby. To help ensure your baby's safety, you will use an electric fetal monitor continually throughout the induction. Depending on the equipment at your hospital, this can limit your mobility. If the contractions do become too strong, the induction may need to be stopped.

3. Induction is associated with increased use of pain relieving medication. This means women who are induced are more likely to request pain medication than women who enter labor naturally.

I always tell my moms when they go over their due date: Ecclesiastes 3:2a says "A time to be born." So wait until God's timing to be born.

Brenda Capp

Methods of Self-inducing

There are a variety of methods women have used in attempts to begin labor on their own. The success rates of these methods have not been studied, with the exception of nipple stimulation which was found to increase the likelihood a woman would begin labor.

The Listening to Mother's II Survey included questions about self-induction. They found 22 percent of the mothers did try to start labor on their own with about one in five actually succeeding at self-induction. The most common methods used by the women of the survey were walking or exercise, sexual intercourse and nipple stimulation (Declercq, Sakala, Corry & Applebaum, 2006).

Though self-induction methods are not medical, they are not all without risk. While many of the methods for self-inducing are things you normally do in everyday life and should continue, others require you to ingest something you would not otherwise eat. Before attempting to self-induce, be sure you understand the risks of entering labor before your body or baby are prepared. God has determined a time for your baby to be born, and intervention with that plan should only be done after much prayer. If you are successful at beginning labor, it is a decision you will not be able to change later.

Considering Induction?
- What makes you believe it is safer for your baby to be born now than to wait?
- What makes you believe your baby is ready to be born?
- What makes you believe your body is ready for labor?

Walking

Walking and other activities that move your pelvis are known to help your baby slide into a better position, which may leave baby pressing lower on your cervix. The increased pressure may help to increase the prostaglandins produced by your cervix, helping your body move into labor. Though walking has been shown to shorten the length of labor, its ability to begin labor remains uncertain.

Regardless of its success at beginning labor, walking is a great late pregnancy activity. The physical exercise can help to lift your mood, keep your body strong, improve your circulation and may help you remain comfortable. Walking is a natural stimulant for your digestive system, which means walking may help to avoid constipation and hemorrhoids. Walking can also be a relaxing activity either alone or with your older children. Some women find an evening walk in the fresh air helps them to sleep better.

Sexual Intercourse

Sexual intercourse is believed to help begin labor in two ways. First, semen is high in prostaglandins, which can help prepare the cervix for labor. Secondly, your uterus contracts during orgasm, which can help to further prepare your body and hormone levels for birth.

For some women, intercourse in late pregnancy is awkward and uncomfortable. It is important to explore new positions and ways to maintain sexual closeness when your growing belly makes your most common or favorite positions unavailable. Though it may not actually start labor, you can at least be satisfied by remembering sexual closeness is important for your marriage.

Nipple Stimulation

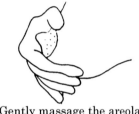

Gently massage the areola, not the nipple.

Nipple stimulation causes your body to release oxytocin, a hormone known to cause uterine contractions. In the first few weeks of breastfeeding this helps your uterus to heal. Before your baby is born, you can stimulate your nipples with your fingers or hand, water from a shower, a breast pump, or let your husband do it for you.

Because nipple stimulation has been known to cause very strong contractions, most recommendations are to stimulate only one breast at a time, and for no more than five minutes per breast per hour. This gives your body time to react to the increased oxytocin before you begin to produce more.

Proper nipple stimulation is actually more of areola (dark area around the nipple) stimulation. You want to be sure the areola is massaged, similar to breastfeeding. It is the stimulation of the areola that triggers the production of oxytocin, not tugging on the nipple.

Acupressure

Acupressure has been used for centuries to help many health problems. Acupressure refers to the use of pressure in certain places to stimulate the body to react in specific ways. If you press the base of your neck or your temples to help relieve a headache, you are using acupressure.

Although its effectiveness has not been studied, there is the possibility it may be helpful. Points on the hand and ankle are recommended to stimulate labor when pressed with a firm but gentle pressure.

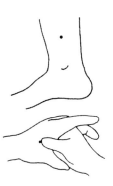

One point is about four finger widths above the ankle bone on the inner side of your leg. Try applying pressure with your thumb or index finger for one minute, then do the same on the other leg after a 30-minute rest.

Another point is between your thumb and first finger. This acupressure point can be used during labor to stimulate stronger contractions.

Castor Oil

Castor oil has been used to begin labor by midwives for years. The basic formula is about 2 ounces of oil in whatever juice you can stomach with it. It tastes unpleasant and will stimulate your bowels to empty. For some unknown reason this bowel emptying stimulates your uterus to empty as well.

Castor oil does have some unpleasant side effects. It can cause abdominal cramping and diarrhea, which may not be pleasant while you are coping with labor. Because of the diarrhea, you can become dehydrated with castor oil, so you will need to drink extra water or juice during labor. Be sure to let your midwife know if you intend to try castor oil, so she can be prepared for the possible side effects.

Herbs

Herbs have been used for centuries by women in all cultures, but have not been studied to show safety of use or to give standard doses for induction. Current methods include use of evening primrose oil and black or blue cohosh. Evening primrose oil works by encouraging the production of prostaglandins. Black and blue cohosh work by stimulating contractions. These and other herbs are available in a variety of formulations from companies that specialize in herb preparation. If possible, speak with an herbalist in your community who can help you prepare a formula specific for your needs.

Methods of Medical Induction

If you are considering a medical induction, your midwife will want to assess the state of your cervix. If your cervix is not "ripe," meaning ready to stretch open, you are more likely to have a failed induction or a long and exhausting labor. Induction with unripe cervix is also more likely to result in a cesarean surgery.

The cervix is rated using Bishop Scoring. During a vaginal exam, your midwife will assess your cervix for effacement, dilation, its consistency and position to determine if it is ripe. There is some evidence using dilation alone may be more predictive of success, so if you score well enough to induce but have not dilated you may want to consider postponing the induction for a day or two.

Know Your Bishop's Score				
Score	0	1	2	3
Position	Posterior	Intermediate	Anterior	N/A
Consistency	Firm	Intermediate	Soft	N/A
Effacement	0 – 30%	40-50%	60-70%	80-100%
Dilation	>1cm	1 – 2 cm	2-4 cm	>4 cm
Fetal Station	-3	-2	-1 or 0	+1 or +2

If the induction cannot be postponed and your Bishop's Score is low, your cervix will need to be ripened before any serious attempts at starting labor can begin. The most successful method of cervical ripening is vaginal doses of prostaglandins. When given vaginally, prostaglandins increase the success rate of induction, decrease epidural use and give a small decrease in the number of cesarean surgeries. Oral doses of prostaglandins and IV oxytocin are ineffective and should not be used for cervical ripening.

Cervical ripening does have risks. Vaginal prostaglandins increase the risk of overstimulating the uterus and fetal heart rate abnormalities. There is a small danger of infection with insertion of the prostaglandin. The procedure can be uncomfortable, and it can be inconvenient to be admitted to a hospital overnight for ripening. In addition, *A guide to effective care in pregnancy and childbirth* states,

> No attempts should be made to ripen the cervix, unless there are valid grounds for ending the pregnancy artificially. None of the successful methods of cervical ripening act exclusively on the cervix.

Sweeping (stripping) the Membranes

Before using chemical methods to induce, some midwives prefer to try sweeping the membranes. During a vaginal exam, your midwife will insert a finger into the cervix, and if it is open enough she will pull the bag of waters away from the uterine wall. This can be uncomfortable during the procedure, and may cause a mild backache and some bleeding the rest of the day.

Sweeping the membranes is successful at decreasing the number of women who use chemical induction methods, and there is no evidence of increased infection rates. However, it does increase the frequency of prelabor rupture of the membranes. There is no information about how it affects other labor interventions.

Amniotomy

Amniotomy is the artificial breaking of the bag of waters. When your cervix is open enough, during a vaginal exam your midwife will insert a thin, hook-ended tool into your vagina to actually put a tear in the bag of waters. Some women find the procedure a little more uncomfortable than a vaginal exam, but it is completed quickly.

Because the bag of waters is broken, there is an increased risk of infection with amniotomy. Also, having an amniotomy means you commit to giving birth within a specified amount of time (24 to 48 hours); however, amniotomy alone has a very poor success rate of inducing labor. Oxytocin is generally used within the first few hours after the bag of waters has been broken to increase contractions. Amniotomy increases your risk of umbilical cord prolapse, bleeding and increases your baby's risk of heart rate abnormalities.

Oxytocin

Oxytocin is a hormone your body produces naturally during breastfeeding and intercourse. Synthetic forms of this hormone are used to stimulate contractions. Like amniotomy, oxytocin alone is often unsuccessful at inducing labor. The likelihood of successfully beginning labor increases when oxytocin is combined with an amniotomy. Oxytocin is administered through an IV, and levels are often regulated by a pump which allows the amount of oxytocin and IV fluids to be better controlled. It is assumed this helps prevent problems; however, no formal research has been done to support this theory.

Though synthetic oxytocin causes contractions, it does not have all the same effects of natural oxytocin. One important difference is synthetic oxytocin does not cause the mothering behavior women experience when natural oxytocin is released. Synthetic oxytocin also decreases the body's production of natural oxytocin, meaning once it is used, its use is likely to need to be continued. For oxytocin to have its fullest effects, it must be released in pulses. Synthetic oxytcin is continuously dripped, which may be why it requires such unnaturally high levels to achieve contractions (Odent & Odent, 2008).

Any medication that causes contractions increases your risk for excessive uterine contractions. This affects the blood flow to and from the placenta which can decrease your baby's access to oxygen. When receiving an oxytocin induction you will be required to use continuous fetal monitoring to track your baby's heart rate and ensure his safety. Uterine rupture is a rare complication with oxytocin. The likelihood of your baby having jaundice increases with use of oxytocin.

Prostaglandin

Your body naturally produces prostaglandins near the end of pregnancy and during labor. The prostaglandins help to ripen the cervix and stimulate uterine contractions. Though several ways of administering prostaglandin have been tried, the most successful method of inducing with prostaglandin is by vaginal application.

Prostaglandin is more effective at successfully starting labor than oxytocin. Although the numbers of women having given birth 12 hours after administration are similar, significantly more women have given birth at 24 and 48 hours when prostaglandin is used. Also, the rate of induced labors ending in cesarean surgery or an instrumental delivery is lower with prostaglandin than with oxytocin.

The risks of prostaglandin induction are similar to oxytocin induction in regards to your baby's heart rate and uterine hyperstimulation. However, when the bag of waters is broken, use of prostaglandin increases the risk your baby will receive antibiotics or be administered to the ICU for more than 24 hours. Because prostaglandins for use in labor are expensive and unstable, it is not always available.

Mistoprostol

Mistoprostol is an ulcer medication containing prostaglandin. It has not been registered for obstetric use, so it has not undergone the extensive testing to determine appropriate dosage or safety in labor. Despite that, it has become popular as a labor inducer because it is inexpensive and easily stored, unlike the prostaglandin preparations made for labor.

When administered vaginally, mistoprostol is more effective at beginning labor than oxytocin. Though it shows promise, mistoprostol use increases rates of meconium staining, hyperstimulation of the uterus and fetal heart rate changes. Because mistoprostol is a tablet inserted into the vagina, it can be difficult or impossible to decrease the dose if a bad reaction happens. Using lower doses decreases the risk of hyperstimulation, but also decreases the effectiveness of the induction. The available research is inconclusive on rates of inductions that end in cesarean surgery. The lack of research on its safety causes concern among many professionals and is the reason its use is not recommended in *A guide to effective care in pregnancy and childbirth*.

Pain Management Options

Medications for the management of pain in labor present a peculiar problem for an expectant mother.

On the one hand, many caregivers and women believe it is cruel and unethical to allow a person to remain in intense pain when you are able to do something to safely alleviate the pain. On the other hand is the fact that there is very little evidence on the safety of pain medications for labor in terms of how it affects the labor process or the mother and baby.

On one hand is the expectation among birth attendants and the general public that less pain in labor equates to a more satisfying experience. On the other hand is the evidence that shows pain and pain relief do not play major roles in childbirth satisfaction.

On one hand is the claim that women have the widest selection of medical ways to deal with labor pain ever possible. On the other hand is the reality that the range of choices for individuals is usually very limited.

Regional analgesia

The most widely used pain medication technique in the United States is regional analgesia, the most common form referred to as an epidural, which is used by 76 percent of laboring women (Declercq, Sakala, Corry & Applebaum, 2006). Regional analgesia is gaining popularity in other parts of the world as well. It is used in 45 percent of vaginal births in Canada (as high as 60 percent in some provinces) and 25 percent in New Zealand (Canadian Institute for Health Information, 2004; New Zealand Health Information Service, 2006). This popularity stems from regional analgesia's very high effectiveness at reducing or removing pain. It provides better and more lasting relief than other forms of pain medication, and mothers who receive it are more satisfied with their analgesia than mothers who choose other forms of medication.

The main difference between an epidural and a spinal is a thin membrane separating the epidural space from the spinal fluid. A spinal will result in faster pain relief, so many hospitals now offer a combined spinal/epidural. To use an epidural, you will need to first receive IV fluids to help prevent a drop in blood pressure. Once you have received enough fluids, an anesthesiologist will prepare your lower back with antiseptic and a local anesthetic. When ready, a large needle will be inserted between your vertebrae into the epidural space. A test dose of the medication will ensure the needle is inserted properly.

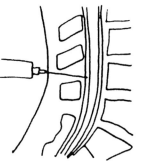

The difference between an epidural and a spinal is one thin membrane.

Once the needle is properly positioned, a small flexible tube will be inserted through the needle. The needle will then be removed and the tube will remain inserted throughout the rest of your labor. The anesthesiologist will tape the tube in place so you do not bump it. You will then be assisted into a comfortable position and the tube will be used to administer medications either continuously with a pump or at regularly scheduled intervals.

Whether or not the benefit of decreased pain outweighs the risks can be hard to determine. Epidural analgesia increases the likelihood of a longer second stage of labor, instrumental delivery and maternal fever. Epidural analgesia decreases the mother's blood pressure, which may be helpful for women with high blood pressure but decreases the oxygen available for the baby in women with normal blood pressure. It is associated with increased use of oxytocin to augment labor and may increase the length of first stage labor.

Epidural analgesia increases the likelihood of fetal malposition and has a possible association with increased cesarean surgery rates. There may also be an association with increased third and fourth degree perineal tears.

Little is known about the affects on the baby because very little research has been done. The current research shows conflicting results. One review of the literature found an increase in fetal heart rate abnormalities while a similar review found no difference (Caton et al., 2002). The data is confusing because most available research is done to determine what method provides the most pain relief, not the safety of the procedure. The research usually compares a regional medication to another type of medication instead of comparing the use of medication to a physiological birth.

Complicating the decision on regional analgesia further is the fact that procedures used differ significantly between hospitals. Some hospitals will provide regional analgesia at any point in labor, while others restrict it to specific progress, such as after reaching 5 centimeters dilation. There are also variations in the distribution of the medication, either a continuous infusion or "topping-up" the medication at intervals or when necessary. Hospitals each have their preferred mix of medications and dosages, so comparing the results of studies is not always possible since you may be comparing two different procedures.

What policies do your local hospitals have about epidurals?

Some hospitals provide lower dose epidurals or combined epidural/spinal analgesia in an attempt to reduce the side effects by using less medication. Unfortunately, there is no difference in operative delivery rates between low and normal dose epidurals. When opioids (narcotic drugs) are used for a combined epidural/spinal, the risks remain the same as a standard epidural but with the additional risks of itchiness, urinary retention and delayed respiratory depression for the mother.

Where the lower dose epidurals are used, women are sometimes told they will be able to move or walk during labor. The reality is most women who receive regional analgesia spend very little time out of bed. This may be due to the drowsiness felt by women who received opioids, fatigue from the labor itself, feeling unstable or weak because of the medication, the presence of wires and tubes necessary for medication confine movements or the lack of assistance with ambulation.

Another factor to consider is the complex interplay of interventions used for regional analgesia. The variety of ways regional analgesia affects labor has led the World Health Organization to state, "If epidural analgesia is administered to a low-risk pregnant woman, it is questionable whether the resulting procedure can still be called 'normal labour'" (1997). While using an epidural you will be continuously monitored by an electronic fetal monitor, receive intravenous fluids which start before administration of the epidural, and may receive more frequent blood pressure and temperature checks. You will have a high chance of receiving synthetic oxytocin to speed labor and also of catheterization to empty your bladder. Each of these interventions has risks of its own that are added to the risk of the epidural medication when they are used.

Many women have an idealized image of labor with an epidural being blissful and easy. However, the actual use of an epidural can look and feel more like being in the intensive care unit than having a baby. An epidural requires a catheter in your back, two monitor leads on your belly and IV fluids attached to your arm–for a total of four wires hooked to your body. Epidurals can often require a blood pressure cuff attached to your arm, a urine catheter, a pulse meter on your finger, an oxygen mask over your nose and mouth, and the external monitors exchanged for internal monitors (meaning they are inserted into your uterus through your vagina)—for a total of eight wires hooked to your body.

How real are these risks?
Percentage of women who experienced based on 19 studies (Caton et al, 2002):
Itching—62% with opioids, 0-4% without
Urinary Retention—28-61% of women catheterized
Sedation—21%
Hypotension—0-50%
No Ambulation—34-85%

If you decide the benefits of an epidural outweigh its risks for your situation, you will want to be aware of a few things that can help improve your satisfaction with this form of pain relief.

1. Regional analgesia requires an anesthesiologist for administration. If your hospital does not provide 24-hour service or if the anesthesiologist is working with another patient, you may need to wait before an epidural can be inserted. For this reason, you will want to be ready to use a few non-medical comfort measures to help you get through until the epidural is in place.

2. Your risk of an operative delivery (cesarean, forceps or vacuum) decreases if you continue the epidural and delay pushing until the baby's head descends enough to be visible. This may also decrease your fatigue. There is no evidence turning off the epidural for pushing is more effective than waiting for the baby's head to appear (sometimes called laboring down).

3. Empty your bladder and have your dilation checked before the epidural is inserted. Emptying your bladder will help decrease the chances you will need to be catheterized and may allow your baby to descend deeper into the pelvis. This may help prevent a malpresentation or may cause you to complete dilation depending on how far in the labor process you are.

4. About 10 percent of women who used regional analgesia found it was not very helpful or not helpful at all. If you find the medication is not having your expected effect, be sure to let the hospital staff know so adjustments can be made.

Systemic Agents

Systemic agents, opioids or narcotics such as pethidine and demerol, are given by injection or through an IV. They provide some relief from pain, but not to the extent an epidural will. Overall 75 percent of the mothers found them at least somewhat helpful (Declercq, Sakala, Corry & Applebaum, 2006). The effects of these medications wear off within one to two hours at which time the pain will return. A technique in which the medication is administered as needed by the mother through an IV provided better pain relief with a lower total dose of medication than standard injections, but is not yet available in all hospitals.

Systemic agents have more visible side effects for mothers and babies than epidurals do, which may be a reason epidurals are considered "safe." Like epidurals, systemic agents can cause a drop in maternal blood pressure, which decreases the available oxygen for the baby, causing fetal distress. Systemic agents have the added side effects of nausea, vomiting, dizziness and delayed stomach emptying.

In addition, systemic agents cross the placenta in high enough concentrations to cause respiratory depression in the baby if given too close to the actual birth. They are associated with lower Apgar scores and behavioral abnormalities. There is concern fetal exposure to opiates during labor is associated with self-destructive and addictive behaviors later in life, although any conclusion about its effects will be difficult to determine.

Despite their risks, systemic agents are used in many hospitals not equipped for epidural analgesia. They are also used to provide immediate relief when an anesthesiologist is not available, since an anesthesiologist is not needed for their administration. If you decide systemic agents provide the right benefits for your needs, be prepared with comfort measures that can make the side effects less frustrating.

Remember, each labor is unique and so is every woman. You cannot know ahead of time how your body or your baby will handle a medication. You will probably experience one or two of the most common side effects, but probably not all of them.

Inhalation analgesia

In the UK, Canada and Australia, inhalation analgesia is widely available. Of the women who use this form of medication, 85 percent rate its pain relief as "good" or "very good" even though it provides incomplete pain relief (Caton et al., 2002). The form of administration may fuel the satisfaction rate; when you want more pain relief you put the mask to your face and inhale. This gives women a sense of control important to a satisfying labor.

The effects of the medication (most commonly 50 percent nitrous oxide) wear off quickly when you stop inhaling it, and it does not appear to interfere with the physiology of labor like an epidural can. There is also less need for other interventions than when an epidural is used. Babies appear to be clinically unaffected by the procedure, perhaps due to the rapid decline in its effects when inhalation stops. Because of this, timing the inhalation with the pain can be difficult.

There is the possibility of nausea and vomiting. The greatest risk is loss of consciousness, which happens rarely and even less when it is self-administered. During self-administration you will hold the mask to your face when you need pain relief. The analgesia will make you drowsy, which makes it nearly impossible to hold the mask at the face. Almost immediately after you remove the mask, the effects of the analgesia begin to wear off.

Sedatives

Sedatives may be recommended early in labor if your caregiver believes you need help to rest or if you are highly anxious. They have no analgesic properties; they simply make you relaxed or downright sleepy. They do cross the placenta and can have profound effects on your baby including poor sucking, breathing problems, decreased alertness and a decreased attention span. In addition, they may cause fetal heart rate abnormalities during labor.

Handling Medication Side Effects

If you experience side effects from a pain medication, these tools might help you manage any discomfort.

Nausea/vomiting
Cool cloths or ice to the forehead or neck
Peppermint lozenges
Peppermint or lavender essential oils
Fennel or ginger tea
Sugar water
Nubain
Mouthwash

Itching
Apply cool cloths to the skin
Use ice packs on the most uncomfortable areas
Narcan/naloxone/nubain IV (reduces pain relief)
Avoid fentanyl in the next dose (reduces pain relief)
Diphenhydramine (Benadryl) (reduces pain relief)

Shivering
Warm IV fluid
Warm blankets
Complete relaxation/ hypnotic state

Fetal Distress (Poor Heart Tones)
Change positions frequently
Change to an upright position (may need assistance)
Use an oxygen mask
Double check the results with a different type of test

Pain Medications and Labor Satisfaction

Though women who use pain medication report satisfaction with the pain relief felt, this does not always translate to overall satisfaction with labor. This is significant because many women and their caregivers mistakenly believe less pain means a better labor experience. In reality, the amount of pain felt is insignificant in the overall satisfaction with labor unless the amount of pain felt was significantly greater than anticipated.

Four factors are strongly related to satisfaction with the childbirth experience (Caton et al., 2002):

1. The amount of support you receive from caregivers

2. The quality of your relationship with your caregivers

3. Your involvement with decision-making

4. Your personal expectations

Caregiver support

It is not enough for your caregiver to be available to you in labor; she must be providing supportive activities. These include both physical and emotional measures to make you more comfortable such as position changes, massage, eye contact, praise and encouragement and help in understanding the purposes of the procedures happening to you.

What sources of support do you have for labor?

Though most women expect the labor nurse to help them through the experience, the reality of hospital work provides for very little supportive contact. Less than 10 percent of a labor nurse's time is actually spent on support. In an evaluation of low risk women giving birth in a teaching hospital, the women were "attended" by 16 different people within a span of 6 hours, but were left alone for most of those 6 hours. On average you may have over six and up to fourteen different staff members participate in your care—but that care will be attending to procedures, not support.

When you use pain medications, your behavior and the behavior of your companions change. Because you will no longer seem "in need," the amount of emotional and physical support you receive decreases. Although you may have relief from painful contractions, that does not reduce the amount of emotional support you will need. When pain medications decrease the amount of support you receive, they can have a negative impact on your overall childbirth satisfaction.

Relationship with Caregiver

If you are unable or unwilling to express concerns, fears, need for comfort or general questions to your caregiver, you do not have a good relationship. You should be comfortable talking with her, leaving your prenatal visits feeling that your questions were answered and she cares for you. If you feel uncomfortable with her during pregnancy, you will feel uncomfortable with her in the same ways during labor. Not feeling free to express concerns or needs can leave you less satisfied with your childbirth experience.

How would you describe your relationship with your caregiver?

The use of pain medication is not likely to change your relationship with your caregiver. On the other hand, your relationship with your caregivers is likely to affect your use of pain medication. At least 10 percent of mothers report having been pressured by their caregiver to accept an induction, pain medication or cesarean section. Only 10 percent of the women refused anything the caregiver recommended (Declercq, Sakala, Corry & Applebaum, 2006).

Decision Making

A sense of control over what is happening is the key component to feeling satisfied with childbirth. Women who feel helpless or unable to affect what is happening to them leave childbirth discouraged. In general, a woman who receives pain medication for labor loses much of her control over the process (unless the control she wants is to have medication as quickly as possible). This is especially true for epidural analgesia, which requires many other interventions and can change the way the labor progresses.

> In what ways can medication reduce your control over labor? In what ways can it increase your control?

Personal Expectations

A general assumption about childbirth is to expect the worst, the belief being that when you are realistic about what is going to happen, you can be better prepared. But it is the women who have positive expectations of childbirth, and their ability to cope with it, who have the most satisfaction with labor (Caton et al, 2002). This may be related to the anxiety felt by women when they assume they cannot handle childbirth. There is a marked difference between being realistic and being overcome by fear. Or it may be because women who are more confident in their ability to work with labor are more likely to work with their bodies in labor and therefore more successful at managing their contractions.

> What expectations do you have about labor?

What is unexplainable is that the personal expectation is consistently more important than the actual pain felt. If it only occurred among Christian women, it might be said to be the result of faith, trust and hope in God. However, the effect of this attitude goes beyond Christianity to all women (at least in developed countries where it has been researched). Is it possible that part of the miracle of faith is that the change in attitude experienced when fear is overcome and actions are in faith make profound differences in the way humans experience life?

The use of pain medications may be related to your expectations of labor. Some women expect to have them available quickly; others expect not to use them. Unless your experience deviates greatly from your expectation, the use or non-use of pain medication is not likely to effect your satisfaction with the labor experience.

Availability of Pain Medications

If you are lucky, you will be given a choice about what type of medication is used for pain. Often the circumstances of your labor leave you with only one option that you must either take or leave. Though there is a wide variety of pain medications that have been used for comfort in childbirth, the most common methods are the three listed previously. Many of the other medical pain management techniques you may read about such as the paracervical block and peudendal block, have disappeared from practice in many areas or are only used in rare situations.

Depending on where you plan to give birth, you may or may not have access to all three types of pain medication. For example, although Canada's statistics for 2001-02 showed a 45 percent epidural rate, the distribution across the country was not equal. In the Northwest Territories only 4 percent of women used epidurals, while 60 percent of women used them in Quebec (Canadian Institute for Health Information, 2004). Smaller hospitals which do less births per year may not devote their resources to ensure every woman has access to an epidural, especially when the World Health Organization states the demand for them is culture driven and, "They are no part of essential care during childbirth" (World Health Organization, 1997).

In addition to the availability of a medication, your caregivers' attitudes about the different types of medication will influence what is available to you. Whatever method your caregivers believe to be the safest or most effective is likely to be what is offered to you in labor. Because women in labor tend to agree with whatever is suggested, your choices for pain relief will consist of whatever your caregivers are most likely to recommend.

Other, less predictable factors will also influence what options are actually available to you once you are in labor. If you are in a busy hospital on a very busy day, or in a small hospital with an "on call" epidural service in the middle of the night, you may not be agreeable to the long wait for an anesthesiologist to administer an epidural. If you decide you need something for the pain when you are dilated to 8 or 9 centimeters, systemic agents may no longer be an option to you because of the risk your baby will be born before the medication wears off.

Alternatives to Pain Medication

There are no easy answers to help you determine if pain medication is a good choice for your baby's birth. However, there are some alternatives to planned pain medication you might want to learn more about before you make any decisions.

The first alternative is use of continuous labor support. Women who receive this type of care are not only less likely to request pain medication, but also less likely to experience the most common problems during labor. Continuous support can be from your midwife or from a doula. You can read about the services of both in the topic on Birth Attendants in the Birth Options section.

Another alternative is water. Women who labor while immersed in a tub report less pain. In fact, the respondents of the Listening to Mothers II survey rated the effectiveness of laboring in water as helpful as an epidural. Depending on where you give birth, you may have the option of laboring or giving birth while immersed in water.

Home birth provides a more comfortable option for labor than a hospital environment. In a hospital, routine, though unfamiliar, procedures, the presence of strangers and being left alone during labour and/or delivery caused stress, and stress can interfere with the course of birth by prolonging it and setting off what the World Health Organization describes as a "cascade of interventions" (1997).

Staying home gives you the freedom to be in control, to stay relaxed and allow yourself to continue normal activities as long as possible. Families who have experienced both home and hospital birth say the experiences are so different they cannot even be compared.

Newborn Care

Once your baby is here, your first question will undoubtedly be, "Is my baby healthy?" To assess your baby's overall health, your midwife will take a look at your baby to ensure all is well. This can take place with the baby near you, or even with you holding your baby for most of the evaluation.

Most important is your baby's breathing and heart rate. If your perineum is left intact, the compression of the perineum against your baby's body causes excess mucus to be spit out the mouth and nose while being born. Your midwife may simply wipe the nose with gauze to clear any residual mucus. If there was a tear or an episiotomy, the perineum will not put sufficient pressure on the baby to expel mucus. In this case, your midwife will use a bulb syringe to quickly suction the mouth and nose. If necessary, your midwife will use a larger suction device to suction excess mucus from your baby's lungs.

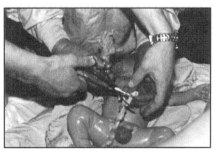
©2002 Jennifer Vanderlaan
Waiting for the cord to stop pulsing before you cut it has benefits.

Many families have someone special cut the umbilical cord. In most cases it is best to wait until the cord stops pulsing before it is cut. Simply place your baby on your chest and wait for nature to take its course. Cutting the cord before it stops pulsing has risks. The first issue is that as long as the cord is pulsing, your baby is receiving oxygen through it. Secondly, allowing the cord to stop pulsing naturally while your baby rests on your chest ensures your baby receives the right amount of blood. When and who will cut the cord is not always an option. If your baby's cord is wrapped tightly around his neck, your midwife may quickly clamp and cut it to give your baby room to be born.

The Apgar rating is a subjective, visual evaluation of your baby's overall health. Your baby will be evaluated at one minute and again at five minutes and given a number between zero and ten. The lower the number, the higher the possibility your baby will need help. Your baby will be evaluated for his skin tone, pulse, response to stimulation, muscle tone and breathing effort. Depending on your baby's condition, he will be given a score between zero and two for each category. The final Apgar score is the sum of the scores for the categories. The Apgar score does not diagnose any problem. Instead it alerts your caregivers to the potential for a problem. Babies with low Apgar scores will be watched closer in the first minutes and possibly days after being born.

Once it is assessed that your baby is OK, attention will turn to other indicators of health. Your baby's weight and length will be measured along with the circumference of the head. The abdomen will be felt to ensure the internal organs seem right. Your baby's mouth will be assessed for any cleft palate. If your baby is a boy, the genitals will be checked to see if the testes have descended. Through these and other observations being performed at the same time, your midwife is able to reasonably establish that your baby is healthy and developed properly for his age.

Newborn babies lose body heat very quickly. To help your baby maintain appropriate temperature, your midwife will put a hat on your baby's head. The baby will then be placed directly on your skin and you will both be covered with warm blankets for the first hours. If you are unable, your husband can do the job. Hospitals have warming bassinets that can be used when no one is able to hold the baby for those first two hours. The bassinets should only be back-up, since they do pose the risk of your baby overheating and do not allow the skin to skin contact both mother and baby need to help adjust hormone levels.

Along with the routine assessment of your new baby, you may have options of other procedures to help ensure your baby's overall health. Although these are options, where you give birth may limit how optional they are.

Many communities require routine administration of one or more of these procedures. However, within the requirements there is the ability to wait a maximum amount of time before having the procedure done. Check with your midwife or hospital to find out your community's requirements and what options you have within the procedures.

You should also be aware that although these procedures can improve the health of newborns, there is some debate about the wisdom of routinely using them on all children. Concerns about the routine administration are included for your review. Some families have peace about using every newborn procedure, others do not have peace even after studying the available research and talking to their midwives. Use your judgment to help you determine what God is telling you about your child, so you can make a wise decision.

Vitamin K Shot

Vitamin K is a factor in blood that causes it to clot (stop bleeding), and is given to newborns to prevent hemorrhagic disease of the newborn. Newborns have a naturally low level of Vitamin K that steadily rises to peak levels at eight days of life and then descends back to normal levels around the tenth day of life. Because of this, babies who may have internal bleeding due to a difficult birth, are premature or will have a circumcision or other surgery performed will be given Vitamin K. In many places it is required by law for all newborns because of its potential to save lives.

There are two ways to administer Vitamin K, orally and by injection. The injection hurts a bit for the baby and provides protection in one dose. The oral dose does not taste good, is given as a series of doses within the first weeks of life and must be given carefully to ensure the baby swallows. Both forms of vitamin K work equally well.

Because of the mandatory vitamin K injection, the natural rate of hemorrhagic disease of the newborn is not known. The last research available from the 1950s shows rates of four babies per one thousand had hemorrhagic disease. However, this may be unnaturally high due to the high incidence of birth trauma and the delay in breastfeeding.

> Frequency of late onset hemorrhagic disease
> 2nd–10th weeks of life (Enkin et al., 2000).
> No Vitamin K—1 baby out of 17,000
> One Oral Dose*—1 baby out of 25,000–70,000
> Injection—1 baby out of 400,000
> *Oral vitamin K is given in several doses

There are two concerns this gives to families. The first is that low levels of vitamin K are normal for newborns, and artificially increasing it may make subtle changes not yet understood. For example, babies who receive vitamin K have an increased risk of newborn jaundice. The second concern is whether it is wise to inject a newborn with a substance that would otherwise have been ingested, especially if the oral dose is able to provide similar success of preventing the disease.

Eye Ointment

Within the first hour after birth, your baby may receive an antibiotic ointment applied to his eyes. The antibiotic is believed to prevent eye infections and blindness from the bacteria that cause chlamydia and gonorrhea. In many areas eye ointment is required even if you test negatively for these bacteria.

Although it is considered required for newborns, there have been no controlled studies to compare the effectiveness of routine antibiotics to the effectiveness of carefully monitoring the baby's eyes and intervening if signs of conjunctivitis appear. Administration of the ointment will cause the baby's vision to become blurry so many parents request it be delayed as long as possible. If you are certain you do not have chlamydia or gonorrhea, you may be able to successfully refuse this procedure.

Blood Testing

If there is concern about your baby's Rh factor, blood may be collected from the umbilical cord to determine your baby's blood type. Other blood tests are done by pricking your baby's foot to obtain a sample. The most common blood test is called the PKU (phenylketonuria) which tests for a collection of rare disorders that can cause problems for your baby. Sometimes blood is tested for levels of bilirubin if there is concern your baby may be jaundiced.

In many areas, the PKU test is required by law to be conducted at least 24-48 hours after birth. The purpose of the test is to determine any issues the baby may have before they become problems. For example, if your baby has phenylketonuria (about 1 in 12,000 babies), certain amino acids will not be digested properly and can lead to poor development or cause mental retardation. If you know your baby will have issues with certain amino acids, a special diet can prevent the problems. You can check with your midwife or hospital to find out what blood tests are required for your area.

Vaccinations

Some vaccinations are given in a series of shots. Find out how many shots are required for the standard vaccination plan in your community.

If your baby is born in a hospital, you will be asked to begin routine vaccinations before your baby goes home. Vaccinations are injections that contain bacteria or viruses in a state that almost always prevents the disease from occurring but tricks your body into fighting off the disease, thereby producing immunity. The number of vaccinations offered to your child will be somewhat determined by the laws where you live. Your pediatrician should be able to tell you which vaccines your child will be expected to have before beginning school and what you may need to do to legally refuse them.

The main concern with vaccinations is the safety of other compounds used to create the vaccine. Depending on the vaccine used, it may contain aluminum, formaldehyde, animal DNA and antibiotics. Until recently, many vaccines included mercury, causing children to receive more mercury in the first six months of life than is considered safe by the EPA. Because it is not fully understood how these substances impact babies, many families choose to delay vaccinations or forego them altogether.

Another concern some Christian families have with vaccinations is the use of fetal tissue in the development of the vaccines. Some vaccines require human tissue to be grown well, and are grown in aborted fetal tissue. Some Christian families find this a double insult for the child whose life was sacrificed through abortion, so although they have no concerns about the safety of the vaccines, they choose not to use them for moral reasons.

Circumcision

There is, perhaps, no more heated debate among expecting Christian parents than whether or not a male child should be circumcised. The conflicting facts, opinions and Biblical references can leave you confused and frustrated. Sometimes it feels you cannot make the right decision because you are not "Christian" enough if your son is intact and you are cruel if you circumcise.

> What pressures have you felt regarding circumcision?

There are generally three factors that go into the decision to circumcise or not to circumcise. Families weigh God's commands in the Bible, medical benefits and risks, and social issues to determine how they will proceed. Your family may put more weight on one factor than another family. Your family may consider all the information and make a different decision than another family. Regardless of how you make your decision, you are only responsible to God and your son for the decision you make.

Circumcision in the Bible

The actual practice of circumcision predates written history, and predates God's covenant with Abraham. Though circumcision was not first practiced by the Israelites, God did require it as part of the covenant made with Abraham. Every boy was to be circumcised on the eighth day of life for the generations to come. The boy received his name during the circumcision ceremony.

Genesis 17:10-14

Luke 1:59

Any male not circumcised was to be cut off from his people. Even slaves that were born into the household or bought were to be circumcised, although they were not necessarily considered Israelites. After the Exodus, circumcision is required to participate in the Passover. It seems circumcision gave a way for a non-Israelite male to convert to following the God of Abraham and made a separation between God's people and the Gentiles.

Exodus 12:48

Though God remained the same, the requirement changed after Jesus' death. Ephesians 2:11-15 says the death of Christ was to render the separation of circumcision no longer necessary because what had been two separate peoples would now be one. Whether or not a Christian needed to first become an Israelite through circumcision was a hotly debated topic.

Ephesians 2:11-15

After much discussion on the need for circumcision, Peter reminds the apostles that God chose to show his favor on the Gentiles without their having been circumcised. It was their faith that purified their hearts, not circumcision. Paul is very firm with the new converts to Christianity that submitting to circumcision was submitting to the law and all of its requirements, and that being circumcised does not help you obey the law, instead it puts the attention on the flesh instead of the heart. Paul states that as soon as you break one part of the law, it is as if you were uncircumcised and goes on further to say that it is not circumcision of the flesh that is important, but circumcision of the heart which can only be done by the Spirit.

Galatians 5:1-4

Galatians 6:12-16

Romans 2:25-29

1 Corinthians 7:17-19

The conclusion of the New Testament, then, is that being intact or circumcised means nothing to God. God cares not about the marking of the flesh but the heart that is willing to keep his commandments. Though God did require the circumcision of every boy on the eighth day, Paul apparently does not consider this requirement of the covenant a commandment.

If you decide your son should be circumcised for religious reasons, you should be sure to follow the religious prescription for circumcision on the eighth day (having a hospital circumcision does not count as a Jewish circumcision). Hiring a Mohel can help you understand the religious ceremony surrounding it and the differences between what is currently practiced as circumcision and the original Biblical cut.

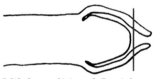

Milah, traditional Jewish circumcision cut location.

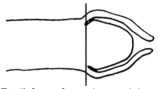

Peri'ah, modern circumcision cut location.

Until about 140 CE, circumcision cut only the tip of the foreskin, leaving a short piece of skin that covered the glans. The procedure, called *milah*, is the original circumcision of Abraham. Though it cut only a small portion of the foreskin, *milah* was looked down upon by Greeks and Romans. Some Jewish men stretched the foreskin in a procedure called *epispastikós* to appear uncircumcised (Schultheiss, Truss, Stief, Jonas, 1998).

The Roman emperor Hadrian forbad circumcision, leading many Jewish men to stretch the cut foreskin to appear uncircumcised. This practice was rejected by orthodox Jews. When the law was lifted they instituted a new circumcision technique. The new procedure, *peri'ah*, stripped the foreskin from the glans for removal making it impossible to appear uncircumcised.

This leaves families with many things to consider before they decide on circumcision for Biblical reasons. If you decide to circumcise to keep the requirements God gave to the Israelites when a baby was born, you may also want to consider redeeming your first born son and observing the purification after childbirth.

Exodus 34:19-20
Leviticus 12

Medical Benefits and Risks

The consideration of medical reasons for circumcision must begin with the understanding that an intact penis is the way God created the male body. The foreskin is a highly specialized functioning organ. It accounts for 80 percent of the penile skin, extending beyond the glans and folding over itself to attach again at the base of the glans. It keeps the glans soft and moist, protecting the glans not only by covering it but by producing oils that help keep the glans healthy and clean.

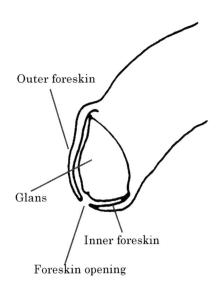

The foreskin provides extra skin to allow for erection of the penis. The foreskin is highly sensitive; when it is removed not only does the man lose the sensation from the foreskin, but the glans also becomes less sensitive without its protection. Removal of the foreskin can change the experience of sexual intimacy for both the man and his wife.

An intact foreskin is not "dirty." In fact, the oils produced by the foreskin help to keep the skin clean and healthy in the same way the cervical mucus helps keep the vagina healthy. The smegma produced is easily rinsed away. There is no need to worry about cleaning under the foreskin until it detaches from the glans naturally. Once it does detach, it is no more difficult to keep clean than vaginal folds. Boys with intact foreskins are perfectly capable of learning to retract the skin in the shower to allow the water to rinse the glans.

Circumcision is an elective surgery; this means you can choose to have it or choose not to have it because there is no medical reason to recommend it routinely be done. Circumcision is the only surgery regularly performed in the hopes of preventing rare conditions. There is no recommendation by any medical body for the routine circumcision of newborns. For the few illnesses in which circumcision may be helpful, the decision should be made on a case by case basis. It does not prevent penile cancer nor the transmission of sexually transmitted diseases.

Recent studies have suggested circumcision reduces the likelihood of a man contracting HIV from a woman; however, the studies were ended early leading critics to point out the difference in infection rate may have been due to the abstinence required by the circumcised men and not the circumcision itself (World Health Organization, 2007). There is no evidence it prevents a woman from contracting HIV from a man. If circumcision can reduce the incidence of HIV, it does not provide complete protection. Circumcised men can still contract HIV, HIV positive circumcised men can infect sexual partners, and circumcision does not protect anyone from the other ways to contract HIV.

Circumcision is a surgical procedure, which means it carries the same risks of all surgery including infection, excessive bleeding, pain and mistake. If you decide your son should be circumcised for medical reasons, be sure the doctor you hire will use an anesthetic to minimize the amount of pain your son feels. Prepare yourself for some behavioral changes, as circumcised boys seem to show an increased sensitivity in the first few months of life, and may have trouble with breastfeeding and bonding while recovering.

Social Issues to Consider

Many circumcisions are done for the sake of family tradition or out of concern the son will not be accepted into society if he is not circumcised. Fathers are sometimes concerned about what the son will think if his penis looks different from dad's. You will need to determine how often you expect your child to see his father's naked body, especially how often he will see it after he is old enough to care about the difference.

Another common concern is how the boy will feel if his penis is different from his friends, if he will be teased. The number of boys circumcised varies from very low to about 75 percent depending on where in the world you live. This means your son has a very good chance of not being the only boy with his particular type of penis in the locker room.

There is another way to look at the social issue, and that is to remember we are not to please other humans but to please God. As a parent, you will most likely teach your child that he is to do what is right regardless of the decisions made by those around him. If you want your child to have the strength to make the right decision even when it is hard, perhaps your decision about circumcision should not be made on ensuring he looks like everyone else. Perhaps you need to be willing to talk with you son about his penis and why it is different instead of deciding it is easier to do what you think everyone else is doing.

Galatians 1:10

At the other end of the circumcision social issue is the belief that amputating a part of a person's sexual organs without their consent is a violation of their rights. Regardless of what you may believe about circumcision, it is your son who must accept the risks. If you do not feel comfortable forcing your child to have this procedure without a medical reason, perhaps it would be best if you waited until he was old enough to be part of the decision making process.

In some cultures, women undergo circumcision around the time of puberty. In a female circumcision, the clitoris, and possibly one or both of the labia are removed. This is done for various reasons that range from opinion to falsehood. In the areas where it is practiced, they say the circumcised vagina is more attractive, helps the woman to stay clean and healthy, prevents her from cheating on her husband and ensures virginity. Unfortunately, it often results in infection, painful intercourse and problems when giving birth. This is a sobering reminder just how much a culture dictates what is considered acceptable to its people.

From Decision to Reality

Having studied the options available to you, you have probably made some preliminary choices about what you would and would not like during labor. The next thing to learn is how to make your choices a reality.

Half the respondents to the Listening to Mother's II Survey agreed with the statement, "Birth should not be interfered with unless medically necessary." Only one out of four of the respondents disagreed with the statement. Presumably, a large percentage of these women had hoped they would have a birth as free of intervention as possible. However, the results show very few of these women actually achieved that goal.

> For every 10 mothers who gave birth vaginally:
> 9 had Continuous EFM
> 8 had an IV
> 7 had an epidural or spinal
> 6 had their membranes broken during labor
> 5 had artificial oxytocin to speed labor
> 4 had a catheter to remove urine
> 3 had labor artificially started (although 4 attempted)
> 2 had an episiotomy

Sometimes an expectant mom begins to think what is happening to her is so unique that things just are not happening properly in her labor, and she must be part of the few who truly need medical assistance. However, these statistics show it is not just a few unlucky mothers. These statistics demonstrate that procedures which should be rare are performed on at least half of all American women.

The World Health Organization (WHO) recommends an overall induction rate of one in ten mothers or less. The Coalition for Improving Maternity Services (CIMS) agrees with them, and *A guide to effective care in pregnancy and childbirth* calls induction, "one of the most drastic ways of intervening in the natural process of pregnancy and childbirth." Yet two out of ten mothers in the United States, United Kingdom, New Zealand and Canada are medically induced. three out ten first-time mothers in Australia are medically induced.

The WHO and CIMS both recommend against the use of continuous electronic fetal monitoring. The Guide to Effective Care in Pregnancy and Childbirth lists continuous electronic fetal monitoring as ineffective or harmful. Yet nine out of ten mothers in the Listening to Mothers Survey received continuous fetal monitoring.

The WHO finds no justification for routine use of episiotomy, and CIMS recommends it be done at less than one out of twenty of births. Yet five out of twenty women in the LTMII survey were given an episiotomy. Seventeen percent of Australian women and 23 percent of Canadian women are given episiotomies. The WHO states there is no valid reason for artificial rupture of membranes during a normal labor. Fifty-nine percent of the women in the LTMII survey had their membranes artificially ruptured.

The WHO and CIMS both agree cesarean surgery should be performed in between 5 and 15 percent of labors. Rates below 5 percent might indicate women who need assistance do not have access to care. Rates above 15 percent indicate cesareans are being done when not medically necessary, which increases the risk to both mother and baby without any benefit. Yet in the United States and Australia, about 30 percent of all births are by cesarean. Canada, the United Kingdom and New Zealand have rates around 23 percent.

Many of the statistics about giving birth in modern hospitals are disturbing. However, understanding the facts about your birth choices is important to making wise decisions. It is unfair and cruel that many women mistakenly believe they can have whatever they like during labor only to find out the decisions are made for them. It is only through ongoing, open dialogue with your midwife that you will truly understand what choices are and are not available to you.

Why do women in labor have medical interventions at such high rates? There are many theories; you will have read discussions of some of these topics in other sections of this book. Although it may never be possible to determine which of the theories are most responsible, the reality is they may all play a part.

Which of these theories have you heard? Do you have reasons to believe one or more play a large part in the birth choices where you live?

- Labor hurts more than women expect and so they decide to have an epidural.
- Though epidural is described as something with low risk, it makes major changes to the birth process.
- The hospital environment itself can cause problems— he intervention rate is much higher when low-risk women give birth in a hospital.
- Because of their need to diagnose and treat abnormality, doctors are not trained in ways to assist normal birth and so must rely on the interventions.
- Fear causes labor to become dysfunctional, and modern culture fears birth.
- Medical systems do not provide the continuous support necessary for labor.
- Women are not interested in natural birth even when they say they are.

Regardless of the reasons interventions are done, there are some ways to help ensure they are not done when you do not want them. There are several things you can do now, although they may not all be effective in your situation and they do all have drawbacks.

Learn how to say, "No"

The value of your yes is strongly determined by the quantity of your no. Unless you are willing to say, "No thank you," to the suggestions you do not want, you are letting someone else make the decisions about how your labor will be handled. This may be OK with you. Choosing to let someone else make the decisions is an option you have about how your labor will be handled. But the majority of women do have opinions, desires and expectations about the care they will receive while in labor. Your caregivers are not able to help you achieve your goals unless you are clear with them what the goals are.

A hard part of saying "no" is the feeling women get that they are somehow being rude or hurtful. Christians strive to be caring and considerate, not wanting to insult caregivers. For some women there is also the concern you must adhere to your midwife's advice since she is the authority. But she is a medical authority, which means she has knowledge and experience in medicine. That does not mean she is in a position of authority over you. In fact, because you are the one who hired her, you are the "master" and she is the "servant." That puts you in authority over her.

> Reflecting on the past week, consider all the requests made of you. Did you respond "yes" when you wanted to answer "no?" Is this good, bad or indifferent?

The other difficulty women often have with saying no is the fear they will be making the wrong decision. They reason that the midwife knows best, so her orders should be followed or you may be doing damage to the baby. Hopefully you have learned enough about your midwife to know if you trust the decisions she makes. If you have, you may feel comfortable following every suggestion she has.

Even if you do trust your midwife and her decisions, you can ask for more information about a recommendation that does not sound right to you. Even if you are positive she has your best interest at heart, you can still ask for more time to make your decision and even say no to what she offers. This does not make you a bad person or a bad parent. Your midwife is offering suggestions of things she thinks might help, but you are the one having the baby and so you are the one who knows what is or is not working for you.

Understand the Normal Birth Process

Obstetrical emergencies are rare, and the problems that occur during labor are usually slow-building issues that do not need immediate attention. By studying the information about labor challenges, you will have most of the information you need to participate in the decision making with your midwife rather than placing all responsibility for the choices on her shoulders. You and your midwife are a team, working together to find the right way to handle your pregnancy and labor. You can only be a team if you are willing to participate in the work of decision making. So ask questions, consider alternatives and take time before you choose.

Hire Continuous Support

Overall, women who hire doulas as continuous labor support have lower levels of interventions. This is very significant if you are considering a low intervention birth. Interestingly, women who use doulas have lower rates of problems with labor, which is significant for every woman giving birth.

Explore Other Options

You may be surprised how little control you have over the options available to you for pregnancy and labor. You may also be surprised how changing caregivers or birth places changes the options available to you. Before you make your final decisions, investigate what other options you may have.

Making Decisions in Labor

Regardless of the specifics of your labor, the decisions you make before labor begins will have a tremendous impact on the decisions you make during labor. Where you labor, who is with you and the type of support you are receiving will all play a part in determining what options are available to you and what options those with you will support.

Though you can work with your care team to make decisions before labor begins, there are still decisions to be made once the contractions have started. The bulk of your decisions during labor will be focused on how to respond to the circumstances of the labor process. You will be choosing comfort measures and determining when interventions might be appropriate. The decisions you make do not control labor. Labor is an involuntary process; you cannot help but give birth. Instead, the decisions will be made with the intention of allowing your body to work with the labor you are having.

Although you cannot know ahead of time if you will have a fast or slow labor, a back labor or a labor challenge, you can prepare to make labor decisions by learning to more accurately predict how comfort measures and interventions will affect the labor process. You make many decisions in your day to day life, and the decisions are all made based on the assumptions and predictions you naturally make about the situations.

As a maturing Christian, you have probably found your ability to make wise decisions improves with experience and maturity. Just as you learn to make better decisions in other areas of your life, you can learn to make wise decisions regarding labor. It simply takes challenging your assumptions to gain a thorough understanding.

Ask Questions

1 John 4:1

Many expectant families fail to question information, especially information given from an authority. 1 John 4:1 reminds us of the importance of questioning every spirit, because there are many false teachings. Though you should trust your caregivers are looking out for your best interests, it is not fair to expect them to be perfect. Your midwife will give you her opinion and let you know about possibilities, but that does not make what she says the absolute truth. Following her advice without exploring other ideas can limit your ability to discover other options that may be just as likely to result in a good outcome.

During labor it can be difficult to gather the mental energy to ask the needed questions before making a decision. Because of this, it is important to understand as much as possible about the options available and the normal process of labor before the first contraction begins.

What questions have you already asked your midwife about tests, options and procedures? What questions do you want to ask but have not?

Many of the options available to you during labor occur more frequently based on where you live. There is disagreement even among doctors and researchers about what is and is not helpful during labor. This means that although one midwife might recommend you handle a situation this way, another midwife might suggest you handle it differently. Often these recommendations are based on the intervention the midwife is most familiar with, so even though there may be another good option available, if you do not seek it out yourself you may not find out about it.

Do Not Rely on Generalizations

Some women make broad generalizations about labor based on one or two stories from friends or relatives. Just because a friend or sister had a particular experience in labor does not mean it is common or even normal. Sometimes even your own previous labor experience is not an accurate predictor of what you can expect during birth. If the situation is different, such as having hired a different midwife, using a different birth place or being in a different state of health, the way your body responds can be different.

Be sure to evaluate labor based on what is happening to you now during this labor, not by assuming from a previous labor. You may be misjudging the progress you are making if you had a difficult labor with your last child. You may also find yourself doubting anything will help you stay comfortable if the first thing you tried was not as helpful as you hoped. There are too many variables to labor to make assumptions about all the comfort measures available based on one small part of your labor.

Think of the birth stories you have heard. How have these shaped your expectations of labor?

Evaluate Common Opinions

Many women have trouble critically evaluating common opinions about pregnancy and birth. Cultural beliefs become part of the general knowledge whether they are true or not. Spend some time before labor begins gathering information and seeking other views to help you determine what beliefs you have that are based on evidence and which ones are based on cultural myths.

What are some common opinions about birth among members of your family? Among your friends? Among your community?

During labor, common opinions you have not evaluated are likely to become a major basis for your decision making. If every woman in your family told you the only thing that helped ease their discomfort was eating chocolate pudding, you would want to try it. Without researching the topic, you might not understand that the chocolate pudding did not contain anything likely to ease discomfort. Unless you asked about the use of chocolate pudding, you would not discover that it was eaten while in the labor tub or while getting a massage, two things very likely to ease discomfort. Lacking any other information about the use of chocolate pudding during labor, you are likely to try it as a means of staying comfortable and find yourself rather frustrated and let down when it does not relieve any of your discomfort.

Do Not Stop at the First Idea

> Recall a time you acted on your first impulse. How might the outcome have changed if you explored other options first?

Oftentimes, women stop at the first idea that hits them, regardless of how many other things may be useful. This is especially true if you are reacting in fear. To accurately determine what is most likely to result in the best outcome, you need to be able to explore other possibilities. You need to be able to accept that your first idea may not be the most helpful.

The work of labor is stressful regardless of how painful a mother says it feels. This stress makes it harder to move beyond the first thing that comes into your head. For example, during active labor it is common for mothers to get "stuck" in the thought that it will hurt too much to move, and so they lie in bed. This is unfortunate since the most uncomfortable way to labor is lying on your back, and the most comfortable way is almost always in an upright position.

Learn to Make Wise Decisions

A good way to gain practice at making predictions during labor is to review birth stories. There are many stories available for you to read freely on the Internet; simply find a site that offers a few, and sit down with a pen and paper to begin working. Or you could ask a friend to share her labor story with you. Start by reading the story out loud, making suggestions for ways the labor experience might have been better. Make a list of what you do and do not like from the story, and how you could change the things you do not like. If possible, go through the stories with a friend so you can benefit from hearing another view of what might have worked.

Another way to improve your ability to predict what might work in labor is to try a labor rehearsal. Trying out different positions and comfort measures gives you the opportunity to know how they feel to your body. Try the labor rehearsals in this book, and the Virtual Labor at www.BirthingNaturally.net.

Labor Rehearsal One
Using Comfort Measures

Practice using comfort measures in labor for 20-30 minutes to gain understanding about how they feel to you. While you are in labor, you will have contractions that are 60 seconds long and 2 minutes apart. Set a stopwatch to alert you every 2 minutes to signal the start of a contraction. If it makes it easier, you can set the stopwatch to alert you every 60 seconds so you have a signal for the start and end of each contraction. Remember that this is a serious time to try out different positions and techniques for labor. You will be practicing the first stage positions, not the pushing positions.

As you try each position, pay attention to what your support persons are able to do for you differently. For example, when you are walking, your support person has to help hold you up and cannot rub your back; the hands and knees position gives full access to your back but some variations of it may be hard on the arms.

As you go through this labor rehearsal, try to spend time:

Walking
Leaning on a wall or support person
Sitting
Using a birth ball
Sitting backwards on a chair
In the bathroom
In hands and knees position
On stairs

Labor Rehearsal Two
Working Through Challenges

Every option you use will change the way you labor and the options you will have to manage your labor. Even the circumstances of your labor may change the options available to you. Refer to the section on comfort measures to determine what can be done in each of these situations. Select the comfort measures you are most likely to find beneficial.

- If you could be anywhere and do anything while you labor for your baby, where would you be and what would you do?
- Now you can do anything; but if you have to be in the hospital while you labor, what would you do?
- Now you have an IV attached and must keep the IV pole with you. What can you do to manage your discomfort?
- Now you have to be monitored and have an IV. These restrict your mobility, but you can still move about 3-4 feet around the monitor. What can you do to manage your discomfort?
- Now you have to stay in the bed because you have received a medication that limits your mobility. You also have a monitor and an IV. What can you do while you labor if the medication is effective at blocking your pain?
- What can you do while you labor if the medication is not effective at blocking your pain?

Labor Rehearsal Three
Making Choices

You can work through this exercise alone or with a labor helper. Try to determine what would best help you in each of these scenarios. To test your labor helper, act out each scenario and have you helper assist you in appropriate ways. Appropriate actions may include: words of support or encouragement; physical touching, massage, leading through relaxation, providing for physical needs or simply by offering companionship.

- The mother is in early labor. She has not had to use any comfort measures yet. On this contraction she tenses and squints while holding her breath at the peak of the contraction.
- Later in the labor, the mother is feeling contractions mostly as a strong backache.
- Now the mother's slow breathing becomes tense-sounding and strained.
- The mother seems to be in active labor. She is moaning, tensing, breathing unevenly, feeling trapped, frightened and overwhelmed.
- The mother breaks down, cries, wants to give up. Contractions are long, hard and close together.
- The mother gets a break in contractions, they seem to space out. On the next contraction she is holding her breath and grunting.
- The mother is feeling urges to push.
- The baby is crowning
- The mother is waiting for the placenta to be expelled.

Labor Rehearsal Four
Wise Decisions

This rehearsal gives you practice in making decisions during labor. Read through the following scenarios and answer the questions. After answering the questions, try to determine how you might like to handle the situation if it happens during your labor.

1. What are the risks to the suggestion?
2. What are other options that may be available?
3. What are potential risks to the other options?
4. What comfort measures could be used in this situation?

- I have been having contractions on and off for a week now. Sometimes they are as close as 8 minutes apart and I think "this must be it," but they always seem to stop within a few hours. At my appointment today my midwife suggested "getting things moving."

- I have been in labor for 8 hours now. It has been back labor for about 5 hours, but the contractions got really painful 2 hours ago. The nurse said back labors are too painful and suggested I use an epidural.

- We have been in the hospital for about 4 hours, and contractions have gone from 5 minutes apart to 3½ minutes apart. At the last vaginal exam I was at 6 (the same as when we arrived at the hospital). My midwife said she can get things moving if she breaks the bag of waters.

- Labor started around midnight, and now it is 8:30 A.M. I am tired and working very hard. My nurse tells me that if I do not do something to get some sleep, I will be too tired to push. She says she can give me something to help me sleep.

- I have been handling late first stage contractions well, but now I feel a sharp pain near my pelvis with each contraction. The nurse says I probably have a full bladder, and suggested we use a bedpan so I can stay in bed.

- My due date came and went 9 days ago. At my prenatal appointment today, I was told that if I did not begin labor on my own in three days I would need to be induced.

- I did not seem to have a transition and suddenly began having a strong urge to push. You get me in the car, and call the hospital as you drive. The nurse you spoke to told you I should not push until we arrive at the hospital.

- As the next contraction begins you see me take a deep breath, hold it for a few seconds and let go to take another breath. My nurse looks at me very frustrated and says I need to push longer.

- The nurse shift just changed, and the new nurse performed a vaginal exam since we had not had one in a few hours. She said I was fully dilated and should push with the next contraction. I whisper to you I just do not feel like I need to push.

- I have been pushing according to my body's urges for about an hour, but the baby seems slow to come. My doctor says he is concerned about the baby being stuck and how long it is taking. He wants to do something to speed it up.

Drawing Conclusions
Review of Section Seven

What would change if . . .

So many times we make our decisions based on what we think we understand, without ever questioning why we think that way. For the next few minutes, spend some time exploring how giving birth would change in your community if some basic assumptions were no longer true.

Most women in modern cultures know they have access to pain medication if they desire it in labor. What would change if pain medication was only available for women who underwent surgical birth?

☙

Many women in modern cultures assume the hospital is the normal place to give birth. What would change if women experiencing normal labor were not admitted to the hospital?

☙

Many women in modern cultures hire a surgeon to attend them during labor. What would change if obstetricians only provided care for women with problems or illnesses during pregnancy and birth?

☙

Many women have never seen a birth before their own baby is born. What would change if women assisted friends and relatives during labor before they became pregnant themselves?

☙

Many women assume a fast labor is the best labor. What would change if women believed the longer a labor lasts the better it is for mother and baby?

☙

Many women assume childbirth will be the worst pain they ever feel. What would change if women expected childbirth to be manageable?

Labor Revisions

The circumstances of your labor can affect the choices you make to respond to your labor. In each of these scenarios, determine what options and comfort measures would be the best for the original and revision.

Original: While laboring at home, you experience strong contractions that are coming relatively quickly. What could you do to be more comfortable?

Revision: While laboring at the hospital, you experience strong contractions that are coming relatively quickly. What could you do to be more comfortable?

ଔ

Original: It is early in the labor. You are handling contractions OK but are very tired. What help do you need?

Revision: It is early in the labor. You are feeling contractions as a backache and are very tired. What help do you need?

ଔ

Original: You have had contractions on and off for a few days, but labor does not seem to be starting. You are tired and emotionally worn out. What can help?

Revision: Your caregiver says that if you are not in labor by tomorrow you will need to be induced. You have had contractions on and off for two days, but labor does not seem to be starting. You are tired and emotionally worn out. What can help?

ଔ

Original: It is transition and you are working hard with each contraction. You do not want to be touched; what can help you?

Revision: It is transition and you are working hard with each contraction. You do not want to be talked to; what can help you?

Home Birth

Marlene Waechter
Certified Professional Midwife

Women have been having babies since Adam and Eve, long before there were doctors and hospitals. Midwives are mentioned in the Bible and other ancient literary works long before doctors make their appearance. Midwives or Traditional Birth Attendants still attend more of the world's babies than doctors. In many countries, (many of which have better statistics than the USA) the doctors are reserved mainly for the high-risk cases in regional tertiary care centers, while midwives attend most normal low risk births in the surrounding countryside. The World Health Organization has declared this method is not only the most cost-effective; it also achieves best neonatal and maternal outcomes. Its research has shown that the number one way to improve infant and maternal mortality rates worldwide is to have more trained attendants. Not more hospitals, more technology, more machines, more physicians or even more licensed midwives. Simply more trained attendants, regardless of their titles.

Every Christian knows that God sent his only begotten Son Jesus into this world to guide us, by his teaching and example, to the next and greater world—heaven. His earthly life is lived as an example to us; every word out of his mouth a lesson for us. Jesus chooses to come to us, as a baby, through the body of the virgin Mary. Jesus, God, comes to us through Mary, a holy but very human handmaiden!

In addition, God could have sent his only begotten Son at any time or place he choose. Think about it . . . Jesus, the most important baby this world has or will ever know. Yet HE is born in a lowly stable in Bethlehem, far removed from the comfort, convenience, and supposed safety of our modern western technological advances. Is God being a negligent Father, sending his only begotten

Son into the world like that? Our almighty God makes no mistakes. "God's way is unerring" He knows everything, down to the number of hairs on our heads. Jesus was born simply. Would that not indicate that God intends birth to be simple?

2 Samuel 22:31 (NAB)
Matthew 10:30

Doctors and technology can surely sometimes save lives, but they can also make mistakes which can cost lives. Many people nowadays assume that because of all the modern equipment and technology, it is safer to give birth in a hospital with a doctor. That has never been proven. It has only been proven that most, not all, very high-risk pregnancies do fare better in the hospital. For the healthy pregnant woman, who has a trained attendant, the outcome is pretty much the same no matter where she births. The World Health Organization (WHO) task force for Safe Motherhood, writes that;

> The care of high-risk women in the hospital was improved by the reduction in numbers of low-risk women, while in the peripheral units [birth centers or homes] time was available to ensure that the low-risk women received the care and attention they needed.
>
> A woman should give birth in a place she feels safe and at the most peripheral level at which appropriate care is feasible and safe.

In other words, for the best outcomes all round, low-risk women should avoid the high-tech hospitals, saving those facilities for those truly in need of those services. The United States spends more per capita than any other country, yet according to the 2004 WHO's maternal and perinatal mortality rates, we rank a shamefully low twenty-third. In most countries that have better statistics, the home birth rates are much higher than they are here in the United States. The Cochrane database has collected many studies proving the safety of home birth for most women. At home it is much easier to maintain the solemn yet joyous air of reverence that should surround every birth. Even with the absence of complications, a pious Christocentric birth can be shattered in a heartbeat, and turned into a medical procedure if there is anyone present that does not believe they are truly witnessing a miracle every time a child is born.

Subject Eight

Labor Challenges

Topics:

Labor Challenges	279
Normal Variation or Emergency?	283
Before Labor Begins	285
During Labor	299
Cesarean Surgery	316
Drawing Conclusions	326
The Miracle of Waterbirth by Barbara Harper	328

Labor Challenges

There are several ways in which you may be challenged during labor. The goal in this unit is to help you understand the difference between a birth emergency and a normal variation of labor, and to give you the information you need to make a decision about how to respond to the challenge.

Labor generally follows a preset order and routine. When a woman experiences differences from the "norm," she is experiencing a labor challenge. There is a wide spectrum of challenges you may experience, ranging from normal variations of the "average" (such as a fast or slow labor) to full blown birth emergencies (such as placental abruption).

Some challenges will reveal themselves before labor begins, such as a baby in a less effective position or gestational diabetes. Other challenges will not be revealed until labor begins, such as a baby in the posterior position or a baby who goes into fetal distress.

Although some challenges are more dangerous to the lives of mother and baby, it is impossible to categorize the labor challenges based on how much they affect the mother. It can be just as stressful for a mother to experience a planned cesarean as it is for another mother to experience a slow labor. How much or how little your labor is affected will depend on the types of challenges you face and your personality.

Why Labor Challenges Happen

There is no one answer to the question of why a woman experiences a labor challenge. While some can occur due to poor health of the mother, such as premature rupture of the membranes which can occur in response to an infection, others can occur because the mother is in perfect health, such as a fast labor, which is usually a sign that everything is working perfectly.

Some labor challenges are not actually problems in labor but can still cause stress and anxiety for the mother based on how her health care team responds. For example, there is no recorded correlation between a shorter pushing stage and a healthier baby; however, some care providers put pressure on a mother to "get the baby out" quickly.

As you review the birth challenges, you can begin to see some of the common themes of birth challenge prevention. Although it is not a guarantee, the healthier you are before labor begins, the better your chances of avoiding many birth challenges. Another way to improve your chances is to be educated about the normal birth process and your options, because some options can change your labor in ways you might not want.

Overcoming Labor Challenges

In the world, overcoming a labor challenge means a malpositioned baby turned, a slow labor sped up or the mother was in some other way successful at changing the undesired circumstances. This is normal for a world in which you are judged by the outcome of your works; where it is your ability and strength that determine your value.

Christians know it is not the outward appearance that God judges, but the heart. When your success is based on your heart, how you handle the situation becomes more important than how it ends. So for a Christian, successfully overcoming a difficult labor is about treating others with love, serving God and following his will in the midst of the challenge.

This does not mean you sit back and do nothing about your circumstances. Many times the Bible shows us individuals who work through difficult situations and

©2002 Jennifer Vanderlaan
Waiting for a slow to start labor to kick in can be a challenge.

1 Samuel 16:7

overcome them. However, the successful overcoming is not about the circumstances changing.

Ruth did not overcome poverty because she married Boaz—she overcame because in the midst of her poverty she continued to sacrificially love and serve Naomi. Abigail did not overcome her husband's disgrace because David found favor in her—it was because in the midst of certain destruction she tried to make things right. The woman with Elijah did not overcome the death of her son because he was brought back to life—it was because in the midst of her sorrow she sought out God. Job did not overcome his trials because God gave him more—it was because in the midst of his pain and sorrow he still sought God.

Book of Ruth

1 Samuel 25

Elijah 17

Book of Job

It is the same with labor. You do not necessarily overcome a labor challenge by removing it. You overcome it by remaining focused on loving and serving God in the midst of the challenge. You do not always have control over what happens during labor, even if you try every technique available. Sometimes the challenge will be removed, sometimes it will not. Regardless of whether or not the challenge is removed, your goal is to labor with God, not for God.

When you approach your labor as something you are doing for God, the outcome of the labor becomes the measure of your success. When you do something for God, it is as if God shows up at the end to see how well you performed, so the only measure of success you have is how everything ended up.

The object is not to show God what you were able to do when the labor is over, but to be with God as labor is happening. When you approach your labor with God, it is the journey, not the destination determining your success. When God is taking every step with you, where you end up is not as important as how you got there.

This is important because when you are dealing with a labor challenge, there are usually several options available to you. There is not always a right or wrong answer, as with any other time in life you will make the best decision with the information you have. Although you can learn many ways to try to change the circumstances of your labor, there is no guarantee you will change what is happening. In fact, with some options you have there is a chance your labor may change, but not the way you had hoped.

As you study the topics in this section, remember to keep a balance between building your knowledge and leaning on God. Like Eve, the combination of your efforts and God's work will bring about the birth of your baby.

Genesis 4:1

Don't Take It Lying Down!

My first suggestion or number one rule for making labour easier is this: STAY ON YOUR FEET.

In the hospital the first thing they do upon admission is issue you one of those ugly backless nightgown-things, and show you to a bed. But you are not like other patients—you don't have an illness and don't need treatment. But you are doing an important job, that of bringing forth a new life. STAY ON YOUR FEET, therefore, because you have a job to do.

STAY ON YOUR FEET and keep walking because sick, weak people are the ones who need to be in bed. Try to think of yourself as a client, using a service, not a patient. Keep upright and keep walking, so you feel freedom to move and not confinement.

STAY ON YOUR FEET, because that raises you up to eye level, where you won't be looked down upon.

STAY ON YOUR FEET, like a capable, *healthy* person, confident and in control.

STAY ON YOUR FEET, because gravity helps the baby to move down the cervix, shortening your labour.

STAY ON YOUR FEET because there is less pain when the weight of the uterus is not pressing on your back.

STAY ON YOUR FEET, because when you lie down, the very bed you lie upon offers resistance to your pelvis, which is doing its best to open for the baby.

STAY ON YOUR FEET, walking, walking, walking through the contractions, rocking, rocking, rocking, easing your baby lower and deeper into the birth canal.

STAY ON YOUR FEET so the doctors and nurses can't keep invading your body with their painful vaginal exams. They have to ask you to lie down for them, and that puts *you* in control! If you STAY ON YOUR FEET they'll only be able to do things when *you're* ready to let them. If you STAY ON YOUR FEET, you can look them in the eye, say no, and walk away.

STAY ON YOUR FEET, walking, refusing a lot of unnecessary vaginal exams, until you realize your body is pushing.

How long can you stay on your feet? Well, if you like, you can push while you are standing, or you can go down into a squat and deliver your baby like that. You don't need to lie down to have a baby!

Sheila Stubbs
Excerpted with permission from *Giving Birth the Easy Way* © 2005

Normal Variation or Emergency?

Most of the challenges you will face during labor will be normal variations of a healthy labor. This means that although it is challenging to you, there is no danger for you or your baby. Some of the labor challenges are normal variations that may indicate a potential for danger. A very few of the labor challenges are emergencies, not normal variations and indicate danger for you and/or your baby. Knowing the difference between a normal variation and a birth emergency is essential for making a wise decision on how to proceed.

Normal variations are challenges that sometimes occur during healthy labors. They usually signal a need for you to change the way you are handling labor but do not mean there is anything physically problematic with the labor process. For example, if you become discouraged you may find additional support or a change of scenery helpful, but it does not signal a potential problem.

It is possible for a challenge that is a normal variation to signal the potential for a problem. For example, a slow labor may simply be a slow labor, or it may be caused by a baby in a poor position, inadequate contractions or cephelo-pelvic disproportion. When a challenge has the potential to indicate a problem, it is helpful to investigate the cause further to respond appropriately.

Birth emergencies are dangerous situations that require immediate medical intervention. For example, a prolapsed cord is dangerous to your baby and may result in death, so help should be sought right away. True birth emergencies are rare, but recognizing a true birth emergency has the potential to save the life of you or your baby.

Once you have determined if your challenge is a normal variation, indicates a potential problem or is an emergency, you can begin to make decisions about how to handle it. You will need to ask yourself what the risks of the challenge may be, and what options are available to you. Usually there are both medical and non-medical options for handling a challenge.

When considering your options, be sure to ask yourself what you hope to achieve by intervening and what risks each option carries. Sometimes it is easy to see the benefits of an intervention outweigh the risks because the situation is dangerous. Sometimes it is easy to see the benefits of an intervention do not outweigh the risks because you are experiencing a normal variation of labor.

The most difficult time to decide how to proceed is when the challenge is normal but may indicate a problem. When you are not sure if what is happening is normal, you cannot accurately predict how the intervention will affect your labor. If this happens, to help determine what is happening you may want to begin by observing how non-medical ways to handle a challenge change the situation. It is possible the non-medical methods will change the course of your labor enough that you will not need medical interventions. It is also possible the non-medical methods will be ineffective and convince you medical interventions are the best option with the least risk.

The following are the recommendations from *A guide to effective care in pregnancy and childbirth* at the time of this writing. Many of these topics are just now beginning to be studied, so while this is a good start for information, be sure to check for more recent research to see if other options are available. Work with your midwife to find the best option for you in any of these situations. Depending on your health, place of birth or other circumstances, some of the options may not be available.

Before Labor Begins

Group B Strep

Group B Streptococcus (also known as beta strep) is a normal intestinal bacteria that sometimes migrates to the perineum. When Group B Strep is found on the perineum the mother is said to be "colonized." About one out of five mothers is colonized with Group B Strep.

The major concern is that during labor, the infection will be passed onto the baby. Group B Strep is the most common bacteria to cause infection in newborns. Though the infection may be passed to as many as one in one hundred or one in two hundred babies whose mother's are colonized, it occurs most frequently among babies who are premature. The other factors related to increased infection in babies are water broken for longer than 18 hours and maternal fever during labor. The most serious form of the infection involves respiratory distress, sepsis and shock, which happens in about one out of a thousand live births to colonized mothers.

Because Group B Strep is a normal human bacteria, and because it comes and goes naturally, there is no proven way to prevent being colonized at the end of your pregnancy. Group B Strep is an infection, so proper diet should be followed to improve immune system functioning and prevent it. You should also be sure to wipe from the front to the back so you do not introduce bacteria from the anus to the vagina. If your midwife feels a vaginal exam is needed during pregnancy, be sure she uses an antibacterial wipe on the perineum and external vaginal skin before inserting fingers. Though midwives have a variety of ways to help prevent infection, such as a regimen of homeopathic penicillin, or use of Echinacea, their effectiveness has not yet been studied. Your local herbalist or naturopath may have other suggestions.

Some midwives recommend trying to remove the infection before labor begins by using oral antibiotics. Because this can result in a temporary removal of the infection, oral antibiotics would need to be well timed so the course of antibiotics is finished before, but not long before, labor begins. Research has found treatment during pregnancy does not change the rate of infection in newborns unless the treatment is continued into labor. Antibiotics given during labor reduce the transmission of infection to newborns.

Risk factors
Water broken 18 hours
Fever of 100.4 or greater
Labor prior to 37 weeks

Prevention of Group B Strep in newborns is most frequently done by determining which mothers and babies will benefit from receiving antibiotics during labor. There are two ways to test for Group B Strep. One is a rapid diagnostic test and the other is the routine test that can take a week for results. This has lead to two different strategies for detecting and managing Group B Strep in mothers.

The first strategy is to use the rapid diagnostic test during labor for any mother who is at risk. This means any mother who is in preterm labor, is experiencing a fever or has had her membranes ruptured for more than 18 hours will be tested. If the test comes back positive, or if the test cannot be given, the mother will receive IV antibiotics during labor.

The second strategy is to use the routine screening test on every mother between 35 and 37 weeks of pregnancy. If the mother is colonized, IV antibiotics will be offered to her during labor. Under this strategy, any mother who has her water broken for 18 hours or shows signs of infection will also be offered antibiotics regardless of the results of the routine screen.

Prolonged Pregnancy

Prolonged Pregnancy, also called post-term, post-dates or post-mature, is a term used to describe a pregnancy that continues after 42 weeks. It occurs in anywhere from 4-14 percent of all pregnancies and is associated with an increased risk of death for the baby. The increased risk of death mainly occurs for two reasons.

> How do you want to handle prolonged pregnancy if it happens to you?

First, prolonged pregnancy results in more deaths because babies who have congenital malformations are more likely to go longer than 42 weeks. In these cases, it is the health of the baby, not the length of labor that is the problem. Inducing to prevent a prolonged pregnancy will not improve outcomes for babies with congenital malformations.

The other reason is asphyxia (suffocation) due to placental problems. It is difficult to know which babies will have problems, as the risk of death increases after labor begins rather than during pregnancy and the risk continues into the neonatal period.

Standard treatment of prolonged pregnancy is prevention by induction of labor. Although there is wide variation in when your midwife may recommend you be induced, there is no evidence inducing before 41 weeks prevents death. Induction after 41 weeks decreases the rate of death (one death prevented for five hundred inductions). Induction after 41 weeks also decreases the risk of meconium-stained fluid, which may be an indicator of fetal distress. Sweeping the membranes at or after 40 weeks decreases the likelihood your pregnancy will progress beyond 42 weeks and decreases the likelihood of a more formal labor induction.

Another possible treatment is to monitor the baby for signs of a problem, acting only if a problem arises. There is no evidence monitoring beyond ultrasound or checking the fetal heart rate improves the outcome of a prolonged pregnancy.

As the due date is no more than an estimate based on averages, it is possible the prolonged pregnancy is simply a variation of normal. In most cases, the outcome is good for mother and baby whether you choose to induce or monitor the pregnancy.

Ultrasound to detect problems

Ultrasound has become one of the most common tests during pregnancy, with many women looking forward to the opportunity to see their babies. Unfortunately, there is very little benefit to having this test done without cause. The only benefits found for routine ultrasound was in early detection of twins and reducing the rate of induction due to prolonged pregnancy. But neither of these benefits came with improved outcomes for babies. The same is true of routine late ultrasound.

Ultrasound becomes most helpful when used for a specific purpose. It can be helpful at confirming a miscarriage, assessing a malformation, locating placental position and confirming a multiple pregnancy. Late in pregnancy, it can help to assess the situation when the growth of the baby may be compromised.

Ultrasound does not help to diagnose feto-pelvic disproportion (the baby not fitting through the pelvis). Likewise, there is no way to predict a shoulder dystocia. Neither early induction or using cesarean for women with large babies showed an improvement in outcomes.

Ultrasound does increase the risk the mother will have a cesarean without any improved outcomes for the baby. There are theories about ultrasound being unsafe for the baby, but there is not yet enough research to determine what harm, if any, it does.

High Blood Pressure

Despite the amount of knowledge about high blood pressure outside of pregnancy, treatment for pregnancy induced hypertension (PIH) is often based on the individual caregiver's experience and anecdotal reports rather than scientific evidence.

There are many suggestions for ways to prevent PIH, but not all of them work. Salt restriction, for example, does not decrease the risk of PIH. Diuretics are able to decrease blood pressure; however, they showed no improvements in outcomes for mothers or babies, causing researchers to question whether excessive water retention should be used to define a risk.

Overall, a mild PIH has very little risk for mother and baby, and there is no evidence to support a policy of bed rest. Anti-hypertensive agents have been shown to lower blood pressure in women with mild PIH, but there is no evidence this prevents pre-eclampsia, how it effects the outcomes for mothers and babies or its safety.

There are many anti-hypertensive agents available if PIH is severe. All anti-hypertensives cross the placenta and so may affect the baby. When pre-eclampsia is feared, anti-convulsant may be used during labor. Their use is more common in some areas than others, and there is no evidence yet that it is helpful when used routinely. If you choose to use an anti-convulsant, be sure you are closely monitored as they can cause cardio-respiratory arrest. They also cross the placenta and are associated with respiratory depression in babies. Magnesium sulfate is the anti-convulsant with the best record and the least amount of risk.

Research is just beginning on expectant management, meaning you watch and wait before doing anything. Though the trials are small and more evidence is needed, so far they show good results for babies but greater risks for moms.

Gestational Diabetes

For many women, the glucose tolerance test is the most dreaded part of prenatal care. If you want to avoid it, there is good evidence it is safe to do so. Overall, test results are not reproducible 50-70 percent of the time which may mean the test is not a valid measure.

The main risk factor for Gestational Diabetes (GD) is fetal macrosomia which increases your risk of cesearean section, shoulder dystocia and the trauma related to it. Up to 30 percent of the women who have abnormal glucose tolerance tests will have a baby over 4000g (8.8 lbs). But a judgement made by observing pre-pregnancy weight, weight gain and length of pregnancy is more predictive of a large baby than the glucose tolerance test. In fact, the majority of macrosomia will be to mothers who tested normal on the glucose tolerance test.

The treatment for GD is diet modification and may include insulin injections. This treatment shows no effect on any outcome other than macrosomia. There is a small increase in death rates for babies associated with abnormal glucose tolerance testing, but that increase can be predicted as much by the indications for the test as the test results. This has lead to very strong language used by *A guide to effective care in pregnancy and childbirth.*

> The available data provide no evidence to support the wide recommendation that all pregnant women should be screened for 'gestational diabetes,' let alone that they should be treated with insulin. Until the risk of minor elevations of glucose during pregnancy has been established in appropriately conducted trials, therapy based on this diagnosis must be critically reviewed. The use of injectable therapy on the basis of the available data is highly contentious, and in many other fields of medical practice, such aggressive therapy without proven benefit would be considered unethical.

Diabetes

Though the risk for death of the baby is still higher for diabetics than the general population, the risk has dropped considerably in the last four decades. There is as much as three times the risk of congenital anomalies, and macrosomia is more common in babies whose mothers are diabetic. Pregnancy induced hypertension is also more common with diabetes. Tight control of diabetes can reduce the risks and is better than too strict or too lenient a regimen.

There is no increased risk of preterm labor and no evidence of long term adverse effects for the baby. When sugar levels are adequately controlled, the only increased risk of waiting for labor to start is shoulder dystocia, which can not be predicted before labor begins and can be anticipated in second stage. When sugar levels are not adequately controlled, lung development may be delayed. This becomes less of a problem when the baby is allowed to mature to a later gestational age.

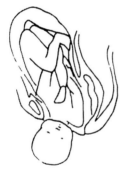

In shoulder dystocia, the baby's shoulder is stuck on the mother's pubic bone.

Cesarean surgery rates tend to be higher for diabetics with little justification. Ultrasound calculations perform poorly on larger babies, inaccurately judging who will or will not have trouble being born. There is no improvement in perinatal mortality when pregnancy is ended through surgery or induction without valid reason other than diabetes.

Baby not thriving

"Baby not thriving" is not the same as a small baby. Small babies will have been small throughout the pregnancy and are a normal variation of the size of newborns that may be related to genetics. The key factor to determining a baby who is no longer thriving is growth that has deviated from its normal progression.

> Determining the health status of your baby before birth is not always an exact science.

When there is evidence growth has faltered, it is referred to as intrauterine growth restriction. It is generally assumed this is caused by inadequate nutrition, a failing placenta or insufficient blood supply. The causes of late pregnancy death are unknown and the ability to prevent it is very limited regardless of the way the pregnancy is monitored.

Detecting a baby in trouble would be easier if there was an accurate way to measure baby's growth and a standard growth curve to compare it to. At present, there is neither. One way to measure your baby, palpitation of the baby through the abdomen, is inaccurate, with less than 20 percent of the guesses falling within 450 grams of baby's birth weight. Fundal height, which measures from the pubic bone to the fundus (top of the uterus) is a good measure of babies who are at a low weight for gestation, but being a small baby is not the same as being a baby whose growth suddenly stopped.

Ultrasound late in pregnancy is done to detect babies who are no longer thriving, but it is limited by the lack of research on what a normal growth curve looks like. Women who use routine ultrasounds are more likely to be sent to and admitted to the hospital, as well as more likely to be induced. Unfortunately, they are no more likely to have a healthy baby. A Doppler ultrasound seems effective for women who are high-risk, but shows no benefit when used routinely.

Fetal movement counting has been suggested as an easy way to measure the health of the baby. To do it, you simply keep track of how long it takes to feel ten distinct movements. It can be done daily, costs nothing and is not inconvenient to most mothers. However, there is no evidence it actually decreases the incidence of fetal death, but it does increase the use of other interventions including elective delivery.

Contraction Stress Test is a technique in which contractions are started while a monitor assesses your baby's heart rate. It has no proven benefits for mother or baby. Instead, it is time-consuming and has the potential to harm the baby. Women who have bleeding, placenta previa, a history of premature rupture of the membranes or preterm labor should not have a contraction stress test because of the risk to the baby. A variation in which nipple stimulation is used was more likely to cause excessive uterine activity.

Non-Stress Test is a technique where your baby is monitored without the use of contraction stimulating drugs. It is associated with increased death rates for babies with no benefits. It may be useful to assess immediate danger to a baby when fetal hypoxia is feared, but should not be used to determine fetal health other than immediate danger.

Biophysical Profile combines a non-stress test with an ultrasound to measure your baby's heart rate, movement and the amount of amniotic fluid. It reduces the false-positive rate of the non-stress test and is a better indicator of an abnormal outcome. Unfortunately, its use is not associated with improved outcomes for babies.

Prelabor Rupture of the Membranes

Pre-labor rupture of the membranes (PROM) occurs in about one out of ten births. Overall PROM is associated with good outcomes for mother and baby with infection being the primary concern. The test used to determine if the waters have broken has a 15 percent false positive rate. Antibiotics may be recommended whether you show signs of infection or not. Depending on the policy where you give birth, your baby may be given antibiotics after birth. Other concerns with PROM include cord prolapse and cord compression.

If the PROM occurs before your baby is at term, concerns about premature labor will be combined with efforts to ensure infection does not occur. You will be offered antibiotics which help decrease your risk of giving birth within one week of PROM. Receiving steroids does help decrease the risk for respiratory distress and does not increase the risk of infection. With early PROM, your baby is most likely to be healthy if you allow your pregnancy to continue as long as possible rather than induce. However, once labor has started, there is no benefit to delaying your baby's birth unless the delay gives time for other changes that may improve your baby's health.

Because infection is the main concern, care must be taken to ensure nothing is inserted into the vagina. Although it may be a sterile instrument or glove, it must touch the labia before it is inserted and so will pick up the normal exterior vaginal bacteria and introduce it to the interior vagina and uterus. Some caregivers recommend against taking a bath, although there is little chance the bathwater will enter the vagina unless you manually separate the labia.

Caregivers differ on how long they feel comfortable with the bag of waters broken before labor begins. Some will recommend induction within 12 hours, others within 24 hours. If you choose to induce, oxytocin has better outcomes than prostaglandins whose administration increases your risk for infection. Seven out of ten women whose water breaks will give birth within 24 hours, and nine out of ten will have given birth within 48 hours. Between 2 and 5 percent of women whose water breaks will not have given birth after 7 days.

> How does your caregiver prefer to handle PROM?

Breech

Breech is the term used to describe a baby who is in a foot or buttocks down position rather than head down. This occurs in about 7 percent of babies at 38 weeks and remains in about 4 percent of babies at 40 weeks. Although most breech babies will do fine, babies in a breech position are more likely to have unfavorable outcomes than babies who are head down regardless of how they are born (cesarean or vaginal). The association between breech position and childhood handicap has led some researchers to believe the head down (or vertex) position for birth is one of a child's first developmental milestones, occurring before sitting up or crawling.

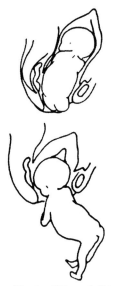

Vaginal Breech Birth

There are reasons breech babies have a reputation for doing more poorly. As the head grows, gravity and normal baby movements tend to move babies into a head down position. Babies who are born early or are small for gestation age are more likely to be breech, since they have not had the time or growth needed to move into the head down position. Babies with neuromuscular disabilities do not engage in the movements necessary to move into a head down position. None of these problems are fixed by having the baby born through cesarean. However, because the poorer outcomes of breech babies have been blamed on damage at birth, cesarean surgery has become the standard method of breech birth in many areas.

Babies in breech position do have increased risks for vaginal birth. In a vertex birth, the baby's head is molded to fit the pelvis by the contractions while it opens the cervix wide enough to allow the rest of the baby to slip through. If a baby in a frank or complete breech position passes through the cervix, the head can be expected to follow without problem. The head also blocks the umbilical cord from slipping through the cervix and becoming compressed. This is most likely when the bag of waters is broken early in labor and breaks with a gush of fluid that could wash the cord through the cervix. Although the risks are higher, skilled midwives are familiar with the techniques used to keep your baby safe during a vaginal breech birth. As more and more breech babies are born through surgery, one of your biggest struggles may be finding a birth attendant who has these skills.

Proper Posture
Imagine a line drawn down the side of you. It starts at your ear, travels to your shoulder, hip, knee and ends at your ankle. Is it a straight line? It should be.

It is believed some breech babies are simply "stuck" in a pelvis that is not allowing them to move head down. To help a breech baby turn to a vertex baby, you can try any one of a variety of positions or postures. The simplest positions are to assure you use proper posture throughout the day, which gives your baby the most amount of room to move. Others involve positions that put your head below your hips to help your baby slide out of your pelvis so he can flip. This can be done by using a hands and knees position with your head on the floor or by lying on your back on an inverted board. One method involves lying on your back with your knees bent and hips elevated while you roll from side to side. Any of these can be tried several times a day for 10 to 20 minutes at a time.

You can schedule a visit with your local chiropractor who can try a maneuver called the Webster Technique. During the session, your chiropractor will make adjustments to your pelvis to help alleviate pelvic constraints that prevent the normal movements your baby should be making. You may also visit a masseuse who is familiar with massage techniques to make it easier for your baby to turn. Other non-invasive techniques to try are acupressure and moxibustion, which involves burning herbs to stimulate acupuncture points. Your local homeopath may also have recommendations to help turn a breech baby.

Types of Breech

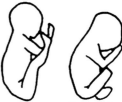

Frank Complete

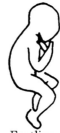

Footling

The Knee-Chest Position

Kneel with your hips flexed slightly more than 90 degrees, but with your thighs not pressing against the abdomen. Do this for 15 minutes every 2 waking hours for 5 days.
From *A guide to effective care in pregnancy and childbirth*

You may have success at getting your baby to turn by using ice, light or sound. Place ice near the top of the uterus so the baby will move away from the cold. Light and sound are placed near the pubic bone because baby will move toward them. Swimming may also allow enough pelvic flexibility to get your baby to move head down.

If none of the non-invasive techniques are successful, you can try an external version. During this procedure your midwife will use a medication to relax the uterus and then using the pressure of her hands, will try to move your baby into a head down position. If this is done before your baby is full term (38 weeks), he is likely to move back into a breech position. Studies found no differences in percentage of breech presentation, cesarean surgery or outcomes for babies when version was attempted before term. There are also more risks for your baby when a version is attempted before 37 weeks.

An external version at term (after 37 weeks) however, can substantially reduce the likelihood your baby will remain breech. It is successful at turning a baby about 58 percent of the time and reduces your risk of a cesarean by

48 percent. Although it can be more difficult to perform a version after 37 weeks because some babies will move into the pelvis, waiting improves outcomes for babies. This is partially because it gives your baby time to turn naturally, and partly because if your baby has trouble during the version, you can immediately have a cesarean.

Transverse Lie

A baby in a transverse lie is in the uterus sideways, with the shoulder or arm presenting at the cervix. Because your baby cannot be born vaginally in this position, you will need to either get the baby to change positions or use a cesarean surgery.

You can try all the methods recommended in the breech section to help your baby change positions. Inverted positions which put your head lower than your hips use gravity to move your baby away from the pelvis and encourage movement. Some women place an ironing board on a shallow slant (either propped on a sturdy stack of books or pillows or leaning against a sofa) and lie on their backs with their heads lower than their hips.

Another position which may be helpful is to lie on your back with your legs leaning against a wall. Put the soles of your feet on the wall and push your hips off the floor, using your legs and shoulders to support your body. This exaggerated bridge position allows you to lift your pelvis higher than performing the same move with your feet on the ground.

Multiple Birth

Families expecting twins (or more) are in the unique position of being faced with decisions on care science has yet to explore. For example, multiples are more likely to be born prematurely than singleton babies. To help prevent this, the mother of multiples may be offered bed rest, cervical cerclage or medication to avoid contractions. None of these have been shown to be helpful in a twin pregnancy and may have risks for the mother and baby. Although there is an increased mortality rate for the second twin, the only trial to assess the use of cesarean found no advantage in terms of injury or death to the babies. As always, cesarean increased the risks for the mother.

What options are available to you in a multiple birth are highly dependant on who you hire as your caregiver and where you live. It is worthwhile to seek out a midwife who is experienced in vaginal birth for multiples. It is also important to focus your attention on excellent nutrition during pregnancy to ensure your babies have every opportunity to fully mature before being born.

No matter what the world says about the challenges and complications that can come with multiple pregnancies, we do not have to experience any negative outcomes. Therefore, don't think of a multiple pregnancy as multiple troubles but that you have been multiply blessed! Change your mindset and see the Lord perform a great work in you. I did and my twin pregnancy was my best pregnancy! While it was more challenging physically because I was a lot bigger than my previous two pregnancies, emotionally, spiritually and health wise it was the best.

Listed below are some of my personal payer points that I prayed during my twin pregnancy, which may help you prepare in prayer for your multiple pregnancy and birth. Just like a single pregnancy, it is important to spend time with God so that the Holy Spirit can quicken any specific scripture(s) for your situation.

- You body will accommodate the growth and development of your babies without any sickness, disease or complication.
- All babies will be in the anterior position (head down and face towards your spine) for a vaginal delivery and with one of the babies' head engaged and sitting firmly on the cervix to help with dilation.
- There will be no obstruction of delivery and that the umbilical cords are not wrapped around the neck or shoulders.
- The placenta(s) will do its/their job efficiently throughout the pregnancy, labour and delivery supplying enough oxygen and nutrients to each baby, without any failure or complications.
- Each baby will thrive without one of them becoming 'greedy' resulting in robbing the other of essential nutrition and growing conditions. Also pray that there will be enough space in the womb for both babies to grow and thrive.
- You will not miscarry or go into premature labour, but will deliver safely at full term.
- Your cervix will remain closed, strong and competent until the proper time for delivery and then dilate quickly and efficiently to the full ten centimeters without any pain or complications.
- All babies will be perfect, strong and healthy and be able to thrive beyond the womb without assistance, that is the lungs being fully developed and sucking reflex perfected for ease of breastfeeding.
- The babies will not be in distress and that the peace of God will be with them during the labour and delivery.

Nerida Walker

Herpes

If you have genital herpes, there is a chance your infant can become infected by an active lesion during a vaginal birth. Though it is possible for you to transfer the virus to your baby without an active lesion, it is rare. Infection of infants happens in one in twenty-five hundred to one in ten thousand births.

It is best to stay as healthy as possible to prevent an outbreak. If you do have active lesions, you may still have the option of a vaginal birth depending on the location of the lesions. Some midwives have reported covering lesions to prevent transmission. Other midwives recommend cesarean to prevent infecting the baby. There is inadequate research to make any definitive recommendation on appropriate treatment.

During Labor

Back Labor

Some women feel contractions as a backache that continues between contractions. Though this was traditionally thought to be due to a baby who was in a posterior position (the back of the baby's head facing mom's back, recent research is showing women also complain of a back labor without a posterior baby. It may be babies whose heads are not ideally lined up for the pelvis put more pressure on the pelvis causing back pain.

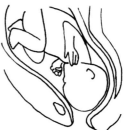

Posterior babies are facing the mother's front.

Regardless of what position the baby is in, back pain during labor is often associated with slower progress through labor and a baby who has a more difficult time navigating through the pelvis. To work with a back labor you need to do two things. First, you need to use positioning to encourage the baby to move into a better position. Secondly, you need to use whatever means available to stay as comfortable as possible.

The medical techniques of using artificial oxytocin to speed up the slow labor and an epidural to relieve the pain may not be helpful during a back labor. Artificial oxytocin may work to increase contractions, but the increase in contractions can force the baby into the pelvis in a bad position causing the slow progress to continue. Epidurals further complicate the problem because they relax the pelvic floor and prevent mom from being mobile—two things necessary to help the baby move into a better position.

Using hands and knees positions with pelvic rocking, walking or asymmetrical positions such as the lunge can help to move the baby into a better position. Counter pressure, hip squeezes and hot or cold compresses can help a mother manage the pain of a back labor. Sometimes back labors continue so long the mother simply needs to rest in a way comfort measures and warm baths are not letting her. In these cases, pain medication can prevent a cesarean surgery by helping a mother sleep so she has the energy to continue.

Prolapsed Cord

When the umbilical cord drops into the vagina before the baby, it is said to have prolapsed. This is a rare and dangerous situation for the baby since any compression on the cord will cut off his only supply of oxygen. Cord prolapse is more common among breech babies or babies who have not yet engaged in the pelvis. It is also most common when the bag of waters breaks with a gush. It is not normal during labor. In the normal labor the head blocks the cord from entering the vagina until after the head is born.

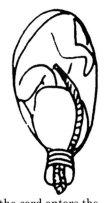

If the cord enters the cervix before the baby it is prolapsed.

If you suspect a prolapsed cord, immediately get into a hands and knees position with your head lower than your hips. This will use gravity to keep your baby's head from compressing the cord. Immediately seek medical help. If you are with a nurse or midwife when it happens, she will probably place a hand into your vagina to hold the head off the cord until help arrives.

Continuing with a vaginal birth is risky with a prolapsed cord, since compression of the cord will prevent your baby from receiving oxygen. Attempts to push the cord behind the head are usually unsuccessful since the hand can only reach so far and a baby's head is so large. A cesarean surgery allows your baby the safest birth if the cord has prolapsed.

Fast Labor

While many women wish they could give birth quickly, the women who do are not always so positive about the experience. Giving birth in only a few hours means your body does all the work in less than half the time. It can be frightening, overwhelming and extremely painful as your body stretches so fast. A labor that lasts less than three hours is called precipitate. Although it generally means everything is working well, a fast second stage is associated with an increased risk of cervical and perineal tears.

In cases of a fast labor, comfort measures and positions that use gravity to slow down the labor process may be helpful. Relaxing in a side-lying position and pushing in a side-lying position can help to slow the baby's descent and help prevent tears for mom. Mothers who experience fast labor may also need exceptional amounts of support to help them cope with fear and stress caused by moving through labor so quickly.

Prolonged Labor

In general, prolonged labor is defined by progress of less than 1 cm dilation per hour in the active phase of labor. This definition of normal was created by Dr. Friedman in the 1950s when he averaged out the length of labor for many women. Subsequent research has found labor more often progresses at half this rate (.5 cm per hour), which more closely equals the 12 to 15 hours women are generally told labor lasts.

For all practical purposes, a prolonged labor is one that is proceeding slower than desired in the active phase of labor. When labor deviates from the average length, it is possible there is a problem that needs attention. It is also possible everything is fine and this labor is simply taking longer than average. Understanding the difference is the key to understanding what to do.

How to respond to a prolonged labor is the subject of much debate. Though many caregivers feel any deviation is reason to intervene, *A guide to effective care in pregnancy and childbirth* and the World Health Organization agree a deviation requires evaluation of the situation but not necessarily immediate intervention. While there is an increase in problems in prolonged births, it is not yet known if it is the longer labor that causes the problems or if the problems cause the longer labor. There are several possible reasons a labor is slow, and to improve the efficiency of labor requires knowing what is happening and what is most likely to bring positive change.

There are several ways of increasing the effectiveness of contractions and progress of labor that have little to no risk for both mother and baby. Hiring a supportive companion to labor with you, such as a doula, not only decreases the likelihood of a prolonged labor, but it also decreases the risk of operative delivery including cesarean and the need for pain medication. Walking and changing positions during labor not only helps the baby to navigate the pelvis, but also helps the mother to remain more comfortable while allowing the contractions to be the most effective possible. Eating and drinking at will help keep mothers comfortable while giving them the strength and hydration their bodies need to keep labor progressing well.

These three techniques should be your first line of defense when your labor seems prolonged. It is best to interview your birth place personnel and midwife before labor begins to ensure you will be encouraged to do them. Not all hospitals allow eating and drinking at will, and some hospitals still employ standard procedures that restrict your ability to move.

Active Management of labor is a program many hospitals have adopted to help prevent prolonged labors. It consists of using an early amniotomy, early use of oxytocin, strict criteria for defining progress in labor and continuous professional support for the mother. In many hospitals, the method has been adopted without the use of the continuous professional support. However, when its components are studied separately, it is only the continuous presence of professional support that shows any improved outcomes for mothers and babies. At this point, the total number of controlled studies is too small to determine any benefit from the program as a whole.

There is no clear understanding of labor progress before active labor, when progressive dilation of the cervix begins (usually around 4 cm). Your cervix can begin to dilate weeks before labor begins in earnest. For this reason, it is important to understand the difference between a pre-labor or false labor and the true start of progressive contractions.

False labor or pre-labor contractions are normal stop and start contractions that help your body prepare for laboring. If you mistakenly believe false labor is a stalled or prolonged active labor, you might decide to use induction agents before labor has actually begun. If part of the induction includes breaking the bag of waters, you will have begun a countdown in which you must give birth within a specified amount of time.

Because induction agents increase the risk to you and your baby, misdiagnosing early labor as active labor increases risks. To avoid misinterpreting labor, be sure to wait until your contractions are showing a progressive pattern of getting longer, stronger and closer together before you consider yourself as in labor. Some women have contractions less than 10 minutes apart for a few hours or on and off for a few days without the contractions moving closer together or getting longer. This is a normal reaction to the changing hormone levels and simply means your body is getting ready to begin labor soon.

If your contractions are strong, your midwife might be concerned your cervix is resisting change. Unfortunately, there is not enough research to determine if any measures intended to decrease cervical resistance are effective.

If your contractions are progressive, meaning they are getting closer together and lasting longer, but your cervix is not dilating, your caregivers may consider the effectiveness of your contractions. As many as half of all women who have slow progress in labor have adequate contractions. If your caregiver believes your contractions are ineffective, you will be offered ways to increase their strength. Women who receive medication for pain, especially epidural medication, have a greater chance of experiencing ineffective contractions.

Artificially breaking the bag of waters (amniotomy) is associated with decreasing labor by one or two hours when done early in labor. It is also associated with a decreased risk of labor progressing slower than .5 cm/hour and use of oxytocin to stimulate contractions. Women who use this method are less likely to consider labor "horrible or excruciating." It comes, however, with an increased risk of cesarean surgery and fetal heart rate abnormalities. Because the bag of waters is broken, you will be required to give birth within a specific time frame and depending on the length of your labor may be asked to use antibiotics to decrease your risk of uterine infection.

Another option is the administration of artificial oxytocin. The effectiveness of oxytocin is still not clear, despite its popularity as a way to speed labor. Only one of three studies showed the use of oxytocin decreased the length of labor, while one showed no difference and the other showed encouraging women to move during labor resulted in shorter labors than using oxytocin did. There was also no difference in Apgar scores or admission to special care nurseries when oxytocin was used. However, 80 percent of the women who received oxytocin felt it increased the amount of pain they felt. Further confusing the issue is the lack of clear information about the dosing that should be used when augmenting with oxytocin.

One of the reasons movement during labor may be so effective at speeding labor is the way it allows for the baby to shift into position in the pelvis. It has been theorized that many slower labors are not caused by inadequate contractions, but by the failure of the baby's head to rest firmly and evenly on the cervix. This prevents cervical dilation, despite the strength of the contractions. In fact, according to this theory, using methods to strengthen contractions may force the baby further into a poor position causing cephalo-pelvic disproportion..

The technical term for a head that does not sit evenly on the cervix is asynclitism. It can occur with or without back labor. In order for the head to line up properly with the cervix, your baby needs to have his chin resting on his chest. There are several movements you can do to help him achieve this: lunging with one foot on a stool or chair, walking up stairs, doing the abdominal lift, pelvic rocking or kneeling with your head lower than your hips. The idea is to get your pelvis moving and to get your baby lifted out of your pelvis enough that he can move his head.

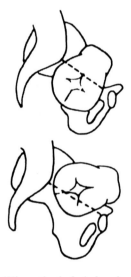

When the baby's head enters the pelvis at an angle, it is called asynclitic.

When Labor Takes Awhile

Moms get weary during labor because of a variety of or a combination of factors including hunger, lack of sleep, prolonged labor and/or a difficult labor. If labor is progressing slowly, mom needs to rest as much as possible. Staying upright to facilitate contractions is only effective if mom is not getting too tired. Her body will expend all its energy on outside activity rather than the hard work of opening and drawing up the cervix. There is absolutely nothing wrong, if mom and baby are tolerating labor well, with taking a rest from labor.

What Mom Can Do

1. Mom can take naps or at least lie down and be completely at rest between contractions or when contractions are lighter. If labor stalls or contractions become inefficient, rest may be the best medicine for mom if she and baby are tolerating the wait well.
2. Mom may continue eating light foods during labor. She should definitely continue drinking vegetable and fruit juices and water throughout labor to maintain adequate hydration. Fruit juices are harder for moms sometimes due to the natural sugar content causing hypoglycemia and resulting nausea and vomiting.
3. A soothing bath with lavender drops added (7-10 drops per full tub of water) can provide relaxation for mom to allow her to gather her reserve strength to continue laboring.
4. She can mix liquid chlorophyll with water and sip a half-cup full each hour during labor.
5. Schisandra, Schisandra chinensis, Schizandra chinensis, liquid extract successfully induced labor in 72 of 80 women with prolonged labor with an administered dose of 20 to 25 drops per hour for 3 hours of a 1:3 extract for 3 consecutive days, and schisandra tincture improved cardiovascular symptoms in hypotensive pregnant women at 30 to 40 drops three times a day of a 1:10 extract.

Enhancing Contractions:

1. StartUp by TriLight Herbs may be used to enhance contractions. This herbal combination, containing Pennyroyal, Hedeoma pulegioides, Mentha pulegium, Feverfew, Tanacetum parthenium, Blue cohosh, Caulophyllum thalactroides, Black cohosh, Cimicifua racemosa, Beth root, Trillium erectum, utilizes herbs that stimulate uterine contractions to assist the body's natural laboring process. 1/2 to 1 teaspoon of the glycerine-based formula may be used every two hours until labor is progressing well.

Shonda Parker
Excerpted with permission from *Naturally Healthy Pregnancy* © 2008.

Meconium Staining

During pregnancy, your baby normally ingests amniotic fluid which travels through his digestive system. This material builds up in your baby's bowel to form a sticky black substance called meconium. Meconium will be your baby's first bowel movements. Sometimes, the first bowel movement happens before a baby is born, so meconium is present in the amniotic fluid when the bag of waters breaks.

The first effect of the presence of meconium stained waters on your labor will be closer evaluation of your baby for fetal distress. By itself, meconium does not mean anything unless there is an abundance of it in the waters. However, it is one sign that your baby may be having difficulty, and so your midwife will be more vigilant about checking for other signs that something may not be quite right.

The second effect of meconium is the concern it raises about the possibility of your baby having some in his mouth or throat when he takes his first breath. Because meconium in the throat can be dangerous for your baby, causing trouble with breathing or pneumonia, your midwife will want to be sure there is none in your baby's mouth. To be sure of this, your baby's throat will be suctioned as soon as the head is born to remove any meconium that may be present.

Fetal Distress

Fetal Distress is a term used to describe a condition in which the baby is not handling labor well. Because it is determined by the baby's heart rate, the terms nonreassuring fetal status or non-reassuring fetal heart tones are more accurate descriptions of what is happening. The importance of the baby's heart rate is based in part on the belief that changes in a baby's heart rate during labor precede brain damage due to lack of oxygen.

Monitoring during labor will assess your baby's heart rate. This may be done by electronic fetal monitoring or intermittent auscultation with a fetoscope. If your baby's heart tones deviate outside a generally accepted safe level, your midwife may recommend taking action. What action you take will be determined by where you are laboring, how much progress you have made in labor and the philosophy of your midwife.

Although the most common treatment for fetal distress is prompt delivery, most abnormalities will resolve with simple measures such as changing maternal position, stopping the use of synthetic oxytocin or giving the mother oxygen. If these techniques are not effective at resolving the issue, drugs called betamimetics may be successful at giving you more time for the baby to be born. If it is believed the heart rate changes are caused by compression on the umbilical cord, an amnio-infusion may help to temporarily relieve the problem.

If the non-reassuring heart tones occur during the pushing phase of labor, your midwife may ask you to change to a more directed pushing method to encourage faster birth. This would involve you holding your breath for 10-second intervals throughout a contraction. If this is not fast enough, your midwife may recommend forceps or vacuum to help move your baby down through the pelvis faster. Cesarean surgery is not always an option if you have already begun to push, because your baby may be to far into the pelvis for a safe cesarean removal.

Depending on the equipment used to assess your baby's heart rate, you may want to reassess the situation with another monitoring procedure. External electronic fetal monitoring, especially continuously throughout labor, is associated with higher rates of cesarean surgery without showing any improvement in outcomes for babies. The number of surgeries for fetal distress decreases when the baby's scalp pH is analyzed through a technique called scalp blood sampling; however, this is a time-consuming and uncomfortable technique that requires a blood gas machine be available. A scalp stimulation test which involves seeing how the baby responds to stimulation of the scalp or a sound may help determine if there is a need to sample the fetal scalp blood.

Placental Abruption

Placental Abruption is a dangerous condition that thankfully occurs very rarely (only about 1 percent of pregnancies worldwide). Women who have hypertension; use drugs, alcohol or tobacco; or suffered trauma; are younger than 20 or older than 35; or who have had an abruption in a previous pregnancy are at greatest risk. You can reduce your risk for an abruption by eating a well-balanced diet with adequate folic acid, assuring you get appropriate sleep and discontinuing use of drugs and alchol.

An abruption can happen as early as 20 weeks into pregnancy. It can be recognized by a contraction that does not go away, pain in the uterus with tenderness in the abdomen and vaginal bleeding. In about 20 percent of cases the blood is trapped behind the placenta and so there is no vaginal bleeding.

If you suspect an abruption, you will want to contact your midwife immediately so the situation can be assessed. It is possible to have an asymptomatic abruption that puts neither you nor your baby in harm. It is also possible to have a severe abruption if a large part of the placenta has become detached and you are bleeding heavily. Depending on the severity of your abruption you may be able to give birth vaginally, or you may require immediate cesarean surgery to ensure your and your baby's safety.

Placenta Previa

In most cases, the placenta attaches itself to the upper part of the uterus in a place that allows placental growth to happen over the growing part of the uterus. Sometimes, the placenta does not attach high enough in the uterus to grow without covering the cervix. When the placenta covers part or all of the cervix, it is called placenta previa.

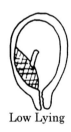
Low Lying

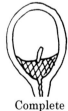
Complete Previa

About one baby in 200 will have a placenta previa at term. Though a low lying placenta may be detected through a routine ultrasound, over 90 percent of early previas grow away from the cervix and are normal by late pregnancy. Your risk of previa increases if you have had a previous cesarean surgery or are carrying multiples. The risk also increases as you age and with each pregnancy. Placenta previa is the most common cause of vaginal bleeding late in pregnancy. It is most commonly associated with painless bleeding in the third trimester that begins light and becomes progressively heavier over two or three weeks.

The main concern with placental previa is the safety of the baby during labor. If the placenta covers the cervix, the baby has no way of exiting the uterus. Even if only a small piece of the placenta covers the cervix, contractions that work to stretch the cervical end of the uterus can detach the placenta from the uterus reducing your baby's ability to get much needed oxygen. Placental detachment can also cause you to lose too much blood.

About 9 percent of previas are also associated with placental accreta, a condition in which the placenta attaches to the uterus in a way that prevents it from detaching. Although babies with accreta are likely to be born healthy, the placenta cannot detach properly, putting the mother in danger of bleeding to death. There are several severities of accreta, ranging from the placenta growing into the uterine wall to growing through the uterine wall and into neighboring tissue such as the bladder. Accreta is a rare condition; however, it is more common in women who have had a previous cesarean. To protect the health of a mother with accreta, caesarean is necessary. Often, a hysterectomy will also need to be performed.

If a previa is suspected, your midwife will recommend an ultrasound to determine the position of the placenta. Depending on how much of the placenta is in the cervical area, your midwife may recommend a cesarean surgery. Your midwife may recommend immediate surgery if you are bleeding heavily. If the placenta is close to the cervix but not covering it, you may have the option to plan a vaginal birth.

Cervical Lip

Sometimes labor progresses well, but at nine or ten centimeters there is a small part of the cervix that did not dilate like the rest. If a cervix dilates unevenly, it is said to have a lip. How the lip is handled will depend on your caregiver. Generally, you would be asked not to push until the lip is gone.

Some caregivers will try to push back the lip during a contraction. Other caregivers might ask you to try pushing gently to see if you can remove the lip that way. A common concern is that pushing against a cervical lip will cause the cervix to swell. If the cervix swells, the opening will decrease in size meaning you will need to wait for the swelling to decrease before your baby can be born.

To prevent a lip, stay as active as possible during labor. This activity will help your baby fit into the pelvis properly. Because the firmness of the pelvic floor helps your baby to align himself properly in the pelvis, you will also want to avoid the use of medications that relax the pelvic floor. Keeping the bag of waters intact as long as possible can help keep even pressure on the cervix, encouraging it to dilate evenly.

Cervical Lip or Swollen Cervix

If mom is 9cm or even fully dilated with a lip left, either the posterior or anterior, and mom is weary, the following may prove helpful. Most of the time, a cervical lip resolves well on its own with no intervention. Having been a woman who had a resistant and quite painful cervical lip in each vaginal birth, I personally preferred the birth in which I held the lip back myself as I pushed baby past. I could feel exactly what was going on and could decide what I wanted to do, without feeling "done to."

What Mom Can Do:

A change of position or moving to another room may give mom a fresh outlook. In fact, some midwives elect to have mom get into the hands & knees position for a few contractions, then switch to leaning on the bed on one bended knee with the other up as if you were trying to stand for several contractions, then switching to the other knee down and other leg up through a few contractions, then lying on left side for a couple contractions, then right side.

- For a rigid cervix, black haw, Viburnum prunifolium, or cramp bark, Viburnum opulus, may be given to relax mom and allow labor to proceed. Dosage: 20-30 drops of tincture or ¼ - ½ tsp tinctract.
- Gently massaging the cervix during early labor just as one would do perineal massage on the perineum during the pushing stage of labor is an option. Since evening primrose oil encourages softening and opening, squeeze the oil from several capsules of the oil and massage the cervix during early labor.
- Make use of water for enhanced relaxation.
- Pray for a gentle opening of the "gate" through which baby will arrive.

Shonda Parker
Excerpted with permission from *Naturally Healthy Pregnancy* © 2008.

Cephalopelvic Disproportion

Cephalopelvic disproportion (CPD) is the term used to describe the condition in which the baby is unable to pass through the pelvis because he is too large. Although measurements of your pelvis could be made in several ways before labor begins, those measurements are not predictive of CPD and so are of little use in preventing this problem. During labor, the bones of your baby's head and your pelvis move to allow the passage of the head through the pelvis. Ways to assess the pelvis before labor cannot determine the extent to which it will stretch or how much your baby's head can mould.

The only way to know if your baby will not fit through your pelvis is to give yourself an adequate amount of time pushing. Your risk of having CPD may be related to the philosophies of your birth attendants, since how long your midwife is willing or able to wait for your baby to be born will determine how long you will push before she intervenes.

In developing countries, CPD is a very real problem. Inadequate nutrition in childhood prevents the proper bone growth, leaving women with misshapen or poorly developed pelvises. The young age at which a woman gives birth to her first child furthers the problem, as a 15-year-old may not be fully grown. Without access to basic medical care, obstructed labor (CPD) is responsible for 8 percent of the world's maternal deaths and leaves many other women severely injured.

Where proper nutrition and basic health care are available, the risk for an obstructed labor is greatly reduced. Though it may be impossible to know for sure, many midwives believe true CPD is very rare in developed nations. They are concerned that women who have slow labors and lack the support needed to help their babies find the best position for birth are inaccurately labeled as CPD. When women are encouraged to stay mobile and change positions during labor and pushing, push only when they have an urge to push and not given arbitrary time limits, the likelihood of a successful vaginal birth is very high.

Perineum Not Stretching

The perineal skin has a remarkable ability to stretch to accommodate the baby's head. In addition to the natural stretch of the skin, midwives have many techniques they use to assist the skin to stretch successfully. Warm compresses, olive oil, massage, support of the perineum and keeping all hands off the perinum are all techniques used to help prevent tearing of the perineal skin.

For most women, the perineum stretches around the baby's head in one or two contractions. Occasionally, a midwife will recognize the signs that the perineal skin is starting to tear. How the tear is handled will depend on the philosophy of your midwife and the location of the threatened tear. Many times the midwife will allow the skin to tear knowing a tear is likely to be less damaging to the skin than an episiotomy. If the threatened tear is near the top of the vagina (close to the clitoris) the midwife may choose to do an episiotomy to encourage the skin to tear down where the tissue is not so sensitive. Even more rarely, a mother has a perineum that resists stretching for several contractions. This can be painful and stressful as you wait for the skin to stretch.

Perineal massage during pregnancy may help prepare your skin to stretch. You can do it yourself or have your husband do it for you. Position yourself comfortably, sitting or reclining in a way that gives access to the skin around the vagina. It can be done for up to 10 minutes a day during the last four weeks of pregnancy. As you become more comfortable with the stretch, you may increase the amount you stretch the skin.

> Wash hands thoroughly. Ensure there are no sharp or long nails that may scratch you.

> Locate the perineum, directly below the vagina. It is the skin between the vagina and the anus. Apply some cold pressed, pure oil (such as olive oil) to this skin.

> Place the thumbs at the base of the vagina, allowing them to slide inside the vagina (to about the first joint) moving some oil with them.

Using gentle but firm pressure, move the thumbs from the base of the vagina up the side walls as if you were making a "U".

Return the thumbs to the base of the vagina, and repeat procedure.

Your local homeopath may have preparations that will help keep the skin elastic. Another option is to spend part of the day (or at least the night) without panties to prevent the skin becoming chapped by the increase in cervical mucus common during pregnancy. Keeping the pelvic floor muscles toned helps your baby to emerge with the smallest part of the head coming first so the perineum can ease open. Choose pushing positions that are comfortable and allow for the most stretch in your perineum, such as squatting or on hands and knees.

Retained Placenta

The placenta will normally be sloughed off the uterine wall within 30 minutes of the baby's being born. As long as there is no excessive bleeding, some midwives consider up to two hours normal. Rarely, the placenta will not detach and is then considered retained. It is also possible for a part of the placenta to not detach properly, and although most of the placenta exited, a piece remains. If other attempts to remove the placenta are unsuccessful, your midwife will need to manually remove the pieces of placenta that remain in the uterus.

There is no way to predict a retained placenta, although it is more common in women who have had several children, have a history of retained placenta or have had uterine surgery. Overall, less than two women in one hundred will have a retained placenta, though your risk may be related to the philosophy of your midwife since manual removal of the placenta may be associated with an active management of the third stage. Proper nutrition during pregnancy may help to ensure the uterus is strong throughout labor and the third stage. In addition, some midwives recommend using red raspberry leaf tea during pregnancy to help strengthen the uterus.

To help prevent a retained placenta, your midwife will want to be sure your uterus continues to contract after your baby is born. Allowing your baby to breastfeed strengthens the contractions naturally, even if your baby only plays with the nipple. If you are unable to breastfeed, you can use other methods of nipple stimulation to encourage contractions. Your midwife may want to use herbs such as red raspberry leaf or tinctures such as blue cohosh to help strengthen contractions. If you are in a hospital, you may receive synthetic oxytocin as routine immediate postpartum care. Manually massaging the uterus through the abdomen is helpful at stimulating contractions, even though it can be very uncomfortable.

While waiting for the placenta to be born, your midwife may put traction on the umbilical cord to see if the placenta has detached. This is not pulling on the cord, no one should ever pull on the umbilical cord as this can cause the placenta to be broken in pieces and can increase the risk a piece will be retained. Traction is holding the cord with only enough support to see if it moves. Another technique to watch for placental separation is to place a clamp on the cord near the vaginal opening and wait for the clamp to "move" further away from the vagina. Once the placenta has been born, your midwife will check for retained pieces.

Hemorrhage

The loss of excessive blood after the birth of a baby is referred to as postpartum hemorrhage. Able to kill an otherwise healthy mother in only a few hours, postpartum hemorrhage is the most common cause of maternal death worldwide. Luckily, it is usually easy for a skilled birth attendant to mange, and most women who receive care make a complete recovery. It is twice as likely in a cesarean surgery as a vaginal birth, and may be more common in women who have had several children.

Your midwife will suspect a postpartum hemorrhage if she sees excessive bleeding, if your blood pressure drops, if your heart rate increases or if she observes pain and swelling in pelvic tissues. Appropriate care will require your midwife to be able to assess the cause of the bleeding and begin treatment. If the cause of the hemorrhage is bleeding due to injury, repair of the injury must happen swiftly. Depending on the location of the injury, your midwife may be able to stitch repairs where you are or will recommend surgical repairs at a hospital.

If the hemorrhage is caused by your uterus not contracting adequately, your midwife will move swiftly to strengthen uterine contractions. Nipple stimulation, either manually or through breastfeeding, and massage of the uterus through the abdomen may be tried. Your midwife may also recommend synthetic oxytocin or herbal preparations to encourage contraction of the uterus.

Replacing lost fluids will be important, so you may be given IV fluids. Depending on how much blood is lost, your midwife will make recommendations on your need for blood transfusion. If you feel dizzy or light-headed an oxygen mask may help.

Cesarean Surgery

Cesarean surgery is the name for the procedure in which a doctor will cut through your lower abdomen and uterus to remove your baby. Though rumor has it the Roman emperor Caesar was born through such a surgery, it is unlikely he actually was. Until recent history, cutting open the mother's abdomen to rescue a baby was deadly for the mother and so reserved for cases in which the death of the mother had already occurred or was obviously unavoidable.

The rate of cesarean birth is highly variable. This means where you live and who you choose to attend you in labor has a large impact on the chances you will have a cesarean. Thirty percent of births in the United States and Australia are cesarean surgeries. In the United Kingdom, Canada and New Zealand the rate is about 23 percent. In parts of South America the rate can be as high as 85 percent. Women giving birth in northern Europe have cesarean rates between 5 and 10 percent. However, even within a country the rate varies widely within regions and even hospitals within the same area.

Women with private health insurance or giving birth in private hospitals are more likely to have cesarean surgery. Women who hire a male obstetrician as a birth attendant have a 40 percent higher chance of having a cesarean than women who hire a female obstetrician. Midwives attending births in the United States have less than 12 percent cesarean rate.

Cesarean Surgery

The World Health Organization believes the appropriate rate of cesarean surgeries should be between 5 and 15 percent. They feel when the rate falls under 5 percent, women may have limited access to necessary life-saving procedures. When it is over 15 percent unnecessary risk is added to birth without improved outcomes for mothers and babies.

> USA Healthy People 2010 has set a target of 15% cesarean for first time mothers and 63% for women with a prior cesarean.

Surgical birth carries more risk than a vaginal birth. Among the risks is increased risk of death for the mother and baby (MacDorman, 2006). Even though the risk of death remains low in developed countries, it is as high as five times more likely with elective cesarean as with a vaginal birth. This means where there is no problem with the pregnancy or labor, surgical birth results in more deaths than vaginal birth.

Other risks include post surgical complications. Post-cesarean infection results in 8 to 27 percent of surgeries. The risk for major complications including severe hemorrhage, need for repeat surgery, pelvic infection, blood clotting, pneumonia or blood poisoning is 4.5 percent. In addition, recovery from a cesarean surgery is painful and takes longer than vaginal birth. Two weeks after the surgery, 15 percent of mothers who had a cesarean to give birth still have difficulty with normal daily activities such as getting out of bed, walking, bending, lifting and tending to the baby. Women who have a cesarean surgery also have an inceased risk of being readmitted to the hospital within 60 days of giving birth (Lydon, 2000). This can interfere with successful bonding and breastfeeding.

Cesarean surgery carries risks for the baby as well. Babies born by cesarean are more likely to have breathing difficulties than vaginal born babies and are three times as likely as vaginal birth babies to be admitted to the intermediate or intensive care nursery. These results are startling because the research compares surgeries done with a healthy mother and baby, not surgeries done for fear of the health of mother or baby.

Women who have a cesarean surgery also have a greatly increased risk of infertility and a moderately increased risk for ectopic pregnancy. There is also an increased risk for injury to other organs with each additional cesarean. The scar tissue from the cesarean increases the risk for placenta previa, placenta accreta and placental abruption. The risks for placental problems increase with each cesarean.

Reasons for Cesarean with Other Options

Prolapsed Cord	Medical emergency necessitating surgery.
Placenta Previa	Waiting for labor to begin increases the risk of the placenta becoming detached. Baby sometimes cannot be born vaginally.
Placenta Abruption	Serious problem for baby, requires immediate surgery.
Placenta Accreta	Because the placenta grows through the uterine wall, this is very dangerous for the mother and requires surgery.
Transverse Lie	Baby cannot be born in this position. Can try to move baby with positions or version before labor begins.
Severe Preeclampsia or Hypertension	There may be other options depending on your circumstances. Epidural can help keep blood pressure down in labor, and magnesium can prevent convulsions.
Large Baby	No real way to tell if baby will fit without a trial of labor. Just as likely to be wrong as right in predicting who will be born, and late term ultrasound is not good at guessing size.
Gestational Diabetes	Major concern is macrosomia in uncontrolled diabetes. Not a valid reason on its own for surgery.
Fetal Distress (Non-Reassuring Heart Tones)	This is a judgment call. EFM has a high false positive rate. Blood Ph can verify before you submit to surgery. If you are already pushing, may use forceps or vacuum instead.
CPD	This is a judgment call, and there is no way to tell without a significant trial of labor. Positioning is another option, as is waiting. Mother's fatigue is an issue.
Failure to Progress	This is another judgment call. Basically means your labor was slower than the caregiver is comfortable with for any reason.
Breech	Can try to turn the baby, vaginal breech may have more risk for baby but cesarean carries more risk for mom. Find a caregiver with breech experience or wait for baby to turn.
Previous Cesarean	Only if you have an indication for surgery in this pregnancy. VBAC is safer for most mothers and babies.
Active Herpes	Judgment call based on the location of the lesions and ability to prevent contact with baby.
Twins	No evidence surgery is safer unless one of the twins has an issue requiring c-section. Find a skilled midwife or doctor with experience in twin vaginal birth.

Even with the risks, cesarean surgery is sometimes the most safe and least risky way for a baby to enter the world. It is important to know your caregiver's philosophy about cesareans because most of the reasons given for cesarean are determined not by evidence based guidelines but by caregiver judgment call.

Procedure

If you do not already have an IV in place, one will be inserted. An anesthesiologist will administer anesthetic, usually an epidural. Using a regional anesthetic allows you to be conscious and see your baby right away. If there is no time, a general anesthetic which will put you to sleep may be used. General anesthesia is only used in extreme situations because it does increase the risks for your baby.

A nurse will shave the hair from your upper pubic region and insert a bladder catheter to collect urine while you are anesthetized. Your abdomen will be washed with a sterile solution to help prevent the risk of infection. A curtain will be used to block your view of your abdomen so you do not watch the cut being made. In addition, your arms may be strapped down to prevent you from accidentally reaching during the surgery. In many hospitals, your husband or a trusted friend or family member can be with you during surgery.

When you are fully anesthetized, the obstetrician, a trained surgeon, will make an incision just above your pubic bone. You may feel tugging, pulling or pressure as the cut is made, but you should not feel pain. The obstetrician will need to cut through skin, abdominal fatty tissue, connective tissue, muscle and more connective tissue before reaching your uterus. After your uterus is cut, the bag of waters can be cut and your baby can be pulled through the opening. You may feel tugging or pulling as your baby is taken out, but it will not hurt.

Birth by cesarean

The curtain may be lowered so you can see your baby as they pull him out, but you may need to wait to hold him. Babies born by cesarean frequently need a little help to stimulate breathing because they missed the stimulation of being moved through the birth canal. When the staff is sure your baby is breathing normally, and if there are no other concerns, your partner may be able to hold the baby. If you request it, a nurse may place your baby near you so you can touch and talk to him.

In the meantime, the obstetrician will remove your placenta and begin the repair of your uterus and abdominal tissues. The entire experience, including the administration of an epidural, will take about an hour. The surgery takes about ten minutes and the closing of the cut will take at least fifteen and up to thirty minutes. When the obstetrician has completed, you will be moved to a recovery area where you will be monitored by nurses. The epidural will be allowed to wear off, and you will receive other medication to help with the post-operative pain. With assistance, you may be able to begin breastfeeding in the recovery area.

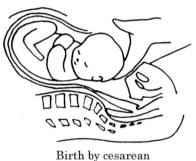
Birth by cesarean

Options You Have

You do have options when you undergo a cesarean surgery. If you know before labor begins that surgical birth will be the safest for you and your baby, you may have the option to choose the day of birth. In some cases, even if you believe your baby should be born by cesarean, you can plan to have the cesarean when labor begins, ensuring your baby is fully ready to be born and experiences some contractions to help prevent breathing problems. If you choose the date of your surgery, you can let friends and family know, or keep it a secret so you can still give the surprise call with the big news.

Most hospitals allow you to have a support person with you during a planned cesarean, giving you the option to invite someone to join you. You can usually have a support person during an unplanned cesarean, but the time factor will limit your choice to those who are already with you in labor. Usually, this is not a problem because the person you want with you during a cesarean is one of the people you want with you during labor anyway. If your baby requires special nursery care, you can choose to send one support person with the baby while a different support person remains with you in the recovery area.

Some obstetricians will describe the events of the cesarean as they are happening to help you feel more comfortable with the procedure and so you do not feel like a bystander. You may also have the option of bringing a camera into the surgical room so your support person can get pictures of the new baby right away. Depending on the reason for the surgery, you may be able to breastfeed as soon as the baby is ready even if you are still in the surgical suite. However this will take considerable assistance from the nurse on duty.

> Which options will make a cesarean surgery a better experience for you?

You may have other options, but this depends on the hospital you choose, the circumstances of your surgery and the philosophy of the doctors attending you. For example, you may be given a choice between different types of regional blocks for pain management. You may be given options about using staples or stitches for closing the cut. If you are under the care of a midwife or doula, she may be able to continue her support through the surgery. You may have the option to complete other uterine surgeries you may be considering such as a hysterectomy or removal of a cyst as part of the same operation.

Emotional Issues

One of the most difficult aspects of a cesarean is the attitude of friends and family. In many areas where cesarean has become accepted as normal, the truth that it is major abdominal surgery is lost. Instead of taking appropriate time to recuperate from the surgery, mothers who have cesareans begin caring for their babies. Complaints and frustrations are often met with hurtful remarks such as: "You are so lucky to have had a cesarean"; or "You should just be thankful your baby is healthy."

If you did not want or anticipate a cesarean, it is hard to just be thankful you underwent unexpected major abdominal surgery. It is possible to love your baby, be glad he is here and be grieving that his birth required you to be cut open. It is also normal to be angry about having a cesarean, especially if it was for reasons that might not have resulted in surgery with another caregiver. No woman would feel comfortable feeling she was cut open for no reason. Many women also feel violated after a cesarean. These are normal and healthy responses to having unexpected major surgery.

Women who were not expecting to undergo surgery are more likely to have an unfavorable reaction to their babies, experience postpartum depression, suffer psychological trauma and have poor overall mental health and overall functioning (Childbirth Connection, 2006). There is healing needed after a cesarean that goes far beyond the physical healing of your body. You need God to heal the wounds on your heart. The disappointment, fear, anger and helplessness many women feel cannot be talked away with shallow words, but they can be healed by a loving and concerned God.

If you experience an unwanted cesarean, be honest with God about your feelings. Let yourself cry to him. Find a trusted friend or loved one who will just listen without trying to make your hurt go away. Give yourself time to grieve your loss. One of the biggest mistakes women make is in assuming they need to just "get over it." The emotional pain will lessen, but only if you truly let it heal. Ignoring or hiding how you feel is not healing, it is avoiding. God is big enough to handle your hurt.

Allow caring friends and family to bring you meals while you recover. Ask for help with the housework so you can focus on healing and caring for your baby. Take it slowly, using your body as your guide. If you find yourself too worn out, then try to do less the next day. Every body is different, and depending on the circumstances of the surgery, you may need a few more days to recover than a woman who had a different cesarean experience.

Take advantage of the lactation consultant in the hospital. She will be able to teach you ways to nurse your baby without putting pressure on your healing abdomen. Practice the rehabilitation exercises before you leave the hospital, and be sure to do them every day to help your physical recovery. Regaining your physical health will not remove the emotional pain, but it certainly will not hurt your emotional state to begin feeling good as soon as possible.

Above all else, do not allow yourself to think of an unexpected cesarean as a failure on your part. Even if you may make different choices in your preparation for your next baby, chances are you did make the best decisions you could with the information you had available. It is not fair to criticize your decision based on information you did not have when you needed to choose. If you believe you should have made a different decision, then you are that much more prepared for your next labor experience.

VBAC

The decision of whether or not to undergo cesarean surgery to give birth can be more difficult if you have had a previous cesarean. The risks of being unsuccessful in a vaginal birth, and the risks of choosing a cesarean should be determined by the present pregnancy, not past experiences. Making a wise decision means carefully considering your unique situation to determine which route is most likely to bring out the best outcome for you and your baby.

Considering a VBAC? Why not make a list of pros and cons before reading this section. Then you can take notes on your list and reevaluate.

When asked their reasons for choosing a repeat cesarean, women share their fear of a failed trial of labor, their concern about the danger of vaginal birth, fear of the pain and the convenience of scheduling (Declercq, Sakala, Corry & Applebaum, 2006). If these are your concerns as well, you may be interested in some facts that can help relieve you of your fears, although they are unlikely to change your level of pain during childbirth or the inconvenience of waiting for labor to start.

Women planning to give birth vaginally after a cesarean have about an 80 percent success rate regardless of the reasons for their previous surgery. Not even having a previous diagnosis of cephelopelvic disproportion is predictive of the need for another cesarean. There is very little difference in the success rate when the mother has had more than one cesarean. Vaginal birth after cesarean also has about five times less risk of injury and four times less risk of death to the mother than another cesarean. Thankfully, the risk of a mother dying while pregnant or in the immediate postpartum is very rare in the developed world.

The most commonly quoted concern with a vaginal birth after cesarean is uterine dehiscence, meaning the scar from the previous cesarean separated. In some instances the scar can rupture, which means it completely opens. Although rupture is dangerous for mother and baby, it is extremely rare. The overall risk for dehiscence during a vaginal birth is less than 2 percent, which is the same number seen in elective repeat cesareans, meaning the dehisancese was there before labor started.

Most cases of a separation of the scar are asymptomatic, which means they cause no problem and heal without the mother ever knowing it happened. Vertical incision scars are more likely to separate than horizontal scars, and the rate of separation increases slightly when there is more than one previous cesarean. Using oxytocin shows no greater risk of separation, and neither does using an epidural.

There is no benefit to searching for a separation after the baby is born. Instead, it increases the risk of infection and runs the risk of ripping the separation into a rupture. Uterine rupture is painful and shows symptoms of abnormal bleeding, so its presence after giving birth is obvious enough to identify without the painful exploration of the uterus. But your chances of a rupture are no greater with a previous cesarean than without. In fact, previous cesarean is a factor in only half the cases of uterine rupture. You have thirty times the likelihood of needing an emergency cesarean for any other reason, so concern for a uterine rupture should be small.

When comparing outcomes for babies, there is no specific improvement in health that comes from an elective repeat cesarean. In fact, babies born by cesarean surgery show more symptoms of respiratory distress than babies of the same age who are born vaginally. All the risks to mothers and babies who have cesarean surgery remain risks, even when the cesarean is by choice, not need.

Even though having a cesarean after a failed trial of labor almost doubles the risks of a planned cesarean, only 20 percent of mothers with a previous cesarean will experience these risks. Speaking straight statistics, you and your baby have the best chances of staying safe with a planned vaginal birth rather than a planned cesarean surgery.

Despite the overwhelming safety and success of a vaginal birth after cesarean, between 30 and fifty 50 percent of women schedule an elective repeat cesarean. In fact, 89 percent of the mothers who had a previous cesarean in the Listening to Mothers II survey had a repeat cesarean. Of those women, 78 percent said the reason for the surgery was the previous cesarean rather than any indication of a problem necessitating a surgical birth for this pregnancy.

Though society says the decision ultimately rests in the mother's hands, where you live may limit your ability to choose between a repeat cesarean and a vaginal birth after cesarean. In many areas of the United States, hospitals have removed the option of a VBAC, leaving women to either agree with a repeat cesarean or search for alternative prenatal care. In other parts of the world, you must have a specific reason for having cesarean surgery, previous cesarean not being considered enough of a reason. It is important to know what the midwives, doctors, birth centers and hospitals in your area offer as options. Be sure to talk to two or three midwives, as practices differ even within the same city.

> "Motherhood is a result of conception NOT delivery."
> *Amy Bookwalter*

Drawing Conclusions
Review of Section Eight

Ten Questions about . . .
Labor Challenges

1. What challenges are you most likely to face in labor?
2. How can you be prepared for those challenges?
3. How are labor challenges talked about in your family?
4. What challenges did your mother face in labor?
5. How does your midwife prefer to handle challenges?
6. What if you have more challenges than you expect?
7. What if you experience no challenges?
8. What support will you need to handle challenges?
9. What support do you have?
10. How can you get more support?

Truth or Fiction?

Births in movies and on television are usually dramatic, dangerous events. The expectant mother, who was casually talking a moment before, is suddenly overcome with the urge to push. By this point, you probably recognize how unrealistic cinematic births are.

However, even reality television can skew the truth. The real business of the media is to entertain, not teach. Normal birth is boring television. The next time you watch a program that shows the birth of a child, pay attention to what is actually happening and answer these questions.

- How many women are likely to have the problem depicted in the show?
- What are some other ways to handle the problem?
- What choices would you make to prevent the problem?

Variation or Emergency?

Understanding the difference between a normal variation and a birth emergency is important to making wise decisions while faced with a labor challenge. Draw a diagram similar to the one below. On one side, list the challenges that are normal variations. On the other, list the challenges that are dangerous or emergencies. Where the two circles intersect, list the challenges that may be variations and may also indicate a problem.

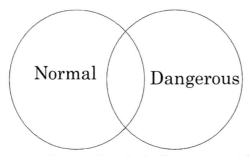

Now that you have placed challenges as either normal or dangerous, take some time to think about the possible responses to the challenges. Make a third circle for the responses so it intersects both the variations and the emergencies. Go through each challenge again. How might a specific response affect your labor if the challenge is a normal variation of labor? How might a specific response affect your labor if the challenge is dangerous or an emergency?

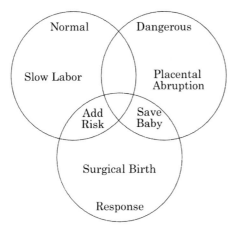

The Miracle of Waterbirth

Barbara Harper
Author
Gentle Birth Choices
Waterbirth International
www.waterbirth.org

When couples ask why I think waterbirth is considered the gentlest of gentle births, I always refer back to the baby. In our effort to help the mother get through the labor we sometimes forget that the baby is having an experience of his own. The entire process of using warm water immersion for labor and birth is a miracle. Water eases the mother's pain, gives her greater mobility, conserves her energy, helps her relax and let go and as a result the baby receives more oxygen, has a better chance to move into the right position for the passage through the pelvis and makes the most gentle transition from womb to room.

Some doctors will argue that mothers who choose waterbirth are being selfish and only caring about their physical and psychological comfort and not thinking about the baby. I have made the very same statement about women who choose epidurals or narcotics to help them with the pain. The effects of the powerful drugs on the baby are much greater than the effects of the water. So, our motivations for caring about the baby's experience of birth are the same as the doctors'.

The most important part of every birth is the connection that mother and baby make immediately after the birth. Connecting is the way humans lay the foundation and the neurological network for all the development that will take place in the brain for the next several years. A baby that is drugged has a much harder time connecting, making his needs known and finishing the forth and most important stage of labor—attaching to the breast. Water babies do not have any problems meeting their mothers eye to eye and skin to skin. Their mothers are usually naked, wet, warm and completely responsive.

The water protects that immediate bond between mother and baby. The warm pool becomes a 'womb with a view' that contains the mother, sometimes the father and the baby together in this dream-like, slow paced, new world into which the baby makes its transition and takes its first breath. There is no hurry, no rush to take baby away or to cut the umbilical cord. For these reasons waterbirth has taught us many lessons in the past 20-30 years. We have seen how important those moments are in the life of the family. Midwives and doctors have often completely changed the way they routinely attend birth after witnessing a number of successful waterbirths.

What caused waterbirth to make an appearance in the mid-1980s at almost exactly the same time in many different places around the world? England, the US, Australia, central Europe all reported places and people starting to offer waterbirth between 1982 and 1984 and a few places even earlier. My own journey discovering the benefits of using water to ease labor and facilitate birth began in 1983 when a woman in the physician's office where I was working told me that she was preparing for a waterbirth. I was intrigued and asked a lot of questions. She handed me a *National Inquirer* article that reported waterbirths in Soviet Russia showing photos of newborns in glass tanks still attached to the umbilical cord swimming between the legs of happy naked birthing women. I was hooked.

As a former labor and delivery nurse, I thought anything that we can do to help mothers have easier births and babies to have a gentle experience had to be good. A year later I, too, was experiencing the powerful, life-changing event of birth in water. I began the organization, Waterbirth International, after researching all over the world in the next few years after my waterbirth. God planted a vision in my heart of sharing information, encouraging couples and teaching about the miracle of waterbirth. For nearly 25 years he has blessed us with the means to instruct, research, assist couples in birth, develop birth pool designs, put on conferences and now offer a credential to doctors and midwives who want to attend waterbirths. God desires that his wonderful children experience loving, gentle births and water is the gentlest birth a mother and baby can have.

Subject Nine

Getting to Know Your Newborn

Topics:

Your Newborn Baby	333
Your Baby as a Person	338
Feeding your Baby	342
Parenting a Newborn	351
Drawing Conclusions	356
The Baby God Gave You—Perfect? by Sharon Tilotta	358

Your Newborn Baby

Your baby will be adjusting to life outside the womb, so these first few weeks are as much about transition to a new state of being for your baby as they are for you. Understanding the changes your baby is going through can help you be prepared to care for him.

There is no "typical" newborn. Babies are as different as the adults they will grow to become. God has made us all unique, each with our own purpose. Who your baby is as a person is as important to your being able to help him adjust to life outside the womb as the "typical" needs of a newborn. For example, all babies get hungry, but some babies experience distress quickly when hungry. How calm or distressed your newborn is when a need is not understood are factors that determine how you will care for your child.

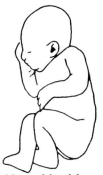

Normal healthy newborns do not look like the Gerber Baby.

Appearance

The normal healthy newborn does not look like the image of the "Gerber Baby." A newborn's head is about two-thirds of the entire body size. The newborn skull is designed to mould under the pressure of birth to allow the head to pass through the pelvis. There is wide variation in how much molding a baby needs, so in the first day or two after birth, your baby may have a pointy head or it may appear quite round. If you touch the top of your baby's head, you will find two soft spots where the bones are not yet joined. These spots are called

A newborn's skull is made to mould during labor.

fontanelles and will become hard as the skull bone grows and covers them. The spot in back takes about six weeks, while the larger spot in front can take up to a year to fully close.

Although babies tend to weigh within a few pounds of each other, there is wide variation in how they look. Some babies are long and skinny, other babies are full and round. In the womb, your baby was scrunched up with arms and legs bent. It may take your baby some time to stretch out his muscles, and in the meantime he may look like a little hunched up bundle. Newborn necks are very short, and it will also take time for your baby to gain the strength to support his head. This tends to make newborns look as if they have no neck, further adding to the look of a hunched up bundle.

Your baby's eyes may appear puffy but will most likely be very alert. Newborns can see, although they are not accustomed to such bright light. Newborn eyes tend to look dark brown, grey or blue. This is only a temporary eye color. You will begin to see what color eyes your child will have around 3 months of age.

Whether your baby is a boy or a girl, the genitals will be swollen, as might the breasts. This normal response to the changing hormone levels of labor will go away in a few days. In most newborn boys, the testicles will have descended into the scrotum before birth. Those that did not tend to do so on their own within the first year of life. It is normal for newborn boys to have erections in response to cool temperatures or before urinating. Newborn girls will sometimes have bleeding from the uterus which ends up looking like a small bloodstain in the diaper. This is a normal, temporary response to the changing hormone levels of the mother during labor. Both boys and girls may experience fluid leakage from the breasts, again a normal and temporary response to labor.

Your newborn's skin may be covered by a white creamy substance called vernix. Vernix helped protect your baby's skin in the uterus and can be rubbed into the skin or wiped off. Some babies are born with downy hair called lanugo hair on parts of their body. This hair was another way your

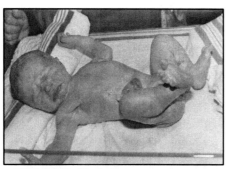
©2006 Jennifer Vanderlaan
The typical newborn has patches of vernix on his skin.

baby's skin was protected in the uterus and will naturally fall out over the first few weeks. Generally, the younger your baby gestationally, the more lanugo and vernix you will see.

Newborn skin is light regardless of race. If your baby will have a darker complexion, you will notice the skin darkening over a period of days or weeks as melanin becomes active. Some babies develop patches of bluish skin that look like bruises where the pigmentation begins. These are called Mongolian spots and disappear on their own within a few years. They are not related to bruises, cancer or any other skin problem.

Most newborns do not have flawless skin; instead, you may see a general blotchiness that looks like a rash; and some babies have bruising from birth. You will probably see tiny white dots that look like pimples on your baby's face. These are called milia and are the normal response to your baby's oil glands starting to work. You may also find your baby has pimples on his face within the first two months of life. This is normal and does not predict future problems with acne. It is common for babies to have dry skin on their hands and feet for the first few weeks.

The umbilical cord will begin to collapse and dry out when it is exposed to air. After it has been clamped and cut, your baby will be left with a short "stump" of cord. It will continue to dry out over the first few days of life, and will fall off within two weeks. Some babies bleed slightly when the cord detaches. In some hospitals, the cord is treated with a blue antiseptic solution, although this is not necessary.

Behavior

Breathing is central to life, and you will probably be concerned in the first few days that your baby is not breathing properly. It is normal for newborns to have an irregular breathing pattern, combining shallow and deep breaths with short periods of no breath. Many babies have a wheezing or gurgle sound with some breaths as their body expels mucus. Most babies also sneeze as they clear the nasal passages. It can take the first 24 hours for your baby to really get the hang of a regular breathing pattern. If breathing and eating do not seem difficult, and if your baby has good skin color, what you are hearing is probably the normal breathing noises of a newborn.

While your baby's nervous system matures, you may find he seems jittery or easily startled, especially when undressed. You will find he is less jittery when swaddled, held or nursing. He will also experience frequent hiccups, caused by a twitch of the diaphragm muscle. Some babies are bothered by hiccups while others do not seem to notice them.

Newborns sleep nearly twenty hours a day, often waking to eat and then falling asleep again in a 2 or 3-hour cycle. Within a few weeks your baby will begin to have longer waking times, but will probably not sleep for longer than 4 hours at a stretch until after 3 months. Newborns have an ability to shut out repetitive sounds while they are sleeping. This skill, called habituation, is why your baby is able to ignore most of the sounds you would expect to ruin a nap.

Eating for some newborns is quick, for others it requires marathon sessions. The speed with which your baby eats will be dependant on your breasts, his appetite and his efficiency at sucking. This is why you can not watch the clock to determine when and how long your baby should eat. While eating, some babies need more help than others to remove extra air from the stomach (burping). Some babies have a tendency to spit out milk when they burp.

Not all newborns like to nurse immediately after birth; some are content to simply cuddle and snuggle mom or nuzzle the breast. Once your baby has begun nursing, you can expect him to nurse eight to twelve times in a 24-hour period. Newborns have small stomachs that can only hold a few ounces of milk at a time, but they need to drink enough milk to double their weight in only a few months. The normal healthy newborn eats frequently through the day and night.

Frequent nursing means frequent elimination. One of the normal reflexes of the human body is the reflex to empty the bowel of its contents when food is swollowed. Because of this, your newborn may need a diaper change with every nursing. At first this will be sticky, black meconium. After the meconium is passed, you can expect breastfed babies to have a watery yellow-green stool. This is normal and not a sign of diarrhea. Bottle-fed babies stools are less frequent and a more formed, tan colored stool.

Newborn reflexes are a normal sign your baby is healthy. When startled, babies stretch out their hands and then bring them back in. The Moro or startle reflex is caused by sudden changes in position or loud noises, and even occurs while your baby sleeps. The grasp reflex causes your baby to hold on to whatever is placed in his hands. A similar reflex in the feet causes him to turn his toes downward. The rooting reflex turns your baby's head toward whatever touches his cheek, helping him learn to breastfeed. The sucking reflex, causing your baby to suck on whatever touches his lips, works with the swallowing reflex to help your baby learn to breastfeed.

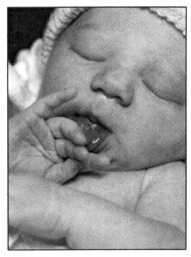
©2006 Therese Franklin
The newborn sucking reflex will cause him to suck on his fingers when they are by his mouth.

Crying is often distressing to parents. It is your baby's signal that something is not right. In most cases, crying is not your baby's first response. Babies do have cues to alert you of a need, and crying is used when the cues are missed. There are differences in babies' personalities, so your baby may respond by crying more or less often than another baby. There are also differences in parenting styles that increase or decrease crying; for example, babies whose parents hold them for at least three hours a day cry less than babies whose parents do not hold them (Hunziker & Barr, 1986). It can be difficult to determine what help your newborn needs when crying, but within a few weeks you will become familiar with your baby's cues and begin to understand the subtle (and not so subtle) differences in your baby's cries.

The baby's skin may become dry and peeling in the first couple of weeks. You can use natural lotion or olive oil, but this will resolve on its own. Many babies also have a series of rashes that are harmless and do not require treatment. Please wait to bathe the baby for a few days, this will help keep the baby from becoming cold and keep the cord stump dry.

Eneyda Ramos

Your Baby as a Person

Sometimes parents get the mistaken idea that babies are mindless lumps who do no more than cry, sleep and poop. Other times parents seem to act as if babies are miniature adults, capable of adult behaviors and thought patterns. The reality is that babies are fully individual humans, capable of communication, emotion and personality, but at a unique stage of development which makes them remarkably different from adults.

Senses

Your baby can see, hear, touch, taste and smell. His senses were all developed before he was born; however, there are some adjustments that need to be made now that he is born. For example, his eyes will need to become accustomed to the bright lights of life outside the womb.

Newborns can see best when an object is 8-12 inches from their faces. The object they prefer to look at most is someone's face. Newborns even know when something is different about a face, such as when mom takes her glasses off. This indicates your baby is learning and forming memory even this early. It may take a few weeks for your baby to gain the ability to hold his eyes on one object. Once he does, you can spend time gazing at each other and imitating each other's facial expressions.

The ability to imitate facial expressions is an amazing thing about newborns. At just a few days old, without an understanding of mirrors and having never seen his face, your baby instinctively knows to open his mouth and stick out his tongue when you do. While you play this imitating game, your baby will probably reach a hand towards your face. These interactions between you and your baby are a great picture of a relationship with God. Although you see and understand only part of who God is, you instinctively respond by wanting to be like God and reach out for him.

1 Corinthians 13:12

Newborns can hear before they are born, and prefer sounds that were familiar from the womb such as the rhythmic beats of a heart or swishing of circulation. Newborns do remember sounds they repeatedly heard such as mom's voice, a piece of music or a story that was read regularly before he was born. Newborns are also able to determine the direction a sound is coming from and will turn their heads towards a sound. Unlike adults, newborns have the ability to block out sounds that disturb them. This allows your baby to sleep even in a noisy environment. In fact, some babies use sleep as a way to prevent sensory overload in loud places.

Communication

While your baby is not capable of speech, he is capable of communication and interaction. Though crying is the most easily understood communication of newborns, they are able to use facial gestures and body movements to communicate needs. Newborns do try subtler ways to interact with their environment before resorting to crying, but you will need to pay attention to notice it.

The other ways newborns communicate include facial gestures, body language, small sounds, turning towards the source of a sound, reaching toward an object of interest and following objects with their eyes. Within a few weeks, you will become acquainted with the faces and bodily movements your child makes when distressed before he begins to cry and can begin to offer assistance before crying begins.

Your newborn is most likely to engage in interaction while quietly alert, meaning he is awake and quietly observing what is happening around him. Be sure you are within his field of vision close enough for him to focus on your face. Once you have his attention, experiment with mimicking his facial gestures or making large facial gestures for him to imitate. Be aware of his body language, allowing him the opportunity to turn away to end the game when he is tired.

Sleeping

Adults sleep in a pattern of light and deep sleep that cycles over a few hours so that in an average 8-hour sleep, you spend 6 hours in deep sleep and 2 hours in light sleep. During the light sleep you might roll over, adjust the blankets, wake up to use the bathroom or get a drink of water. Your baby sleeps differently.

The first major difference between adult and newborn sleep is that babies spend about twenty minutes in a state of light sleep before they gradually begin to enter deep sleep, which is why babies always seem to wake up if they are put down immediately after "falling asleep." As your newborn matures, the amount of time he will need to spend in light sleep before drifting into a deep sleep will decrease. But in those first months, he might need a lot of help to settle into a state of deep sleep.

Another difference is that newborns have a light and deep sleep cycle that lasts half as long as adults, meaning the opportunity for your baby to wake at night happens twice as often as an adult. Additionally, babies spend more time in light sleep than adults do. This is built in protection for the baby, who requires help to do any of the simple things you do without waking. If your newborn is too cold or too hot, he needs help adjusting the temperature. If your newborn is uncomfortable, he needs help to reposition herself.

There are strong physiological needs for your baby to wake at night as well. If your newborn has to use the bathroom, he requires help to change the diaper. If your newborn is hungry, he needs help to get food. He will need to eat at night because his stomach can only hold a few ounces at a time and he has to double his body weight in just a few months. God has designed babies in a way that as nighttime needs become less intense, his sleeping patterns will change, allowing him to spend more time in deep sleep and wake less frequently.

Personality

A major part of your newborn's personality will be how sensitive he is to stimuli. Some babies easily adapt to changes and comfortably accept new experiences. Other babies find excessive stimulation uncomfortable and may need help making things "right" again. As you begin to understand who your child is, you will be able to adapt your responses to meet his specific needs. For many parents this is easy. For other parents this is a struggle, especially if the newborn has a personality somewhat opposite of the parent.

Recognizing personality traits in your newborn will give you your first glimpses at who God made him to be. There are benefits to being highly adaptable and there are also benefits to being highly sensitive. God created some people to be strongly determined and others to be flexible in their approaches to problem solving. There is no right or wrong; it is simply understanding who God made him to be. As he grows older, you will help him learn how to properly employ his strengths and improve weaker areas.

One of the major differences between personality in an adult and personality in a child is that as an adult, you have had many years to mature in your understanding of how your personality shapes the way you interact with people. You have had time to learn patience, trust, discipline and sacrifice—the things that make it possible for you to overcome your initial responses to stress, fear or pain. You may also have worked to change the most extreme parts of your personality so they conform to social norms, such as overcoming shyness or learning not to react in anger.

Your newborn has not had the time or experience to control emotions, patiently wait for needs to be met or understand how his interactions affect the world around him. While continually demanding things as an adult may be seen as bullying or manipulating, newborns do not have either the understanding to try manipulating or the ability to temper their initial reaction even if they did understand. Maturity happens slowly; it cannot be forced or rushed.

Feeding Your Baby

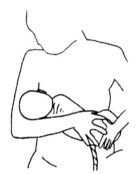

One of your first parenting tasks will be to feed your baby.

One of the first decisions you will be making as a parent will be how to feed your child. Though the ways you accomplish the feeding may be many, your choices are actually few. You can feed your baby breast milk, artificial milk or a combination of both.

The factors that go into making the decision vary from family to family. While friends may suggest one thing, your family may be recommending another. The information available can make it hard to discern truth from opinion. Recommendations for one feeding method say the other is just as good. The mixed messages can be confusing, leaving you more frustrated than you were before you began the work of making your decision.

Once you decide about the type of food your newborn will receive, you must then make decisions about how your child will receive that food. Again, mixed messages and competing philosophies vie for your loyalty, claiming to be the most healthy and spiritual way to feed your child. How do you begin to make a decision about the feeding method that is right for your family?

When making your decision, you will need accurate information about the benefits, drawbacks, prodedures and support you will have for a feeding method. With that information in hand, it is much easier to determine what is most likely to meet the needs of your family.

The History of Infant Feeding

Isaiah 66:10-11

Rejoice with Jerusalem and be glad for her,
 all you who love her;
rejoice greatly with her,
 all you who mourn over her.

For you will nurse and be satisfied
 at her comforting breasts;
 you will drink deeply
 and delight in her overflowing abundance.

The ancient Hebrews breastfed until the child was three years old. It seems the entire ancient world extended breastfeeding beyond two years, using wet-nurses when the mother was unable or unwilling to nurse the child. In the Bible, breastfeeding is talked of as nourishing and comforting, normal for the infant even though the Bible also places a sexual emphasis on the breasts as seen in Proverbs 5:19, "A loving doe, a graceful deer—may her breasts satisfy you always, may you ever be captivated by her love."

Proverbs 5:19
Song of Songs 4:5; 7:3
Ezekiel 23:2

Today, breastfeeding is met with mixed feelings at best. How did breastfeeding change from something so normal, expected and praised to something controversial, inciting shame and making women feel like failures? Slowly, over 2000 years of human history, superstition changed the understanding of breastfeeding. The spread of misinformation made it difficult for women to successfully breastfeed, and the poor success rates were seen as proof of the superiority of artificially feeding infants.

Kathleen Huggins shares an in-depth history of western breastfeeding practices in her book, *The Nursing Mother's Guide to Weaning*. She explains that although breastfeeding was the norm for most of history in Africa, Asia and Latin America, the western world began to become distrustful of the breastfeeding process. As early as the Roman civilization, concerns about breastfeeding being too difficult for the mother led doctors to recommend alternatives. The Romans also began the practice of regulating feedings, believing overfeeding caused the baby to be sick.

By medieval times, wealthy Europeans hired wet-nurses for their babies. While poor women had no choice, wealthy women and their husbands found it unfashionable to nurse as they believed it prevented them from wearing the popular clothing styles, caused breasts to sag and delayed the return of their fertility. Lack of understanding the way milk is produced caused restrictions on nursing behavior. A woman who was pregnant, menstruating or had engaged in sexual intercourse was believed to have bad milk, so even those who chose to breastfeed weaned their children early. The practice of using a wet-nurse began to lose popularity in Europe in the seventeenth century amid fears the child would take on the vices of the wet nurse through her milk. Wet-nursing fell out of popularity in the United States by the early 1900s due to fears that without constantly monitoring the health and morals of the wet-nurse, the milk could be hazardous to the baby.

Although babies had been fed a variety of solid foods mashed, sauced or dipped in broths since Roman times, people began seriously experimenting with artificial baby foods around the eighteenth century. The disastrous results of feeding newborns foods that could not be properly stored to prevent bacterial growth or that were so nutritionally poor as to starve the infants were illness or death.

Not understanding the true causes of illness and death, they were blamed on overfeeding the infants and feeding schedules were born. Since breastfeeding was commonly combined with artificial foods, breastfeed babies continued to suffer the same gastrointestinal illness as artificially fed babies. Doctors began to see breastfeeding as too demanding and of no benefit to the baby. They believed it was only healthful in rare cases and most women had inadequate or bad milk. They believed nursing could cause all types of health problems for the mother and began preferring the use of artificial infant foods.

The fears about the dangers of breastfeeding continued into the 1900s, when science became the standard by which everything was measured. Breastfeeding was seen as uncontrollable and unscientific. The prevailing attitude was to control everything about the baby, from scheduling feedings and sleeping to bowel movements and crying behavior. Women were advised not to trust their instinct but instead to become trained in the domestic sciences. When birth moved to hospitals the policies of placing babies in nurseries, sterilizing everything including the mother's breast and feeding from a bottle regardless of need caused delayed or limited milk production. Many women gave up breastfeeding from the start due to "bad" or insufficient milk. Artificial feeding became normal and was the method passed down from mother to daughter.

The Blessing of the Breasts

Within the last thirty years, the modern world has become aware of the many benefits of breastfeeding. The nursing relationship between a mother and her baby is one of the most beautifully intricate and amazingly useful designs God has bestowed upon creation. It is more than just the perfect nutrition for your baby. Breastfeeding benefits the mother and the baby so much so that nutritionally, developmentally and emotionally, breastfeeding is the best choice for babies and mothers. Perhaps this is why God considers breastfeeding the "blessing of the breasts." *Genesis 49:25*

Through breastfeeding, the baby receives not only nourishment for the body but also the ability to prevent illness and allergy, increased intelligence, proper development of the jaw, the touch needed for bonding and the emotional comfort of being held. The composition of your breastmilk changes to meet his specific nutritional needs as your baby ages.

The mother who breastfeeds receives the immediate benefit of prevention of postpartum hemorrhage, regular release of oxytocin (a feel good love hormone), a break from the menstrual cycle, protection from cancer and osteoporosis; she is more likely to rest during the day and sleep more at night than her bottle-feeding friends. In fact, the very act of breastfeeding causes mothers to be more "mothering" of their babies. This may be due to the prolactin hormone produced in the mother while she nurses her baby. Once you get the hang of it, breastfeeding can be done with one free hand for talking on the phone or playing with your toddler. You can even breastfeed your baby while lying in bed.

Families benefit from the economy and convenience of breastfeeding and the milder smells produced by a breastfed baby as compared to bottle-feed babies. Breast milk can be stored and served from a bottle when mom is away. Breastfeeding also helps prevent problems of inaccessibility to formula or water while traveling.

Modern Breastfeeding Reality

The legacy of distrusting breastfeeding and lack of understanding how to be successful at it continues to cause problems. Some mothers attempt to breastfeed expecting it to be easy, only to find the process is more difficult, painful and frustrating than they expected. Others find their attempts to breastfeed are met with anger or criticism by friends and family. Many women find even their doctor has a natural distrust of breastfeeding, recommending they instead use artificial feeding methods.

Breastfeeding is time-consuming work. Without proper support through the first few weeks, it can be difficult for a mother to work through a problem with latch or a baby who does not seem to nurse well right away. Other mothers run into problems because of the type of birth experience they had. Certain medications or procedures can make it difficult to establish a good breastfeeding relationship.

Not all families are supportive of a woman's decision to breastfeed. Some family members have been misinformed about the benefits of breastfeeding; others are jealous of the mother's time with the baby when breastfeeding. When friends and family do not trust a mother's decision to breastfeed, subtle and not so subtle comments add stress and frustration to an already difficult task.

Although breastfeeding is usually the safest method for feeding a baby, it is not always possible due to the health of the mother or the baby. Women who have had breast surgery may be unable to nurse due to severed ducts; however, the only way to know for sure is to try breastfeeding since the ducts can heal. Some mothers

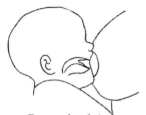

Proper latch is important for successful breastfeeding.

Do you have adequate support to be successful breastfeeding? How can you get the support you need?

(less than 2 percent) have insufficient glandular tissue which can be detected before the baby is born, although in this case breastfeeding may be successfully combined with artificial feeding.

If you become ill, your choices of infant feeding may be limited. Some illnesses are mild and with good support you can be successful at breastfeeding. However, other illnesses can prevent you from being able to nurse, pump your breasts and sometimes even care for your baby. In those cases, artificial feeding will need to either supplement what milk you have or be used solely to keep your baby alive and healthy. Mothers with an illness or condition requiring medication may need to adjust medication or avoid breastfeeding to prevent side-effects for the baby. Some babies have illnesses that make them unable to nurse, meaning the child will need expressed milk or artificial milk.

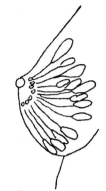

Milk is formed in mammary glands, and travels through ducts to your baby's mouth.

HIV infected mothers may be able to transfer the infection to their babies and should carefully consider the risks before making decisions. The risk is higher when breastfeeding is mixed with artificial feeding. When mixing breast and artificial milk, the risk of your child becoming infected is about 4 percent for every 6 months nursed (Coutsoudis, 2005). If you are HIV positive, get extra support to help prevent cracked nipples, mastitis or other problems that may increase the risk of transferring HIV to your baby.

In response to the needs of mothers who want to be successful at breastfeeding, women have begun to train as lactation consultants. Usually nurses, lactation consultants work with new mothers to help them understand the importance of position and latch. Knowing how to breastfeed prevents most of the problems a new mother may face with nursing. When a problem does arise, the lactation consultant can help the mother figure out what is happening and how to improve the situation.

Modern Artificial Feeding Reality

While women of the past chose not to breastfeed based on fashion, a large number of modern women choose not to breastfeed so they can continue in their employment.

Some mothers begin breastfeeding, switching to artificial feedings or a combination of breast and artificial feedings when they return to work. Others believe it is best for the baby to start artificial feeding from the start. In these cases, mothers try to make the bottle feeding experience (whether breast or artificial milk) as similar to the breastfeeding experience as possible.

Artificial feeding has an undeserved reputation for being the most convenient method for feeding a baby. In reality, artificial feeding is only easier if someone else does the feeding for you. Breastfeeding requires you to sit comfortably and make the breast available to your baby. Artificial feeding requires the sterilization of bottles and nipples, mixing of formulas and heating to the proper temperature. Nighttime artificial feeding means preparing a clean bottle at the right temperature before you are able to feed your crying baby. When traveling, the equipment needed to bottle feed must be brought with you, and a way to prepare the artificial milk must be found.

In some communities, there is a belief that artificial feeding is the best method to feed the baby. This is partly due to the history of artificial feeding being available only to the wealthy, and partly due to the history of misinformation about what causes childhood illnesses. Although formula companies continually try to improve their product, artificial milk can never provide everything available in breast milk. Breast milk is a living fluid, containing not only the most complete nutrition for babies but also immunities to help prevent the baby from getting sick.

Many families are unprepared for the costs of artificially feeding their infants. The San Diego Breastfeeding Coalition calculated the cost of artificial feeding in 2001. Using the costs for Enfamil®, one of the most popular formula brands, they calculated the cheapest way to artificially feed is using powder in one pound cans, which will cost $1,188 for one year. If you use the 13-oz concentrate cans you will pay $1,512 for 1 year. The 32-oz ready to feed cans cost $1,728, and the four packs of 8-oz ready to feed cans cost $2,376 for one year San Diego Breastfeeding coalition, 2001). These costs only included the formula. You still need to have a supply of bottles, nipples, and the appropriate equipment to transport the formula while you are out.

Artificial feeding does not prevent a difficult adjustment to life with a newborn. It does not prevent flabby breast tissue since the breast changes happened during pregnancy. Because some women's bodies will hold extra fat until they are done breastfeeding, artificial feeding may allow you to initially drop weight faster. However, breastfeeding mothers lose more weight between three and six months after birth, have slimmer hips and weigh less than women who exclusively formula feed. It is important to remember weight loss after pregnancy is a more complicated issue than just whether or not you breastfeed.

Though it is possible for families who feed from a bottle to cuddle, hold and show love to their babies at feeding times, they tend to do less of it than breastfeeding families. Even less frequently will families hold their bottle feeding babies next to bare skin to simulate the body contact of nursing. Though many bottle feeding families expect the father to help with nighttime feedings, how likely this help is to continue after the first two weeks varies widely.

Making Decisions

As you make your decision about how you will feed your baby, here are some things to consider.

1. Looking beyond the idea of immediate convenience, which method(s) of feeding really serves the needs of the members of your family? If needs are likely to be unmet with a method, how can you ensure those needs are taken care of in another way?

2. There are consequences and hidden costs for all the decisions you make. Realistically, what are the hidden costs of the options you are considering? How can you minimize those hidden costs?

3. Pay attention to the reasons you give for the choice you are making. Is your decision being made on truth and accurate information, or is your decision being made on opinion? Is your ability to honestly weigh the options clouded by desires or fears? How can you find more information to help you fully understand your options?

4. Making a Godly decision is about more than just doing what someone else did, even someone in the Bible. It is

not about abdicating your need to make a decision; it is about choosing to follow wherever God leads. Do you have peace that you are following where God has led you with your decision? Does your decision bring glory to God?

If you are sure God is calling you to bottle-feeding (whether breast or artificial milk), try to make the bottle-feeding experience as much like the breastfeeding experience as possible. This can help you and your baby benefit from the closeness and skin contact that happen naturally during breastfeeding.

If you are sure God is calling you to breastfeeding, begin to identify the sources of support available to you. The first few weeks with a new baby are difficult, and it is often beneficial to have the reassurance of someone experienced in breastfeeding to help answer any questions you may have.

Regardless of which method God leads you to, praise him for his ability to provide nourishment for your family.

> Many women have lost a considerable amount of their pregnancy weight gain by six weeks postpartum but there will undoubtedly be more to loose. It took nine months to gain the weight so allow several months to loose it. Being active and continuing to eat healthy combined with breastfeeding should be all you need. If you remain sedentary and go back to eating junk food and soda, it's likely that you will not loose the remaining weight, but actually gain more. A bowl of ice cream after the baby is asleep can seem like a reward for the fatigue and hard work but don't turn to food for your comfort. The Lord is our sanctuary and only He can provide what your soul is longing for!
>
> *Lori Luyten*

Parenting a Newborn

Many people are accustomed to thinking of parenting a newborn as a series of diaper changes, baths, feedings and rocking the baby to sleep. These physical tasks are important, but they are not the main purpose of parenting. The purpose of parenting your child is to help your child grow to become the person God made him to be, so he can fulfill the purpose for which God made him. As part of this parenting you will change diapers, give baths, feed and rock the baby, but those things are never the goal.

One of the dangers of focusing your parenting on the small physical tasks to care for your baby is how easy it is to measure your parenting by how infrequently your baby gets a rash, how quickly he falls asleep or how long he can go between feedings. Never lose sight of the truth that these tasks are a small piece of accomplishing a much larger goal; they are temporary and they are not an accurate measure of success.

It is very similar to the problem Christians sometimes have with Bible reading, quiet time with God and other spiritual disciplines. These are important components for having a growing relationship with God—in fact, it is nearly impossible to grow a relationship with God without them. However, if the focus becomes the disciplines instead of God, it is very easy for us to allow these tasks to replace a growing relationship with God. It is possible to go through the motions of the disciplines without ever giving God your full heart.

The needs of your baby go much deeper than clean diapers, frequent feedings and undisturbed naps. Even before birth, your new baby is fully human with spirit and flesh. He will have both physical and emotional needs. God has uniquely equipped you to meet these needs, so you can enjoy parenting your baby.

Need to Adjust

All of your baby's senses work before he is born, which means immediately after birth he is suddenly taking in great amounts of information. Depending on his ability to manage this transition, he may need help becoming accustomed to the world around him. New sights, sounds, smells and being constantly touched are all important to your baby's learning, but can be overwhelming at times. Babies have a built-in mechanism to shut down when they become over-stimulated. In technical terms, they go to sleep. But not all babies are able to fall asleep to escape the stress; some experience great distress and express it through uncontrollable crying.

Even if your baby is calm in familiar surroundings, you may find he reacts intensely to new situations. Some babies are laid back, whether they like or do not like something they let you know gently. Other babies are more intense, whether they like or do not like something, they let you know forcefully. There are also differences in how much assistance babies need in soothing, themselves when they become upset. Some need only the reassurance of a familiar face, others need to be held and rubbed and talked to before they feel comfortable again.

Need to find purpose

All of these little nuances of your baby's behavior are a part of his personality. This is who God made him to be, and by paying attention you can start to get glimpses of the person God will grow him into. God designed your child for a purpose, and by recognizing who he is, you can help him discover the job God has prepared for him to do. Is he reserved around strangers, or does he light up the room by cooing and smiling for everyone. Is he sensitive to change, or does he go with the flow? Is he self-determined and persevering towards his goal, or is he content with what he has? It is exciting when you start discovering your child's strengths.

One of your child's biggest needs is to know who he is, who God made him to be. Although he is immature now, as he grows you can help him learn to use his strengths well so he can accomplish the work God prepared in advance for him to do. This newborn and early parenting time gives you the opportunity to know who your child is without him wearing the masks of proper social communication. As he gets older, the manners and social customs you teach him can make it more difficult to see his unique make-up.

Ephesians 2:10

Need to Trust

While your baby is becoming accustomed to this world, he is also learning how to trust. As an adult you might accept the reality your baby will be fed; however, your baby is not born with that understanding. All he knows is he is uncomfortable and he needs help. Even the adult rational brain has trouble trusting. Though you know God is always in control, you still become impatient with God. You should not expect any less from a newborn who has not yet learned his needs will be met.

Numbers 21:4-5

A key to helping your baby learn to trust will be successfully communicating with him. God created mothers so their bodies physically react to their babies' cries. When you hear your own baby cry, the blood flow to your breasts will increase and you will get an urge to pick him up. This reflex is stronger in some women than others. In some women it is so strong they begin to leak breast milk in response to their babies' cries. This is normal and helps you learn to understand your baby.

Contrary to popular belief, babies have more ways to communicate than just a loud cry. Babies use eye contact, body language and non-crying sounds before they cry. Crying is the last resort when help does not respond to the other signals. If you miss one of your baby's non-crying signals, the crying will alert you to a need. After a few times of witnessing the body language and non-crying sounds that precede crying, you will start to catch on to what your baby is asking for before the crying starts.

Even if you have not figured out what he wants, picking up your baby will reduce the amount of crying. Babies who are picked up within 90 seconds of beginning to cry cry less often than babies that are not picked up (Hunziker & Barr, 1986). This may be because touching decreases stress hormones and helps achieve bonding. It is also related to your baby learning to trust you will respond when he needs help. As your baby gets older, is better able to use non-crying communication and learns ways to sooth himself, his trust that you will come helps him wait until you can meet his need.

Newborn babies have an abundance of red blood cells that were needed in the womb to get oxygen. This amount of red blood cells is excessive once the baby is out and breathing. So the blood cells are broken down after birth until the level of cells is appropriate for breathing. During this process a substance called bilirubin is produced. Some babies get slightly yellow a few days after birth, this is called physiologic jaundice and is normal and it goes away on it's own. Exposing the baby to sunlight through a window can be beneficial.

Concerns: Baby gets yellow within the first 24 hours, or it is increasing rapidly, if your baby is excessively sleepy, irritable, or does not nurse.

Eneyda Ramos

I remember the first contractions and thinking, "I do not want to do this." But it was too late. My water broke and so we went to the hospital. My contractions were slow at first and then stopped. Even thirty-four years ago they gave you pitocin.

So contractions picked up and I felt them in my back, he was probably posterior. I felt like I was riding a wave and the pain would reach a point that I thought would never end—and then it did. I got a para-cervical block and got one hour of relief. At 10 centimeters his head was not engaged and they sent me for an X-ray (no ultrasounds in Germany). He was a brow presentation, but my measurement was good. So I pushed for five hours. I didn't feel any pain after I was pushing, just got tired. After all that, I had a cesarean surgery.

Now the second birth twenty-one months later was so different. I was scheduled for a cesarean surgery because there were no VBAC's then. My water broke again so I went to the hospital. I was 1 centimeter with no effacement and a high baby—so they put me in a room until they delivered two other ladies.

I was having contractions fairly regular, but no real pain—like period cramps. A floor nurse was coming in to see me so I told her when one contraction stopped the next one started. An hour or so later the charge nurse came in to check me, I was 5 centimeters dilated, 100 percent effaced and zero station. Still no pain, just pressure.

She went to get the doctor who also checked me and said I was 7 centimeters so he sent me to the operating room. On the way he checked me again and I was at 9 centimeters so they took me to the delivery room instead and used forceps to help get my baby out. No pain meds were used until the doctor sewed me up (forceps are wicked on your bottom).

I was just feeling sorry for myself because I was in labor again and going to have another cesarean surgery. I had a rash all over my body which meant I would need a general anesthesia. So I just laid there on my side listening to soft music. I was so relaxed, having my pity party. I did not have a cesarean because I had no pain that anyone could visually see. When they paid attention to me everything happened so fast they forgot to get my husband and I didn't think to ask for him!

Patsy V. Seay

Drawing Conclusions
Review of Section Nine

Ten Questions about...
Becoming a Parent

1. How will you and your spouse make parenting decisions?
2. In what ways will your spouse be a good parent?
3. In what ways will your spouse need to change to be a good parent?
4. In what ways will you be a good parent?
5. In what ways will you need to change to be a good parent?
6. What issues involving parenting concern you?
7. How do you know you and your spouse will be good parents?
8. What preparations are you making for the necessary adjustments of parenthood?
9. What adjustments do you expect will need to be made to parent this child?
10. How will the entrance of this baby to your family affect your family?

Sleeping Like a Baby

Make a 24-hour schedule on a piece of paper. Knowing what you know about newborn sleep habits, draw up a sleep schedule to represent the normal sleeping and waking patterns of a healthy newborn. Indicate the time spent in light sleep both before and after a period of deep sleep.

Using your simulated schedule, how can you realistically ensure you will get enough sleep until your baby is mature enough to sleep for longer periods of time? How can you adjust your daily routines to better fit the new schedule you will be working with?

Feed the Baby

Normal, healthy newborns will eat eight to ten times in a twenty-four hour period. Some babies cluster several of those feedings around a particular time of day; others spread them out evenly both day and night. Some babies nurse quickly, spending less than ten minutes on each breast or bottle. Other babies nurse leisurely, nursing at least twenty minutes on each breast or bottle.

Based on what you have learned about infant feeding, draw a sample 24-hour schedule that represents one way a normal, healthy newborn might eat throughout the day. Using your simulated schedule, what can you do to ensure both your newborn's need for food and your family's other needs are all met?

Sample Schedule

	Sleeping	Feeding
12:00 am		
1:00		
2:00		
3:00		
4:00		
5:00		
6:00		
7:00		
8:00		
9:00		
10:00		
11:00		
12:00 pm		
1:00		
2:00		
3:00		
4:00		
5:00		
6:00		
7:00		
8:00		
9:00		
10:00		
11:00		

The Baby God Gave You–Perfect?

Sharon Tilotta
First Birth Ministries
FirstBirthMinistries.com

It's celebration time! A baby is born; the family cheers as the first cries are heard. The new mother asks if the baby is alright and sighs with relief when it is confirmed there are, in fact, ten fingers and ten toes. The baby is a miracle!

The miracle begins long before birth; it begins at conception. The baby's first "home" is the womb, a place God describes as an environment of love, compassion and mercy. His marvelous works begin creative knitting to fashion together a baby until this new form is fearfully and wonderfully made. The very breath, food and song of the mother become the incubator of God's creative design. When fully fashioned, the mother does some of the hardest work that she will ever do by travailing to give birth to this new miracle.

As Christian parents, we understand and acknowledge that a newborn baby is a gift that God has given. We know that God's gifts are good and true; children are a heritage and a reward from the Lord. Recognizing our children to be God's blessing enables our hearts to receive whom God has given to us.

Our expectations are high as we start this miraculous journey. This is a journey that beckons the family to embrace the sacrificial nature of God's perfect love. The new road traveled will prove to be a path that leads us to greater understanding of our own Heavenly Father and how he parents us.

It is natural to have a preconception regarding this new baby. Women in the Bible often did as well. The name given to a child reflected the mother's impression of the child. For example, if labor was difficult, she might choose a name that meant pain or sorrow. Christian mothers tend to be more positive, believing that they have given birth to a perfect child. However, unknowingly, parents label the new baby according to how many or how few needs the baby expresses. If the baby sleeps a lot and cries little, the baby is tagged as a "good" baby. Nowhere in scripture do we see such a description. In fact, we are told to bring comfort indicating that our child will cry out in a time of need. When we receive the comfort of the Holy Spirit, we have the same heart of compassion to comfort our little one in trouble. Our Heavenly Father lavishes us with his everlasting love giving Jesus, the ultimate sacrifice. If we allow God's love to flow through us, we can embrace our children with unconditional love, resisting the temptation to label or to manipulate them to become our ideal gift.

God's perspective is so different than our natural desires. The new father has visions of the football games that he will share with his son or the achievements that will promote his son to wealth or fame. The new mother imagines the daughter that will shine brilliantly accomplishing the dreams of the American woman. However, God envisions a life that he can use to manifest his life.

Our earthly ambitions and needs must surrender to the way God chooses to accomplish his purpose. As we understand his vision for the child's life, it will move us to grow past our own personalities and become the parents our child needs. The "macho" man suddenly has a new desire to learn sensitivity to parent his new baby. The strong-willed child may require a mother to let go of her passive nature to stand firm with love and wisdom. With God's help, we can become the Godly parents our children needs. He has entrusted us to shape the life of these babies. The challenges can motivate us to grow in the knowledge of God's Word knowing it will benefit our sons and daughters.

God has an assignment for your child's life. Deposited in this little baby are gifts and talents like hidden treasures that we sometimes take years to discover, but when found, will enrich the lives of the parents, grandparents, and most of all the body of Christ. So yes, the baby that God gives you is PERFECT!

Subject Ten

Your New Family

Topics:

God's Design for Family	363
Mom's Needs	366
Dad's Needs	374
Sibling Adjustments	377
Drawing Conclusions	382
Adjusting to Life with a New Baby by Tina Ellis	382

God's Design for Family

God is the mastermind behind family. It was one of the ways in which he could ensure the well-being of his new creation. Not only does family provide for a safe environment in which to grow the population. Family also provides for the community humans need. Even God does not exist in isolation but in three parts. It is through relationships with other humans that Christians are able to demonstrate and grow our love for God.

Genesis 2:18

A new child forces changes in the family. There are new tasks to be done, new timelines to adjust to and new relationships to build. If this is your first child, you will also be undergoing the identity addition of mom and dad. If you are experienced with childbearing, you may also be assisting your other children as they go through the changes associated with enlarging your family.

The goal of Christian parenting is to help your little ones fall in love with God while you continue to fall deeper and deeper in love with God. Just like any other part of life, there is variation in the way it will look when families wholeheartedly put God first. There are as many theories about how to raise your children as there are families. To love and serve God through your family, you need to be focused on the roots instead of the flowers.

There are many similarities between an artificial flower and a living flower. They both have green leaves and colorful petals. From a distance they both may look the same, the artificial plant may even look better because real plants deal with issues such as insects, drought, too much water and seasons. However, a real flower has roots and a stem. Although it may not always look the best, it is able to come back after challenges because it is firmly planted in soil and able to use the nutrients to feed and repair all its parts.

Artificial flowers do not have roots, so when left on their own in the elements for several months, the artificial flower will not stand a chance of coming out looking like the real flower. Artificial flowers have no way to repair damage done by animals, wind, bleaching from the sun or the effects of rain. It may look like a real plant, but it cannot maintain its perfect appearance for long. Once the damage is done, the plant cannot be repaired.

It is a danger in modern society to live as an artificial flower, focusing on the outward appearance instead of ensuring you have strong roots. No one wants to start as a root, seed, or bulb. They are ugly and look lifeless. So instead, people put on a mask to look the way flowers are supposed to look, all the time oblivious to the fact that without proper roots they cannot survive.

Before you decide what your family is supposed to look like, live like and love like, take the time to root your family in God. It means you will not jump on the bandwagon with parenting techniques and programs just because they are popular at your church. It means you may end up parenting differently than your parents, siblings, neighbors or friends did. It means you may spend time as a lifeless looking root while you nurture each other. You may take longer to develop into a flowering family unit, but in the long run, you will be stronger.

Proverbs 31:10-31

It is easy to confuse traditional with Biblical. Many things are traditional in our society that cannot and should not be supported by the Bible. For example, many believe the idea that a woman should not work outside the home is Biblical. Yet, Proverbs 31 paints a picture of a wife who is considered Godly. This woman owned her own business and dabbled in real estate. There are no details of her life listed, if she was a work at home mom, or if she cared for the children until they were in school before starting her business. It does not say how much work she did in a day or in a year. It simply explains her family was taken care of, and she used her time to contribute to the community. She lived her everyday life honoring God through her actions.

Rooting your family in God means reading the Bible not only to learn more about how the world should work, but also in regards to how it is relevant to your life. Certain Biblical passages were written to certain groups of people. There are admonitions to husbands that they are to love and serve their wives and to wives that they are to submit to their husbands. But nowhere does the Bible give wives the right to demand to be waited on or for husbands to subdue their wives. There are also directions for children to obey their parents. You may be tempted to believe this gives you as the parent the right to demand perfect obedience. Instead, it should be speaking to you as the child to right any problems you have in your relationship with your parents.

Ephesians 5:25
Colossians 3:19
Ephesians 5:22
Colossians 3:18
Colossians 3:20
Ephesians 6:1

Finally, understand the Biblical principles that should be the basis for your actions are just as relevant with your child as they are with strangers. Jesus said the greatest command was to love God, and the second greatest was to love others. In that way we fulfill all the law of God. Understand Biblical love means you sacrifice your wants to meet the needs of your child. Newborns have lots of needs and they are unable to fill any of them on their own. Through filling your baby's needs not only is your baby able to learn to trust and love, but God is also able to use the experience to grow you.

Matthew 22:36-40

1 John 3:18
1 John 4:9
1 Corinthians 13:4-7

Mom's Needs Postpartum

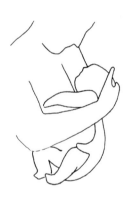

You sometimes see the image in books or stories of women in undeveloped countries giving birth easily and then going about their normal routine. Although it is a nice story, it is not exactly the truth about a healthy postpartum. Giving birth is a normal, healthy event in a woman's life. Yet there are some important changes going on in your body after you give birth, and working with your body to stay physically and emotionally healthy should be at least as important to you now as it was while you were pregnant.

Physical Healing

Recovering from birth is about more than fitting in your jeans or getting back to work. Your body is physically changed, and you need time to adjust to the changes. You cannot ignore the importance of your physical healing to make a smooth transition from expectant mother to new mother. Good quality nutrition, getting plenty of rest and appropriate exercise are essential. Not only will ignoring these cause your physical healing to delay, they will also increase your risk of postpartum mood disorders (Baker, Mancuso, Montenegro & Lyons, 2002).

Within a few days of giving birth, you will find your body undergoing many physical changes. Your milk will come in, possibly leaving you feeling engorged. The normal pregnancy swelling will go away, causing an increase in urination as you eliminate the extra fluids. Your abdomen will be mushy and if you had a surgical birth will require extra tenderness as the wound heals. You may have an increase in the number of hairs you lose each day. You will be very tired from the new schedule of feeding.

The process of the uterus returning to its pre-pregnancy state is called involution. It involves the healing of the site where the placenta was attached, the shrinking of the uterus and the expulsion of the remaining tissue. The most obvious physical change you will experience will be the lochia (the flow of blood from the uterus). Lochia consists of the blood, mucus and tissue that is in the uterus after your baby is born. As your uterus returns to its pre-pregnancy state, the lochia is expelled. Your uterus does not scar over at the site of the placental attachment. Instead it heals like new, allowing placental attachment in the next pregnancy.

For the first three to five days after your baby is born, you can expect a very heavy bright red discharge because it contains a high volume of blood from the placental site. Around the tenth day after giving birth, the lochia will turn pink or brownish and thin out a bit. Sometime after the second week it will change again to a yellow or white discharge that can last up to six weeks.

Being aware of your lochia can help you know your body is healing properly or alert you to a problem. If the lochia has a foul odor, it can mean you have contracted an infection. If the lochia suddenly becomes heavier again, or if you begin to have red spotting after the lochia has thinned, it can mean you are overdoing it and need to get more rest. It is normal to have a heavy flow or some small clots upon rising after lying or sitting for awhile since the blood will collect in your vagina while you are lying down. If you experience large clots, it can be an indication of a problem.

Lochia and Levitical Law

Leviticus 12:1-8

What may be most interesting about lochia is its treatment in the Levitical laws. According to Leviticus 12, a woman who has given birth is unclean for 7 days if she gave birth to a boy and 14 days if she gave birth to a girl. This period of impurity is the same as being unclean during menstruation. Following the initial time of being unclean, she will be purified from her bleeding in 33 days for a boy and 66 days for a girl.

Sacrifices are no longer needed for purification from sin; the blood of Jesus has purified us. Giving birth does not somehow overpower the Holy Spirit. Though Christians do not live under the law, this law brings up intriguing questions about the immediate postpartum period.

When a person is unclean, many of the things she touches become unclean. This means if a woman who has recently given birth cooks food for her family and they eat it, her family may also become ceremonially unclean, because "uncleanness" was able to be passed on. Was a new mother separated from her family? Was she not allowed to cook or clean, depending instead on the generosity of the other women in her community? If she was limited in her duties, did this promote healing? Did the time of separation give her the time to establish a strong breastfeeding relationship and learn to read her baby's cues?

If she continued with her normal routine, the entire family must have been unclean, so did the family separate from the greater community as a whole? Did they require a woman who had just given birth to relax and be waited on until she could be purified, or did the uncleanness make no difference if they did not need to go to the temple?

Did designating the new mother as different increase the amount of support she received, or did it decrease the amount of support available to her? Did the other women avoid her until she could be purified? Was the time of separation isolating, decreasing the help she had for the other children and increasing her chances of suffering depression?

There is no physical reason why a woman would need longer to recover after giving birth to a daughter rather than a son. Why does it take longer to be purified after having given birth to a girl? Why did it require both a burnt offering and a sin offering to be purified? What about giving birth did God consider related to sin? Is there a deeper spiritual significance to giving birth or mothering a newborn?

These are all great questions, and the sad truth is you may never get answers to them In the end, it may not matter if you know how the Israelites interpreted these laws because it would only tell you their cultural understanding of them. The relationship between Jesus and the Pharisees shows how the cultural practice of laws is subject to change with time, and sometimes ends up looking vastly different from what God commanded or intended.

Matthew 23:13

Separation after Birth

According to Kathleen O'Grady, The Temple Scroll required special places in every city for women to go during menstruation and after childbirth (O'Grady, 2003). The women themselves were separated to prevent the other members of their households and the entire community from becoming ceremonially unclean. However, God does not say that the woman is to be isolated or removed from her home, just that she is not to touch anything sacred. God does not even say it is bad for the other members of her household to become ceremonially unclean with her—just that it will happen.

As early as the mid-fourth century, churches required women to go through a purification ceremony to allow them to reenter the church after a postpartum period of separation (Roll, 2003). Though women were not separated from their families, they did enter a time of confinement in their homes. Despite prominent leaders of the church stating women were not unclean after having given birth, the practice continued up until the 1950s, at which time women refused to continue it.

The main lesson to learn from this is that there is often a difference between what God expects of you and what your culture expects of you. Trying to fulfill the demands of a culture designed by imperfect humans is setting yourself up for failure. The weeks after having given birth are hard enough on a new mother without imposing on her the unrealistic expectations of a culture that does not value the things God values.

A new mother may not be seen as impure anymore, but she is still met with cultural expectations that separate her from her community and God. The demands of caring for a newborn make it hard to entertain company; and yet the company comes with expectations only of cooing over the baby. The conflicting emotions, feeling letdown or overwhelmed and struggling to learn how to best meet the needs of your baby can leave a new mother feeling like a failure; and yet she will be told these should be the happiest days of her life. There is general agreement that caring for the next generation is one of the most important jobs to be done; and yet new mothers are continually asked when they will be returning to their real work. Despite the fact that glamour and fashion are of little importance to the successful raising of a baby, a new mother is expected to quickly return to her pre-pregnancy body and style, which frequently takes more time than the mother has to devote to hair and makeup.

All these conflicting expectations combine to create an environment in which the new mother cannot win. You need to decide now how you will handle the unwritten expectations society has for you and that you may have accepted without realizing it. How will you prevent yourself from becoming overwhelmed? Who can you go to for help or just to be honest about what you are feeling? Where will your sources of support be, and what type of support can they offer? Answering these questions before your baby is born will help you make a smoother and healthier transition to motherhood.

Emotionally Healthy

After your baby is born, you suddenly have much less estrogen and progesterone. These hormonal changes may be what cause the "baby blues" experienced by about 80 percent of all new mothers. Many women are sensitive to this change, causing them to feel anxious, sad, exhausted and tense. In addition, it is common to have changes in appetite and in your ability to sleep. The baby blues start between the second and fifth day postpartum, and for most women, these symptoms tend to resolve themselves within a few days as the body adjusts to the normal level of hormones. Other women take up to two weeks to fully adjust to these changes. If you experience symptoms for longer than 2 weeks, seek help.

Between 10 and 15 percent of new mothers will not recover well emotionally and will experience postpartum depression. There is evidence the hormonal changes may affect the functioning of the thyroid causing depression, although the causes are not yet fully understood. Mothers who have a personal or family history of depression are more likely to experience depression after the baby is born. Postpartum depression generally starts between 4 and 8 weeks postpartum and if not treated can last for 6 months or more.

There are several things you can do to help your body adjust, reducing your risk of developing postpartum depression. Getting adequate rest and proper nutrition will help your body adjust physically. Appropriate levels of activity allow you to begin the healing process without overworking yourself, which will result in more risk. Lack of social support has one of the strongest correlations with postpartum depression, so be sure to identify your sources of support before your baby is born.

Baby Blues
Tearfulness
Confusion
Insomnia
Anxiety
Irritability

Postpartum Depression
Doubt, guilt, anger or irritability with no clear source
Unable to concentrate
Confusion
Lack of interest in baby
Overly concerned about baby
Fear of harming baby
"Dreadful" thoughts

Communicating with Baby

Your baby will communicate with you through a variety of signals or cues. One of your first tasks as a parent is to become sensitive to these cues so you can respond appropriately. This is good for you and your baby. Babies whose mothers are more sensitive to their cues mature faster in their ability to think and learn. Mothers who are more sensitive to their baby's cues are more likely to be successful at calming their newborn and feel more confident in their mothering ability

How confident you feel in your ability to calm your baby affects your ability to actually calm your baby. This confidence does not come from having a feeling of control over your baby. In fact, mothers who feel they are in control of their babies' crying are less likely to discern the differences in their babies' cries and more likely to struggle with soothing them. Instead, the confidence comes from understanding who your child is and what response your child needs when distressed (Leavitt, 1998).

The fastest way to build your confidence in your mothering ability is to respond to your baby's cries as quickly as possible. Babies who are responded to within 90 seconds of beginning to cry sooth quickly, while those who are responded to after 90 seconds take considerably more time to sooth after being responded to (Hunziker, & Barr, 1986). Seeing the immediate results not only helps to improve your confidence in your ability, but it also helps you to further your understanding of who your child is.

Another great tool to boost your confidence is a sling or baby carrier. Babies who are held close to mom in a carrier for three hours a day cry significantly less than babies who are left alone while quiet or sleeping. The most significant decrease in crying is during the evening hours, a time when many babies tend to have a fussy period. Using the baby carrier allows you to hold your baby and still keep your hands free for playing with your other children, putting away laundry, reading a book or other simple task.

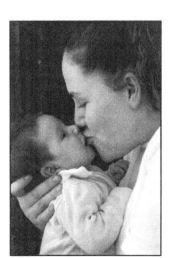
©2000 Erin Lowery
Playing with your baby helps you build confidence in your mothering skills.

Social Support

Lack of support is one of the leading risk factors for postpartum depression. Find a way to get assistance with daily chores and meal preparation for at least 3 to 4 weeks after your baby is born. This helps to reduce your stress level, gives you more time to heal and gives you uninterrupted time to get to know your baby. The help can be a family member, friends or hired help such as a doula or a mother's helper.

It is important that those who assist you understand it is your job to take care of the baby. Gaining confidence in your skills requires you have the opportunity to get to know what it takes to meet your baby's needs. There are plenty of chores that will need to be done in the first few weeks such as washing dishes, preparing meals, laundry, sweeping, mopping and scrubbing the bathroom. These are all tasks that are easily completed by most adults.

Do not be afraid to ask for help when friends or family come to see your new baby. Most friends and family will ask if you need anything before they come, so take them up on the offer and request a few groceries or ask if they will stay long enough to vacuum or wash some dishes. The people who really care about you want to help you and are excited to be a part of your new baby's life.

If you are unable to request help from friends and family, consider hiring professional help. A postpartum doula can do chores, prepare meals and answer your baby care questions for a very reasonable rate. A postpartum doula is a great new baby gift from family members who are not able to help themselves.

Breastfeeding Support

There are mothers and babies for whom breastfeeding comes naturally. With little effort the baby latches on and is quickly satisfied with a hearty meal. There are also mothers and babies for whom breastfeeding is an exercise in patient trial and error. Feeling unsuccessful at breastfeeding can destroy your confidence in your ability to care for your baby, putting you at greater risk of postpartum depression. Feeling unsuccessful at breastfeeding also puts your baby at risk, since any interference with a good breastfeeding relationship diminishes the quality of nutrition available to him.

For breastfeeding success, nothing is more important than accurate information. Fortunately, accurate information can be easy to find. Most hospitals have lactation consultants on staff to help new mothers. You can access the lactation consultant even if you did not give birth in the hospital. Some consultants work privately; check your local phone book to see if any are in your area. La Leche League is based on mother to mother support, helping you get the information you need to make your decisions. In addition to monthly meetings, some local groups have lending libraries and a 24-hour hotline. Other good sources of information are doulas and midwives, since both require training in breastfeeding support. It is a good idea to have a book about breastfeeding available to troubleshoot the most common problems and provide reassurance.

Dad's Needs Postpartum

Though fathers are not recovering from the physical exertion of having given birth, they do have needs that must be addressed as they build a relationship with their new babies. Just like mothers, fathers bond with their newborns, and the way the father is treated can either encourage or discourage the bonding.

A father is someone distinct with a vital role to play in the family and a fundamental component of the parenting team. Fathers are just as good as mothers at parenting. They are just as anxious about leaving their infants. They are able to identify their infants while blindfolded. They respond to infant cues and even spontaneously change their speech patterns when talking to their babies. What fathers usually lack is the time spent as primary caregivers to help build on these skills.

There are many factors that prevent a father from spending time with the baby. Long hours at work, caring for other children and the new mom can all divert his attention. There are a few things within the control of the family that can help provide the one-on-one time a father needs to bond with his baby.

First and foremost, you must accept that you are just as much a parent as your wife. You are not a babysitter, nor are you a second-rate caregiver. Men who are given time alone with their new babies during the first 24 hours of their lives spend significantly more time with them in the next three months. You may do things differently from your wife, but that only means they are different, not wrong. Take the opportunity to spend time with your baby, caring for him. Give yourself the freedom to make mistakes and learn from them just like your wife will. It is only through trying something new that it can ever be mastered.

You will also need to be secure with your marriage. Men who are more satisfied with their marriages have better attitudes about their babies than men who are in a failing marriage. If you are having struggles, seek help now so you begin working through them before the baby is born. Not only will this improve your bonding with the baby, it may help prevent postpartum depression for your wife.

Men tend to be more physical in their relationship with their infants than women, even when they are providing normal day to day care. Play is an important part of the daddy–baby relationship. Your baby will seek out your attention and even give you cues to continue playing. This can be a great source of joy for both your baby and you. It does not mean the baby likes you better than your wife. It just means your baby likes to engage in the type of play you provide as much as he likes to engage in other types of communication. It is OK to have fun with the baby.

Just like mothers, fathers need time to feel confident in their parenting abilities. You did not get the wash of oxytocin your wife's body received from giving birth to help you bond with your baby. You are not getting the reassurance of a budding breastfeeding relationship. If you are not able to take time off work; you are trying to learn to parent in just a few short hours a day. These can be big hurdles, especially if you feel you cannot do anything right for the baby, and your wife looks like she knows what she is doing. Continue to try, especially if you feel uncomfortable with the baby (Pruett, 1998).

Strengthening your marriage and giving yourself the opportunity to build your confidence in your parenting ability will help build the strongest relationship possible with your baby. In the process, it will give your wife the support she needs to recover both physically and emotionally from the experience of pregnancy and giving birth.

The roles of mother and father should be complementary and build upon each other. As each parent cares for the child and each other, the family grows closer. The Bible refers to God as our Father—giving us glimpses at times of the things fathers do or should do. However both male and female are made in the image of God. God does "motherly" things as well as "fatherly" things. God has some "mother" in him. When determining who will do what, it should not be seen as the father's job is this and the mother's job is that. Instead, parenting involves all these things, and between the two of you they get done.

Genesis 1:23
Isaiah 66:13
Matthew 23:37

Stay in your gown and robe and visitors won't stay as long or expect you to wait on them!
Lori Luyten

Sibling Adjustments

There are no hard and fast rules for helping your children prepare for the arrival of a new baby. There are too many variables for any suggestion to always work. Younger children need different information than older children. Sensitive children will need more reassurance than laid back children. You simply need to know your child and how much assistance she will need.

Some of your preparation for birth will be decisions that affect the older children. Consider how much participation in the decision making your child needs. Is she old enough to have an opinion about where she stays or what she does? Does she react better when she knows what options are available for her? Is she unlikely to care what decisions are made?

Whether or not your older child attends the birth of her new sibling is a decision you need to make together based on each individual child. Does your child have a desire to attend the birth? Does your child posses the self-control to handle the long hours it may take to give birth? Young children will need someone to assist them with basic needs during labor. Can you arrange for a caregiver to stay with her during labor? Does your child have the freedom to change work or school plans for a labor? Will your child be a help to you in labor?

Your child is likely to have many questions about pregnancy, birth and babies. Be honest with your answers; do not be tempted to believe lying to your child is easier. Listen carefully to the question to discern what it is your child wants to know. Chances are you can easily answer the question without giving extra information she is not interested in.

Some parents find involving young children in a birthday celebration helps prepare them for the arrival of the new baby. Young children can pick out a small present to share with the new sibling, pick out or help make a cake and plan a small family party. Other parents find having a small gift for the older sibling from the new baby helps make the new baby welcome.

Once the baby is born, pay attention to the older sibling to determine how much special time she may need from mom and dad. Scheduling alone time with one parent gives the other time to gain confidence in parenting the new child. Using a sling to carry the new baby gives you at least one hand free to play with or read to a preschool sibling. Eating meals with the older child can help create special time as well.

Young Children

Young children have many questions about new babies. It is important for you as a parent to understand the things that make sense to you are not automatically understood by young children. Talking about what the new baby will be like can help prevent some disappointment and misunderstanding when the baby is born.

Babies are very small

Young children do not necessarily understand sizes yet. To help them realize how little a new baby is, compare the size of a baby to familiar things in your home. You could say, "Our baby will be smaller than the radio, but bigger than your toy truck."

Babies cannot play with toys

The inability of new babies to control their bodies can be frustrating to young children who just want to play with them. It can be helpful if you show your child how to play with the baby, or give suggestions of games such as Peek-a-Boo.

Babies cannot use words to talk

Crying can be as frustrating to toddlers as it is to parents. Help your child understand crying means baby needs help. Your toddler may become an ally in deciphering baby's cries.

Babies cannot use the bathroom

Depending on your child's age and how often she is around babies, she may not realize how often a newborn needs a diaper change. Some older children enjoy participating in diaper changes by gathering supplies when needed.

Babies drink milk from mommy

Newborns take a lot of "lap" time from an older child. Helping your child understand nursing is the only way the baby can get food may help her be more understanding. Feeding your newborn while sitting on the floor or while using a sling can make it easier to play with an older child while the baby is eating.

Babies need help from the whole family

If your child is young, she may not realize the intense needs of a newborn are temporary. Some siblings really enjoy helping the baby learn the things he will need to be independent and can celebrate each milestone with the baby.

Babies are people and have likes and dislikes

Young children do not have the capacity to understand the entire world is not like them. Point out differences between your child and friends or family members such as "you like to sing, but I like to draw." This can help your child understand that it is OK when baby does not like to play with the toys your child thinks are great.

Handling Stress

Having a new baby in the house can be as stressful for your older child as it is for you. While adults have learned many ways to handle and control their stress, children have not. Young children have an especially difficult time dealing with stress.

When a new baby is introduced to the home, the older child has new schedules, less parent time, more noise, more visitors and a new resident of the house. As your older child attempts to handle the stress of the new baby, you may notice sleep pattern changes, clinging behaviors, bathroom "accidents," changes in eating or even increased anger. Be patient with your child as she adjusts to the new patterns of your home. If possible, help your child learn ways to express her stress before the baby is born.

Look for opportunities to model good stress management to your older child. When you are tired and frustrated, it is OK to be honest with your child and say, "I'm feeling frustrated. I'm going to pray that God will help me to figure out what to do." Then pray. If possible, have your child pray with you. Making it normal to be honest about feelings opens you up to ask your child if she is feeling frustrated and offering to pray with her.

If you have a child who does best with routines, it may be helpful to start introducing new routines before the new baby is born. A routine is not the same as a schedule, bedtime every night at 8:00 is not a routine. A routine is the things you do regularly, not the time you do them. Consider what will and will not be possible with a new baby in the house. If your normal bedtime routine is a 2-hour process with baths, stories and snuggle time, you may want to consider readjusting the schedule or breaking it into two separate routines to make it easier to continue all parts of the routine after the baby is born.

I think too often as women we forget that we are not the only ones experiencing the labor. My great grandmother used to always tell me that the best way to forget your own troubles was to listen and help with someone else's. The baby is working and communicating with the mother—moving and shifting and turning and working to be born—just as much as the mother's body and mind are.

And very honestly, birth is just the beginning of a series of jobs that little life is going to do over the next few moments; breathing air for the first time, having a heart go from two chambers to four and learning the job of breastfeeding. I think it would be good to focus a bit on what our babies go through. Then our own job of birthing might become a bit less significant in comparison.

Maribeth Glenn

With my first, I was induced with Cytotec (7 hours). It felt like tightening everywhere from my ribcage to my mid-thighs. It was intense—like a huge muscle cramp that was not able to be massaged away. Uncomfortable, but not painful.

With my second, she was persistently posterior—and it was my only truly "PAINFUL" labor (11 hours). She felt, as horrible as it sounds, like someone was trying to dislocate my spine from my body with a hot grip around it.

With the twins, I was induced with pitocin for medical reasons and it was INTENSE, but not painful (5 hours). There was great discomfort as the contractions didn't gradually increase, peak and wane off. Instead, they came on suddenly and intensely, only to go away just as abruptly. I felt them low, from my pubic bone to my coccyx bone, like a hammock between my legs and up to my belly button. It was like intense internal pressure that expanded at the same time it balled up all of this energy in my womb to the point that I thought it could not tighten and ball any more. At that point, it would inevitably release me. It was intense.

My last was a 21 hour labor (my longest labor and biggest baby) and was exquisite. It was my least uncomfortable labor. Very similar to the balling of energy and expanding pressure of the twins contractions, but it came on gradullay and left gradually. Very "wave-like" and was all in my belly. None in my back and non in my buttocks.

Nicole Deelah

Drawing Conclusions
Review of Section Ten

Sources of Support

Think about the people in your life who are supporting you now and those who you expect will support you after your baby is born. Make a diagram representing the support you have. Draw a circle in the center of the paper for you. Add a circle for each person representing how much support you feel they will give you. A larger circle means more support or assistance for a longer amount of time. A smaller circle means less support or assistance for a shorter amount of time.

Sample Diagram

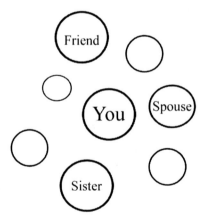

Ten Questions about...
Expectations of Family

1. What is positive about your relationship with your mother?
2. What is negative about your relationship with your mother?
3. What is positive about your relationship with your father?
4. What is negative about your relationship with your father?
5. What is positive or negative about your relationships with siblings?
6. In what ways are you ready to be a mother or father?
7. In what ways do you feel unprepared to be a mother or father?
8. What is your ideal for your family relationships?
9. What would need to change for that to become a reality?
10. What will help or prevent that change?

Newborn Family Needs

Families with newborns have many needs, but they are not filled with items from a gift registry. Make a list of all the chores that absolutely must be done regardless of how easy or hard life is with a newborn. These chores might include making meals, taking older children to school or events, housework or laundry, yard work or other needs your family has.

Once you have your list, determine which needs are best met by your family and which needs are best met by caring friends and relatives. Keep a list of those items that can be filled by friends and relatives handy. That way, when someone calls and asks what you need, you can quickly look at the list and pick something appropriate.

If possible, ask your close friends and family to help you prepare for baby by accepting responsibility for some of the items before the baby is born. It helps to reduce stress if you know ahead of time your family meals will be prepared and your children will make it to soccer practice.

Adjusting to Life with a New Baby

Tina Ellis
Author
Pregnancy = 40 Weeks of Preparation.

The moment you have been anticipating for months has finally arrived. The baby room is decorated and awaiting a new arrival. You have survived childbirth and now are ready to take your next big step. Each phase of life is a stepping stone for the next. You have prepared for 40 Weeks; now you are officially entering the stepping-stone of parenthood.

The first few weeks of parenthood may seem like a roller coaster ride. Remember, it is okay to take baby steps—that is the best way to learn. This roller coaster ride may remind you of the emotional ride you experienced during pregnancy—big swings of happiness followed by an overwhelming feeling of sadness. The incredible joy you feel while holding your delicate treasure along with the misery of sleepless nights. New mothers go through an adjustment period and this adjustment period comes with no instructions or directions. A new mother has to find herself and deal with the changes of being a happy woman to becoming a happy woman with a baby. This adjustment is being made from having a new baby. Please know you are not alone and you should not be alone. If you do not already have one, find a buddy to talk to, maybe a close friend or sister or even mother-in-law. As time goes by, you will soon forget the roller coaster ride.

Privacy is something that has to be thrown out the window at least until your children are 18 or so. Privacy is a valued commodity and one that sometimes needs extreme measures. One mother I know actually went in the bathroom and locked the door so she could have 2 minutes in peace. The space you once knew as your own has officially been invaded. If you get through a day and your clothes are still clean at the end of the day, it is amazing. It never fails that the perfect time to spit up is when no burp towel is available.

Grooming time is something that will need adjustment. The key here is to be flexible and accept that your schedule as you once knew it will need a little modification. Grooming time is well and fine, but what you once did in an hour will amazingly be condensed to 20 minutes or so. And this reduction will show off your hidden talents as not just anyone can take a shower while entertaining a 6-month-old sitting in a bouncy seat. Or how you are able to make supper, take care of the baby, and still find time to work out.

Honey time is also an area that takes a turn—sometimes a wrong turn, but if your focus is on God, all turns can be corrected. The time you and your spouse used to spend together is now different. It is no longer the two of you. But remember as you work through this transition that you should always be husband and wife. Together you can accomplish anything including raising a child. Together you can cry in joy when he says his first word. Together you can cry in sadness when he tells his first lie. Together you can raise him to be a servant of God and stand proud at the job you have done. So take time for your relationship. Have a date night and have some alone couple time.

Privacy, grooming time, and honey time are just a few areas that will need adjustment in your new life as a parent. But with God's direction you can and will succeed.

As you have completed a very special time in your life, a new phase has begun. Remember to take each day as an opportunity to prepare for the challenges that may arrive tomorrow. If you do not buy a fire extinguisher today, you will not be able to put out the fire tomorrow.

Appendices

A1	Sample Menus	389
A2	Overcoming Fears	392
A3	Birth Planning Checklist	393
A4	Comfort Measures Check List	394
A5	Midwife Interview Questions	395
A6	Birth Place Checklist	396
A7	Breastfeeding Questions	397
A8	Childbirth Verses	398
A9	Global Birth Issues	399
A10	Resources	400

A1: Sample Menus

If you enjoy cooking at home, and have the time to cook, planning nutritious meals is probably not an issue for you. However, if you work, have children or volunteer your time it may not be as easy to ensure you are eating well.

The following sample menus have been included to help you find simple ways to adjust your eating that will greatly improve your nutrition. They are based on the guidelines for good eating from the Brewer Pregnancy Diet. You can learn more about pregnancy nutrition in the Healthy Pregnancy section of this book or through the nutrition.birthingnaturally.net website.

Included with each menu are hints and suggestions so you can tailor them to your specific needs. Good pregnancy nutrition does not require you to follow a strict diet. Instead, there are guidelines you can use to get the required nutrients from the foods your family enjoys.

These menus were taken straight from the Birthing Naturally website. On the website you will find recipes for some of the foods as well as other recipes that may help you eat healthy during pregnancy. You will also find more sample menus and other tools to help you make the best nutritional decisions at the website.

Limited Cooking:

Breakfast
Bowl of fiber cereal
1 C milk
1 C of fresh fruit

Snack
Cottage Cheese
Whole Wheat Crackers

Lunch
Egg Salad on 1 slice Whole Wheat Toast
Cup of Milk

Snack
Peanuts

Dinner
Beef and Vegetable Soup from a Can
Whole Wheat Freezer Roll or whole wheat toast
Dinner Salad with Cheese
Instant Pudding

Snack
Fruit and Yogurt

Making this menu work for you

- Keep healthy snacks such as yogurt, nuts, whole wheat pretzels and fresh fruit and vegetables on hand.

- Keep a variety of frozen foods (like vegetables, bread rolls and bagels) on hand so you can whip up a meal with very little preparation time.

- Try mixing frozen fruit with yogurt and juice to make a smoothie. It takes very little time but is nutritionally packed, especially if you add protein powder.

- Keep salad greens washed and ready to eat in a container in your refrigerator so you can have a salad as a snack instead of chips or cookies.

- On days that you feel better and can cook, cook a double portion of your meal and freeze the second half. It will come in handy on a busy day or when you don't feel up to cooking later in the pregnancy.

Flexible Cooking

Breakfast
Amish Baked Oatmeal
Slice of Whole Wheat Toast
1/2 Grapefruit
8 oz Glass of Milk (8oz = 1 Cup)

Snack
Blueberry Muffin

Lunch
Broccoli Bacon Quiche
White Bean Salad

Snack
2 Deviled Egg Halves

Dinner
Parmesan Chicken
Emerald Rice
Steamed Carrots
8 oz glass of Milk

Snack
Chocolate Pudding

Making this menu work for you

- Instead of cooking Amish Baked Oatmeal, follow the stovetop or microwave directions on a package of oatmeal. Most can be made in five to 10 minutes.

- If you have at least half an hour to bake one morning a week, use that morning to bake a batch of muffins. Store them in your freezer in sealable freezer bags. Thaw in the microwave. Another option is to buy muffins from your grocery store bakery.

- Many foods are able to keep well refrigerated for 2 or 3 days, so you can cook once and eat twice.

- If you have one day a week to cook a few dishes, you can have them prepared and in the freezer for the whole week.

A2: Overcoming Fears

Philippians 4:8 — Finally, brothers, whatever is true, whatever is noble, whatever is right, whatever is pure, whatever is lovely, whatever is admirable—if anything is excellent or praiseworthy—think about such things.

My fear or concern is:

What is true?:
   (What is true about you or your situation?)
What is noble?:
   (How can you handle this situation in a noble way?)
What is right?:
   (Is there a righteous response to this fear?)
What is pure?:
   (How can you respond in a way to keep your heart devoted to God?)
What is lovely?:
   (How can this fear be worked for good?)
What is admirable?:
   (Who has overcome a similar fear; how did they do it?)
What is excellent and praiseworthy?:
   (How can you respond in a way that keeps you from sin and brings praise and glory to God?)

A3: Birth Planning Checklist

Did you include information about:

	The environment you hope to achieve/
	Who you do or do not want with you?
	How you want to manage pain?
	The positions you want to try?
	How you prefer to have the labor monitored?
	How you want to handle normal variations?
	How you want to handle complications?
	How you want to handle a possible cesarean?
	Your choices for care of your newborn?
	Any other points important to you?

Is your birth plan:

	Easy to read?
	Organized with important points at the top?
	One page (two at the most)?
	Proofread by someone you trust?
	Already discussed with your midwife?
	Copied, so you can hand them out to nurses?

A4: Comfort Measures Checklist

Use the following checklist in labor as a quick glance guide to the most common comfort measures for labor.

Positions for Labor

Upright:
Dangle
Labor Dance
Walking and Swaying
Leaning on someone
In shower
Squatting
Lunging

Hands and Knees:
Head down, bottom up
Leaning over ball
Kneeling over bed
Kneeling over a chair

Sitting:
Recliner Chair Sitting
Toilet Sitting
Rocking
Sitting on ball

Reclining:
Side Lying
Reclining in tub

Techniques for Labor
Abdominal Breathing
Aromatherapy
Acupressure
Basic Massage
Close Eyes
Cool Compresses
Darken the room
Eat
Effleurage
Encouragement
Foot massage
Hand massage
Hip Squeeze
Ice Packs
Listen to book or music
Meditation
Nipple Stimulation
Perineal Massage
Relaxation
Rhythmic Breathing
Rocking or Swaying
Sing with music
Stroking
Vocalization
Warm compresses
Water in tub or shower

A5: Midwife Interview Questions

The following is a list of sample questions you may wish to ask before hiring a caregiver to attend you in labor.

1. Under what circumstances would you recommend I be induced?
2. What is your preferred method of induction?
3. What treatments do you recommend to clients who are diagnosed with gestational diabetes? or Group B Strep positive?
4. In what ways do you support a woman who wants to have an unmedicated labor?
5. Under what circumstances would you recommend that I not attempt an unmedicated, vaginal birth?
6. Under what circumstances would you recommend I not use an epidural? or other medication?
7. What are some reasons I might have to labor in bed as opposed to walking around?
8. What are some reasons I might need continuous fetal monitoring?
9. What indicates to you that an IV is necessary during labor?
10. What indicates to you that an episiotomy is necessary during labor?
11. How will you help keep my perineal skin intact?
12. What are the benefits you have seen from squatting for second stage? or changing positions during second stage?
13. How much time do you spend with a laboring mother?
14. Where do you recommend I give birth?
15. What has your experience been with doulas at labors?
16. What has been your experience with friends and family at labor?

A6: Birth Place Checklist

Use this checklist to ensure you gather the information you need about possible birth places.

Environment:
I can include the people I want.
I feel comfortable here.
I feel safe here.
I have access to the food and drink of my choice.
I have access to the options for care I want.

Care:
I feel supported by the staff.
I know the options available to me here.
I have the right to make decisions about my care.
I am comfortable with the support I receive from the staff.
I know the rates of cesarean surgery.
I know the rates of other interventions.
I am comfortable with the philosophy of care.
I am comfortable with the options given to me.

Emergency:
I know the planned response to an emergency.
I am comfortable with the options for emergency care.
I know the reasons I may be separated from my spouse.

Newborn:
I am in control of my baby's care.
My baby will not be separated from me against my will.
I am comfortable with routine newborn care.
I will have support for immediate breastfeeding.

A7: Breastfeeding Questions

If you plan to breastfeed, you should be able to answer these questions before your baby is born. You can learn the answers in a book, through a class, at a La Leche League meeting or by personally speaking with a lactation consultant.

1. How do you position a baby properly for breastfeeding?
2. How do you ensure your baby is latched on properly?
3. What can you do about engorgement?
4. What can you do about sore nipples?
5. How can you tell your baby is getting enough to eat?
6. What can you do if your baby is not getting enough?
7. How often does a normal newborn eat?
8. How often should you feed your baby?
9. How long should you feed on each side?
10. When is it safe to begin using artificial nipples?
11. What can you do when your baby suddenly feeds all day?
12. When do babies sleep through the night?
13. Where can you find immediate help if you have questions?

A8: Childbirth Verses

Here is a collection of verses you may find helpful during labor. Memorize them or write them on cards so you can meditate on them during labor.

For Strength:
Psalm 18:31-33
Psalm 28:6-7
Psalm 29:11
Psalm 59:17
Psalm 86:16
1 Corinthians 1:25
2 Thessalonians 2:16-17

For Patience and Perseverance:
Psalm 139:13
Ecclesiastes 3:2
Jeremiah 1:5
Galatians 5:22-23
Colossians 3:12
Hebrews 10:35
James 1:4
1 Timothy 2:15

Children as Blessings:
Genesis 49:25
Psalm 127:3
Proverbs 17:6

For Peace and Rest:
Psalm 22:9-10
Psalm 62:1-2
Psalm 71:6
Psalm 91:1-2
Isaiah 66:9
Matthew 11:28-29
Colossians 3:15

For Wisdom:
Isaiah 55:8
Proverbs 2:6
John 16:13
Romans 15:5-6
James 1:5-6

For Praise:
1 Chronicles 16:9
Psalm 7:17
Psalm 28:6
Psalm 86:12
Luke 5:26
Colossians 3:2

A9: Global Birth Issues

In developed countries 99 percent of women receive prenatal care and are attended by skilled health personnel during labor. In Burundi only 25 percent of births are attended by skilled health personnel. In Rwanda only 10 percent of mothers receive adequate prenatal care, and only 31 percent give birth with a skilled attendant. Both Rwanda and Burundi have less than one midwife per 10,000 people.

These statistics are deadly. The World Health Organization estimates 533,000 women die during pregnancy or childbirth each year. This is the equivalent to one woman every minute. These deaths are distributed unequally around the globe, with women in parts of Africa and Southern Asia having one hundred times the risk of dying compared to women in developed countries. Their children are at least six times more likely to die within the first year of life; five times more likely to die within the first week after birth; and four times as likely to not live long enough to be born.

At least 75 percent of these deaths are preventable with basic health care. By creating a system in which women have access to skilled birth attendants during pregnancy and childbirth, many lives could be saved. When skilled birth attendants are able to refer at-risk women to hospitals for care, even more families can be spared.

You can be part of the solution to global birth problems. Every year, May 5 is set aside as the International Day of the Midwife. Consider hosting a prayer event on that day to raise awareness about global birth problems. You will find more information on the Global Day of Prayer for Childbirth at www.birthingnaturally.net.

A10: Resources

There are a variety of Christian (friendly) resources available to help you prepare for childbirth and parenting. More resources are listed in the Christian section of the Birthing Naturally website.

Above Rubies
www.aboverubies.org
A ministry designed to encourage women in their calling as wives, mothers and homemakers.

Apple Tree Family Ministries
www.appletreefamily.org
Apple Tree provides training for Christian childbirth educators and offers resources for families expecting a new baby.

Association of Christian Childbirth Professionals
www.christianbirth.org
The ACCP is a membership organization that provides referrals to families.

Birthing the Easy Way. . .by someone who learned the hard way
By Sheila Stubbs
Explains why "luck" has nothing to do with an easy labor.

Blessing God's Way
www.blessinggodsway.com
Celebrating the changes throughout a woman's life.

Breastfeeding and Catholic Motherhood
By Sheila Kippley
Combining the writings of Catholic leaders with sound advice about parenting.

Cascade Christian Childbirth Association
www.christianchildbirth.org
CCCA provides training for Christian birth professionals and resources for expectant families.

Celebration of Pregnancy
By Doran Richards and Susan Tederick.
Description of meaningful ways to celebrate pregnancy and go beyond the traditional baby shower.

Christ Centered Childbirth
By Kelly J. Townsend
Information and encouragement to prepare for birth.

Christian Midwifery
By Betty A. Peckman
Midwifery text covering all aspects of birth care.

Christian Midwives International
www.christianmidwives.org
CMI is a membership organization for childbirth professionals.

Christian Nurses and Midwives
www.cnm.org.uk
Fellowship of Christians in nursing and midwifery professions.

Christian UC
www.christianuc.com
Web forum offering support for families considering an unassisted home birth.

The Complete Book of Christian Parenting & Child Care
By Dr. William and Martha Sears
Wisdom and encouragement as you learn how to parent your child.

Couple to Couple League
www. ccli.org
Volunteers provide education in natural family planning.

Cutting Edge Press
www.cuttingedgepress.net
Pregnancy, birth and postpartum bookstore.

The Dabbling Mum
www.thedabblingmum.com
A place for parents to learn, grow and dream.

Eve Becomes Mother: Childbirth as a Positive Spiritual Event
By Coralee Murray and Kathy Nesper
Review of prevailing Christian views of birth, and their effects on women (audio-recording).

Family Life Today
www.familylife.com
Information for families at all stages of life.

First Birth Ministries
www.firstbirthministries.com
Providing Christian childbirth education.

Focus on the Family
www.family.org
Resources and information for families.

Gentle Birth Choices
By Barbara Harper
Explores gentle options for labor and birth.

Gentle Christian Mothers
www.gentlechristianmothers.com
Online newsletter and forums to discuss mothering.

Great With Child
By Debra Rienstra
Reflections on becoming a mother.

Grief and Grace
By Amanda Axelby
Help for families experiencing pregnancy loss.

Hearts at Home
www.hearts-at-home.org
Encouraging and equipping women for the profession of motherhood.

I'm Pregnant . . . Now What?
By Ruth Graham and Sara Dormaon, Ph.D.
Written to encourage and inform pregnant teens and their parents.

In His Hands Birth Supply
www.inhishands.com
Birth supplies, books and other materials.

The Joy of Natural Childbirth
By Helen Wessel
Classic review of what the Bible says about birth.

The Lord of Birth
by Jennifer Vanderlaan
Bible study exploring what the Bible says about fertility and motherhood.

Midwifery Today
www.midwiferytoday.com
Magazine for midwives and those interested in birth.

Ministry of Midwifery
By Patti A. Barnes
Handbook for those who wish to study midwifery

Mom Sense
www.christianitytoday.com
Online and print periodical for mothers.

Mothers of Pre-Schoolers (MOPS)
www.mops.org
Support for mothers of young children.

Mother to Mother
mothertomother.tripod.com
Periodical discussing pregnancy, childbirth and new parenting.

Myth of the Perfect Mother: Rethinking the Spirituality of Women
by Carla Barnhill
Dismiss cultural ideals of perfection and find worth in a relationship with God.

Natural Family Planning Blessed Our Marriage
By Fletcher Doyl
Exploring the use of natural birth control.

The Naturally Healthy Pregnancy
by Shonda Parker
Information and advice to help you stay healthy and comfortable during pregnancy and birth.

Naturally Healthy, Birth and Beyond
www.naturallyhealthy.org
Focusing on the natural things you can do, and how they might work with more traditional medicine.

New Life International School of Midwifery
www.midwifeschool.org
Training for midwifery missions.

Nighttime Parenting: How to get your baby and child to sleep through the night
By William Sears
Practical advice for families.

New Life Ministries
www.newlifeministries.com.au
Support network for prayer, encouragement, and the knowledge of God's will in any area of childbearing.

Nine Months and Counting
By Alice Chapin.
A small guided journal for pregnancy with encouraging verses and suggestions from other moms.

Out of the Valley Ministries
www. outofthevalley.org
Support for pregnancy mood disorders.

Pregnancy = 40 Weeks of Preparation
By Tina Ellis
Collection of encouraging writings to help you prepare for motherhood the first or tenth time.

Supernatural Childbirth
By Jackie Mize
Seeking out the promises of God for fertility.

Titus 2 Birthing
www.geocities.com/titus2birthing
Offers certification for childbirth educators and doulas.

Waterbirth International
www.waterbirth.org
Support and information for families considering waterbirth.

40 Weeks
By Jennifer Vanderlaan
Weekly devotional guide to pregnancy.

References

Baker, J., M. Mancuso, M. Montenegro, & B.A. Lyons. 2002. Treating postpartum depression, 26(10): 37-44.

Birch, E. 1986. The experience of touch received during labor. *Journal of Nurse-Midwifery,* 31(6): 270-276.

Brewer, G. S. &. Brewer, T. 1985. *What every pregnant woman should know.* New York: Penguin Books.

British Nutrition Foundation. 2007. *Healthy eating.* Retrieved September 28, 2007 from http://www.nutrition.org.uk.

Campbell, D., Scott, K.D., Klaus M.H., & Falk, M. 2007. Female relatives or friends trained as labor doulas: Outcomes at 6 to 8 weeks postpartum. *Birth: Issues in Perinatal Care* 34(3):220-227.

Canadian Institute for Health Information. 2004. *Giving birth in Canada: A regional profile.* Ottawa.

Caton D., Corry M.P., Frigoletto F.D., Hopkins D.P., Lieberman E., Mayberry L., Rooks J.P., Rosenfield A., Sakala C., & Simkin P. 2002. The nature and management of labor pain: Executive summary. *American Journal of Obstetrics and Gynecology.* 186(5): S1-S15.

Centers for Disease Control and Prevention. 2007. *2005 National Hospital Discharge Survey. Advance Data from Vital and Health Statistics*, 385.

Childbirth Connection. 2006 *What Every Pregnant Woman Needs to Know About Cesarean Section* 2nd ed. New York: Childbirth Connection.

Coalition for Improving Maternity Services (CIMS). 1996. The Mother Friendly Childbirth Initiative. 1996. Available electronically at www.motherfriendly.org.

Coutsoudis, A. 2005. Current status of HIV and breastfeeding research. *Breastfeeding Abstracts,* 24(2):11-12.

Declercq E.R., Sakala C., Corry M.P., & Applebaum S. 2006. *Listening to mothers II: Report of the second national U.S. survey of women's childbearing experiences.* New York: Childbirth Connection.

Dick-Read, G. 1959. *Childbirth without fear.* New York: Harper.

Doering, S., Entwisle D., & Quinlan, D. 1980. Modeling the quality of women's birth experience. *Journal of American Psychiatry,* 45(5):825-837.

References

Enken, M., Keirse, MJNC, Neilson, J., Crowther C., Duley L., Hodnet, E., & Hofmeyr, J. 2000. *A guide to effective care in pregnancy and childbirth.* 3rd Ed. Oxford: Oxford University Press.

Field, T., Hernandez-Reif, M., Taylor, S., & Quintino, O. 1998. Labor pain is reduced by massage therapy. *Journal of Psychosomatic Obstetrics and Gynecology,* 18(4) 286-291.

Fraser, W., Hatem-Asmar, M., Krauss, I., Maillard, F., Breart, G., & Blais, R. 2000. Comparison of Midwifery Care to Medical Care in hospitals in the Quebec Pilot Projects Study: Clinical Indicators. *Canadian Journal of Public Health* 91(1)I5-11.

Goer, H. 1999. *The thinking woman's guide to a better birth.* New York: Perigee.

Government Statistical Service. 2005. *NHS Maternity Statistics, England: 2003-04 Bulletin 2005/1.* London.

Harper, B. 1994. *Gentle Birth Choices.* Vermont: Healing Arts Press.

Health Canada. 2007. *Canada's Food Guide.* Retrieved September 28, 2007 from http://www.healthcanada.gc.ca/foodguide.

Huggins, K. 1994. *The nursing mother's guide to weaning.* Boston: Harvard Common Press.

Hunziker, U.A.& Barr, R.G.. 1986. Increased carrying reduces infant crying: A randomized controlled trial. *Pediatrics,* 77(5): 641-649.

Johnson, K. C. & Daviss, B.A.. 2005. Outcomes of planned home births with certified professional midwives: Large prospective study in North America. BMJ, 330:1416-1423.

Klaus, M.H., Kennell, J.H., & Klaus, P.H. 1993. *Mothering the Mother.* Massachusetts:Perseus Books.

Klaus, M. H., &. Klaus, P.H. 1999. *Your Amazing Newborn.* Cambridge, MA: Perseus.

Kozak L.J., DeFrances, C.J., & Hall, M.J.. 2006. National Hospital Discharge Survey: 2004 annual summary with detailed diagnosis and procedure data. *Vital Health Stat* 13(162). National Center for Health Statistics.

La Leche League International. 1997. *The womanly art of breastfeeding.* New York: Penguin Group.

Laws P.J., Grayson, N. & Sullivan, E.A.. 2006. Australia's mothers and babies 2004. *Perinatal statistics series* 18(34). Sydney:AIHW National Perinatal Statistics Unit.

Lederman, R., Lederman, E., Work, B., & McCann, D.. 1979. Relationship of Psychological Factors in Pregnancy to Progress in Labor. *Nursing Research,* 28(2):94-97.

Leavitt, L. A. 1998. Mothers' sensitivity to infant signals. In *New Perspectives in Early Emotional Development.* Johnson & Johnson Pediatric Institute.

Lydon-Rochell, M., Holt, V.L., Martin, D.P. & Easterling, T.R.. 2000. Association Between Method of Delivery and Maternal Rehospitalization. *Journal of the American Medical Association* 283:2411-2416.

MacDorman, M.F & Singh, G.K. 1998. Midwifery care, social and medial risk factors, and birth outcomes in the USA. *Journal of Epidemiology and Community Health,* 52(5): 301-317.

MacDorman, M.F., Declercq, E., Menacke,r F. &. Malloy, M.H. (2006). Infant and Neonatal Mortality for Primary Cesarean and Vaginal Births to Women with "No Indicated Risk," United States, 1998-2001 Birth Cohorts. *Birth: Issues in Perinatal Care* 33(3):175-182.

Melzack, K., Taenzer, P., Feldman, P., & Kinch, R.. 1981. Labor is still painful after prepared childbirth training. *Canadian Medial Association Journal,* 125:357-363.

References

Mohrbacher, N. & Stock, J.. 2003. *The breastfeeding answer book*, 3rd ed. Illinois: La Leche League International.

National Health and Medical Research Council. 2003. *Dietary Guidelines for Australian.* Retrieved September 28, 2007 from http://www.nhmrc.gov.au/publications/nhome.htm.

New Zealand Health Information Service. 2006. *Report on Maternity Maternal and Newborn Information 2003 – 2006.* Wellington.

Odent, M. & Odent, P. 2006. *Drips of synthetic oxytocin.* Retrieved February 15, 2008 from http://www.wombecology.com/oxytocin.html.

O'Grady, K. 2003. The semantics of taboo: Menstrual prohibitions in the Hebrew bible. In *Wholly Woman Holy Blood.* Harrisburg, PA: Trinity Press International. .

Oxorn, H. 1980. *Oxorn-Foote Human Labor & Birth* 4th Ed. New York: Appleton-Century-Crofts.

Peckmann, B. A. 1997. *Christian Midwifery* 3rd ed. Illinois: NAPSAC International.

Pruett, K.D. 1998. Attachment: Role of the Father. In *New Perspectives in Early Emotional Development.* Johnson & Johnson Pediatric Institute.

Porter, L. 2007. All night long; understanding the world of infant sleep. *Breastfeeding Review.* 15(3):11-15.

Roll, S. K. 2003. The old rite of the churching of women after childbirth. In *Wholly Woman Holy Blood.* Harrisburg, PA: Trinity Press International.

Rooks, J.P. 1997. *Midwifery and childbirth in America.* Philadelphia: Temple University Press.

The San Diego Breastfeeding Coalition. 2001. *Infant feeding costs.* Retrieved February 10, 2008 from http://www.breastfeeding.org/bfacts/costs.html.

Sears W, & Sears, M. 1993. *The baby book: Everything you need to know about your baby from birth to age two.* New York: Little, Brown and Company.

Schultheiss, D., Truss, M.C., Stief, C.G. & Jonas, U. (1998). Uncircumcision: A Historical Review of Preputial Restoration. *Plastic and Reconstructive Surgery* 101(7):1990-1998.

Simkin, P, Whalley, J. & Keppler, A. 2001. *Pregnancy Childbirth and the Newborn.* New York: Meadowbrook Press.

Simkin, P. & Ancheta, R.. 2000. *The Labor Progress Handbook.* Oxford: Blackwell Publishing.

Taylor, C. 2002. Giving Birth. New York: Perigee.

US Department of Agriculture. 2005. *Dietary Guidelines for Americans.* Retrieved September 28, 2007 from http://www.mypyramid.gov.

U.S. Department of Health and Human Services. 2000. Maternal, infant and child health. In: *Healthy People* 2010, 2nd ed. Washington DC: U.S. Government Printing Office.

Wesson, N. 1999. *Labor pain: A natural approach to easing delivery.* Vermont: Healing Arts Press.

White, M. Focusing on the senses: The amazing "sensational" abilities of newborns. *International Journal of Childbirth Education*,18(4):14-17.

World Health Organization, Maternal and Newborn Health / Safe Motherhood Division of Reproductive Health. 1997. Care in normal birth: A practical guide. Geneva.

World Health Organization. 2007. *New data on male circumcision and HIV prevention: Policy and programme implications.* Programming Montreux, 6-8.

Index

A

active labor, 73-75, 169, 189, 190, 191, 266, 269, 303
active management, 107-108, 302
adrenal glands, 28
alignment, 40, 123
amniotic fluid, 27, 32, 33, 292, 306
anesthesiologist, 240, 241, 246, 319
antibiotics, 235, 251, 252, 286, 292, 304
Apgar, 214, 241, 249, 304
aromatherapy, 190
asynclitism, 304

B

back labor, 263, 270, 299-300, 304
backache, 70, 173, 233, 299
   pregnancy, 37, 40
bag of waters, 59, 64, 77, 170, 225, 228, 233, 235, 293, 294, 300, 306, 310
   artificial breaking, 108, 233, 303
   see pre-labor rupture of the membranes
biophysical profile, 292
birth canal, 60, 62, 80, 319
birth centers, 218
birth plan, 93-104, 393
birth stool, 173
Bishop Scoring, 232
blood volume, 31-33, 84

bloody show, 67, 70
breastfeeding, 83, 84, 342-350
   cesarean, 317, 320
   hormones, 57, 234
   nutrition, 34, 38
breathing,
   abdominal, 184-185
   shortness of, 27
breech, 293-296, 318

C

calcium, 32-33
cephelopelvic disproportion, 304, 311, 318, 323
cervical checks, 59, 225
cervical mucus, 67, 255, 313
cervix, 8, 25, 28, 58-84, 88, 89, 126-127, 132, 144-145, 227-235, 294, 302, 303, 304, 308-309
cesarean surgery, 219, 259, 314, 316-325
   doulas, 214
   place of birth, 220
   risk factors, 224, 232, 235, 238, 240, 294, 296, 298, 300, 303, 307-3096
circumcision, 250, 253-257
coccyx, 80, 172, 173
colostrum, 67
comfort measures, 75, 134-141, 147, 155-192, 202, 240, 241, 263-270, 394
   massage, 135, 137, 138, 161-166, 170, 177, 178, 181, 190, 214, 224, 244, 265, 269, 295, 312, 315, 394

music, 189, 194
confidence, 137
constipation, 37, 229
contraction stress test, 292
contractions, 28, 55-84, 131, 294, 299, 304, 314, 315
    Braxton-Hicks, 28, 66, 69
    comfort measures, 162, 165, 166, 168, 190
    inducing, 228, 230-234
    pain, 122, 126, 139-145, 147
coping strategies, 140
corpus luteum, 25, 26
crowning, 81

D

dehisancese, 324
dehydration, 223
descent, 80, 81, 301
diabetes, 228, 290
    gestational, 289
dilation, 40, 59-61, 67, 70, 76, 77, 86, 108, 174, 226, 232, 238, 240, 301, 302, 304
double hip squeeze, 164
doula, 100, 115, 136, 179, 204, 208, 214, 215, 247, 302, 372, 373
due date, 287
dysfunctional labor, 132

E

early labor, 65, 69 -73, 87, 122, 191 , 303
effacement, 59, 61, 232
electronic fetal monitor, 108, 224, 225, 239, 259, 306, 307
epidural, 178, 212, 220, 223, 232, 236-247, 299, 303, 319, 320, 324
episiotomy, 103, 208, 219, 223, 224, 248, 259, 312
exercise, 23, 36-38
expectant management, 107, 108, 289
external version, 206, 295

F

fast labor, 272, 280, 301
fatigue, 34, 37, 123, 177, 238, 240
fear, 5, 8, 11, 94, 128-133, 139-144, 172, 190, 203, 216, 245, 261, 266, 301, 322, 323
fear tension pain cycle, 134, 135, 183
fetal distress, (fetal heart rate abnormalities) 145, 232, 238, 241-243, 287, 304, 306, 307, 318
fetal malposition, 238
fetal malpresentation, 240
fetal movement counting, 291
fetoscope, 224, 225, 306
flexion, 81
folic acid, 32
fontanelles, 334
foreskin, 254, 255

G

gate control theory, 134
genital herpes, 298
gestational age, 227, 290
glucose tolerance test, 289
Grantley Dick-Read, 8, 131
group B streptococcus, 285, 286

H

hands and knees, 41, 162, 169, 171, 175, 267, 294, 300, 313
hemorrhage, 314-317, 345
high blood pressure, 228, 237, 288
home birth, 87, 202, 215-218, 275
hormones, 25-28, 59, 66, 69, 74, 76, 89, 123, 131, 135, 228, 354, 371
    catecholamines, 131, 132
    corticotropin-releasing hormone, 66
    cortisol, 28

endorphins, 37, 74, 76, 122
estrogen, 25- 28, 66, 67, 69, 370
follicle-stimulating hormone, 25
human chorionic gonadatropin, 26
lutenizing hormone, 25
oxytocin, 28, 56, 66, 76, 83, 84, 108, 205, 206, 213, 219, 230, 232-235, 237, 239, 293, 299, 302-304, 307, 314, 315, 324, 345, 375
progesterone, 25-27, 69
prolactin, 74, 122
prostaglandin, 28, 67, 69, 206, 229-235, 293
relaxin, 27
hospital, 171, 187, 188, 191, 192, 211-220, 221-226, 246, 247, 250-252, 260, 291

I

immunity, 227, 252
heartburn, 27
induction, 4, 108, 205, 220, 227-235, 244, 259, 287, 290, 293, 303, 395
   amniotomy, 233
   mistoprostol, 235
   sweeping the membranes, 233, 287
infection, 59, 225, 232, 233, 292, 293, 317, 319, 324, 367
informed consent, 104, 205, 209
inhalation analgesia, 241
intrauterine growth restriction, 291
intravenous fluids, 213, 223, 237, 239, 240, 315, 319
ischial spines, 81

J

jaundice, 234, 251, 252

K

kegel exercises, 39, 176

L

labor, 53-85
labor challenge, 94, 227-325 327
labor environment, 129, 131, 135, 187-195, 220, 247, 260
labor pain, 117-151
labor position, 167-173
labor tub, 169, 177-180, 247
lactation consultant, 322, 347, 373, 397
lanugo hair, 334
lightening, 67

M

macrosomia, 289, 290, 318
mammary glands, 26
meconium, 235, 287, 306, 337
meditation, 6, 185, 186
midwife, 16
   certified nurse midwife, 212
   certified professional midwife, 212
   direct entry midwife, 212
milia, 335
modesty, 128, 178, 226
Mongolian spots, 335
multiple birth, 296

N

nipple stimulation, 229, 230, 292, 314
nitrous oxide, 213, 217, 242
non-stress test, 292
nutrition, 27, 31, 33, 35

O

obstetrician, 34, 211-220, 316-320
occiput anterior, 62
occiput posterior, 62

opioids, 238
ovulation, 61

P

pelvic floor, 39, 40, 169, 170, 299
pelvic rocking, 41, 175, 300, 304
pelvis, 27, 56, 164, 168, 311, 333
   alignment, 123, 144, 296, 299, 304
   movement, 168, 170, 174, 229, 302
   position, 61, 62, 126, 163, 240, 294-295
perineal massage, 312
perineal tears, 224, 238, 301
perineum, 61, 81, 181, 224, 248, 285, 286, 312, 313
PKU test, 252
placenta, 25-28, 31, 66, 67, 83, 84, 227, 234, 241, 242, 287, 289, 291, 367
   abruption, 144, 279, 308, 317
   accreta, 309, 317
   previa, 292, 308, 309, 317
   retained, 313, 314
posterior position, 279, 299
postpartum depression, 371
posture, 40, 167, 294
pregnancy induced hypertension, 288, 290, 307
pre-labor rupture of the membranes, 280, 292, 293
premature, 250, 285, 292
presentation, 62, 295
professional labor assistant. *See* doula
prolapsed cord, 300
prolonged labor, 108, 301, 302
prolonged pregnancy, 228, 287
pubic bone, 67, 80, 81, 168, 181, 295
pushing, 40, 41, 56, 62, 77, 79-82, 122, 138, 145, 172, 173, 181, 224, 240, 301, 307, 311

R

red raspberry leaf tea, 180, 313, 314
regional analgesia, 236-240
relaxation, 129, 135, 165, 166, 169, 170, 177, 178, 183-186
retained placenta, 313
rotation, 80, 82

S

Sedatives, 242
self-induction, 229
   Acupressure, 230
   castor oil, 231
   cohosh, 231, 314
   intercourse, 230
   nipple stimulation, 230
shoulder dystocia, 145, 289, 290
skin to skin contact, 83, 249
spinal, 237, 238
squatting, 41, 80, 172, 173, 313, 394, 395
station, 59, 61, 189, 225
sterile water injections, 182
symphisis pubis, 127, 168

T

transition, 63-65, 76-78
transverse lie, 296

U

ultrasound, 288, 290, 291
umbilical cord, 233, 248, 251, 294, 300, 314, 335
uterine hyperstimulation, 235
uterine rupture, 234, 324
uterus, 25-28, 39, 56, 59, 61, 62, 83, 123, 126, 132, 144, 231, 232, 235, 308, 309, 313-315, 316, 319, 320, 324, 367

V

vaccinations, 252
vagina, 25, 28, 39, 59, 61, 67, 70, 76, 80, 81, 126, 223, 239, 312
vernix, 334
vertex, 206, 293, 294

Vitamin K, 250

W

walking, 175, 229, 267, 302
Webster Technique, 295
weight gain, 30

CPSIA information can be obtained at www.ICGtesting.com
Printed in the USA
239895LV00002B/115/P